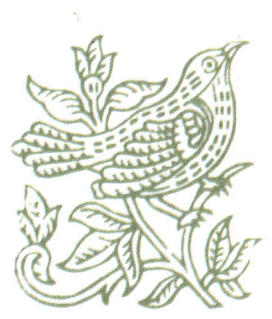

THE
HERBAL
SUTRA

DISCLAIMER

Consultation with a qualified medical professional before using or consuming these herbs is advised. The information provided in this book is for general educational purposes only and does not seek to substitute medical advice. Individual health conditions, allergies and potential interactions with other substances must be taken into account for safe usage.

ISBN: 978-93-92130-35-9

First published by Roli Books in 2023
M-75, Greater Kailash II Market
New Delhi-110 048, India
Ph: +91-11-40682000
E-mail: info@rolibooks.com
www.rolibooks.com

COVER DESIGN: PALLAVI AGARWALA
CONCEPT: PALLAVI AGARWALA
DESIGN: SNEHA PAMNEJA
ILLUSTRATIONS: ANITA VERMA
PRE-PRESS: JOYTI DEY
PRODUCTION: LAVINIA RAO

Printed and bound at
Naveen Printers, New Delhi

THE HERBAL SUTRA

INDIAN WISDOM & WELLNESS
THROUGH 100 HERBS

MADHULIKA BANERJEE

ILLUSTRATIONS BY
ANITA VERMA

Lustre Press
Roli Books

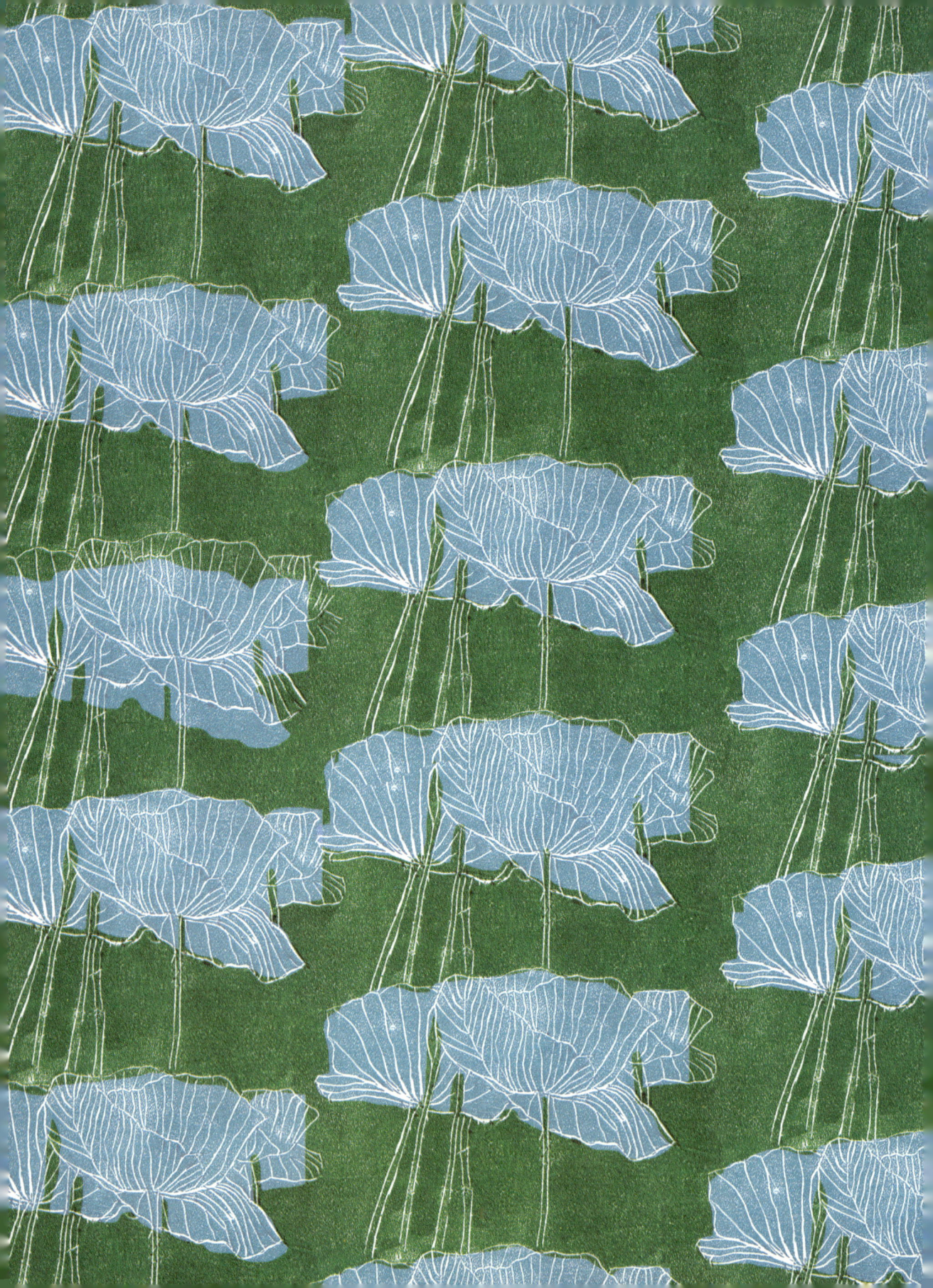

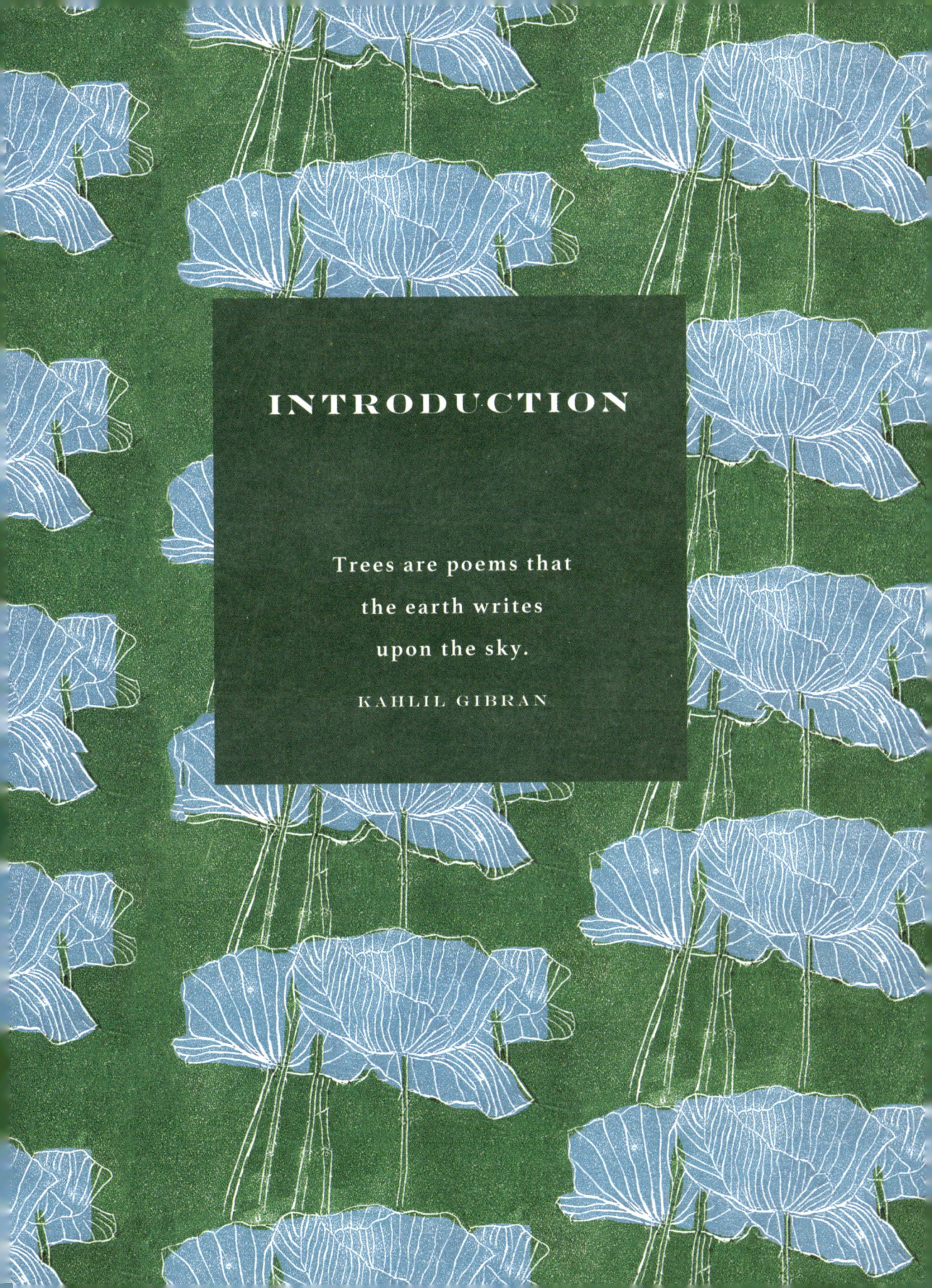

INTRODUCTION

Trees are poems that
the earth writes
upon the sky.

KAHLIL GIBRAN

This is the story of a hundred herbs that are deeply connected to our everyday life in myriad ways. This book, a careful and intimate study of herbs, is an attempt to discover how utterly fascinating their world is. We hope that *The Herbal Sutra* is able to peel away the element of the exotic around them, by bringing the age-old uses of these plants, as well as how they are being adapted today in different ways.

Let me take you through the different elements in each page of the book. Firstly, it is important to note that we have taken a very broad meaning of the term from the Latin word 'herba', referring to any part of a plant like the fruit, leaf, seed, flower, bark, stem etc., and not to the image of a small-size plant that the word evokes. So we have included as many varieties of trees or shrubs that had deep significance, in varied ways, for the lives of ordinary people. To begin with, the different elements of the very design of this book seeks to reflect that significance. The special aesthetic of the drawings of the plant is to represent the herbs artistically, while complying with its actual appearance. The design of the book draws upon and reflects something we take completely for granted – that there is a deep complementarity between nature, knowledge and culture in most practices in our society.

Each plant in this book is listed with different categories of names. This is followed by the English name and then the Latin name of the herb. The Latin name denotes how botanists classify it naming each variant separately. The local names of these plants are often used in different parts of the country a little loosely – so sometimes, plants with broadly similar characteristics might have the same name. On closer analysis, it has often been noted that they aren't the same, and this proves to be a problem when medicines have to be made with them. Latin names help avoid this kind of confusion. But of course, given how much we still don't know about the natural world, there can still be mistakes in identification.

The final category is its names in many languages. This indicates their widespread prevalence – after all, it is only when communities know a plant and have use for it, would they also have a name! It also indicates how widely known and used some herbs are, while others are lesser known; that some are powerful, valuable herbs that grow only in the lesser talked about parts of the country. In this book, we attempt to talk about all kinds of herbs – the well-known and others not so; some whose names roll easily off the tongue and for others, it trips over. They all belong here, to these varied ecosystems that make up the Indian subcontinent.

THE MEDICINAL AND THERAPEUTIC USES OF PLANTS

The herbs are listed in terms of their qualities and how they have been traditionally used. So, a part of or the entire plant itself is used for making medicines, and/or cosmetics, is cooked, or processed for other household uses, and also used in rituals. While some herbs are common across the country, those specific to certain regions have a few special qualities that have been identified in addition to the stated purposes.

What is unique in the knowledge about herbs amongst common people is that, apart from nourishment, they are most often the first source of medicine for everyday ailments. At the very foundation, is the familial knowledge that people have about them, especially women, responsible as they are for the health of their household. Knowledge is passed on amongst women in families and communities, including all aspects of women's health during childbirth, antenatal and postnatal care. Then there is knowledge held by local healers – a much underestimated category of healers, vilified by modern urban society as quacks and charlatans. Often, they carry great knowledge of plants, know how to access and collect them and make medicines from them. Both categories of knowledge are carried in the form of what we call the 'oral tradition'. Additionally, a significant amount of knowledge of medicines made from plants is available in thousands of texts in Indian knowledge systems such as Siddha, Swarigpa, Unani, Ayurveda and others; these comprise the 'textual tradition'. Healers trained in these systems, learn not just how to administer these medicines but how to identify the plants that are used and the complex processes by which they are made. In the section on the medicinal uses of each plant, we share a tiny sliver of information and knowledge that we have about these plants.

What is also interesting is that a great proportion of people around the world still depend on plant-based medicines for two reasons. First, indeed because those are the only kind of medicines they have access to, given that biomedicine still has not fully reached them. Equally important is the reason that they believe that these medicines 'understand' their bodies and are compatible with their food and living habits. In recent years, those that had moved away from plant-based medicines have begun to discover the value of these herbs and are incorporating them back in their everyday lives. The difficulty there is that they expect them to be available in 'ready to use' and 'quick to deliver remedy' forms!

As you browse through the wonders of these hundred herbs, you will notice how one single plant can do so many things. As each plant is constituted by a complex set of chemicals, modern pharmacology identifies its 'active principle', that is, the one most powerful or representative of the central action it is capable of, and develops it to make medicines for specific conditions. But this approach of extracting and singling out a herb's quality in isolation is *not* the way it works in perspectives of earlier medical knowledge, where they use most plants in combination with others, that either enhances the positive qualities of one herb or cancels out any possible negative impact of the other. This is how each herb can be put to use in a large number of conditions. This basic difference in the approach between the two makes for the differences in use by traditional healers and modern medicinal and pharmaceutical markets.

One of the common properties in many of these herbs is that they are antioxidants. A commonly-used word today, antioxidants are substances that can prevent or slow down damage to cells caused by unstable molecules that the body produces as a reaction to environmental and other pressures, sometimes called 'free-radical scavengers'. It is important to remember that they do this not by themselves, but in combination with other inputs that we give our bodies, along with the atmosphere and context in which we work our minds. This is in fact the real meaning of holistic. This is also why the herb cannot always serve its best purpose if its form is changed to suit convenient packaging, as indicated earlier. While we have listed many of their uses, they are meaningful only in context, and we need to understand and operationalize it if we want the benefits.

With climate change knocking on our doors, it is sobering to note that a great many of these herbs are on the endangered lists of several international conservation agencies. The irony is that they became endangered precisely when they were converted into mass-produced cosmetic and health products, which increased their popularity. And there lies the rub. For the modern market system to make a product that is optimal in quantity and viable to produce, sell and profit from, it needs to be produced in large quantities. And if producers increase, then there are larger number of buyers of the herbs, with only two possible outcomes – greater quantities are widely collected from the wild so that the prices of the products remain low, or small amounts are collected, which makes the product expensive and exclusive. Either way, it does not consider the regenerative cycle of the plant because that does not match the production cycle of manufacture. Inevitably then, the more cosmetic products or medicines made from these plants become available, the more endangered the plants are likely to be. So even as we endorse the use of herb-based medicines or herbal cosmetics, we need to keep in mind the negative impact of producing them in the current large-scale system of production. For a balance between the two – demand and supply that does not endanger the plant-base – a different system of production and distribution needs to be worked out. Simply put, things need to be produced locally and consumed locally, with the focus on the good quality of the product, and not fancy packaging and marketing. Some people are already doing this in small ways and we should encourage them by buying form them. Nature provides bountifully and if we focus on what we already have, and want a little less, we would use it sensibly, and sustainably.

An amazing feature of the uses of these plants is their astonishing similarity across different regions, even those which might not have had much communication. Ambolakpa, for instance, is an engendered orchid from the region of Ladakh but also found in the alpine regions of the state of Uttarakhand. Comparisons of the practices of Amchis and of the local vaidyas (names of local practitioners of these regions) show that they use it for the same disease or health conditions. Further, when studied in laboratories to validate their claims, they are found to be sound and practical. So, clearly, similar knowledge about plants developed in different places, and systems of credible medical knowledge emerged from them, even when their ways of knowing were very different from those of modern medicine and science. However, wherever they are not found in textual traditions, they were either not taken seriously by modern medical practitioners and scientists for a long time, or that only if their efficacy was established by 'scientific' parameters, would they be considered legitimate. Some Ayurvedic practitioners crafted clinical trials based on Ayurvedic parameters and this could be a way of establishing evidence for the 'oral' knowledge traditions as well.

Some scientists, however, have systematically collected information about the uses of almost all the herbs listed here on the basis of traditional knowledge. Thus, they have given credence to that knowledge and carried out analysis and experiments on these herbs along the lines of biochemical parameters and documented them accordingly, with the aim of bridging the knowledge systems. Many such scientific sources have been used in this book, and are listed at the end. But here, I must point out a glaring omission. While all scientific papers are required to acknowledge whatever information/knowledge they use that is not their original work, through citations of some kind, none of the scientific papers documenting the traditional knowledge about medicinal plants ever record the sources from where they learned them. So the irony is that local healers, home-makers and any other sources remain unknown and unacknowledged, even while their knowledge gains some legitimacy.

THE RITUAL USE OF PLANTS AND FLOWERS

In Hindu and tribal practices across India, the integrity of nature – that human beings, their belief systems, plants, animals and the five elements of air, water, earth, fire and space, all belong in one connected whole – has been observed consistently. One of the manifestations of this is that there are specific plants and flowers that are used as offering for different gods and rituals. This is usually based on particular virtues or qualities that the plants are known to have, that match or complement those of the gods being worshipped.

Sacred groves are an idea emblematic of a notion of integrity with nature. They were a means to make sure that some plants and herbs remained in their natural habitat and were not accessible for use in any way. So even in non-modern societies that followed non-exploitative systems of using nature, it was recognized that special care and efforts were required if plant variety and biodiversity was to be preserved.

Finally, for several herbs, we have listed some common uses, and a highlight, which draws your attention to a significant aspect of that plant that is not commonly known.

By way of acknowledgement, I would like to thank Chirag Thakkar for persuading me to take up this project, Abhishek Handa, Akshay Bhambhri, Niranda Karam, Princi Verma and Priyanka Sharma for research assistance, the University of Delhi for leave of absence and The New Institute, Hamburg for the Fellowship in 2022–2023 to have the space to complete this book. I'd like to thank Anita Verma for working so meticulously through the beautiful illustrations, maintaining a balance between the aesthetic and the accurate. I would also like to thank the editorial team at Roli Books for their constant support and understanding. The errors remain mine alone.

MADHULIKA BANERJEE
Delhi/Hamburg 2023

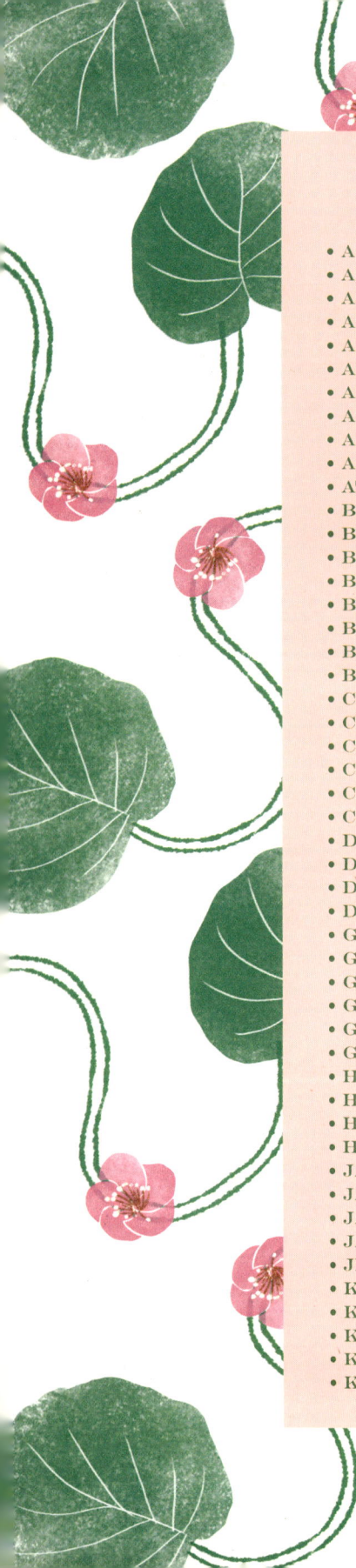
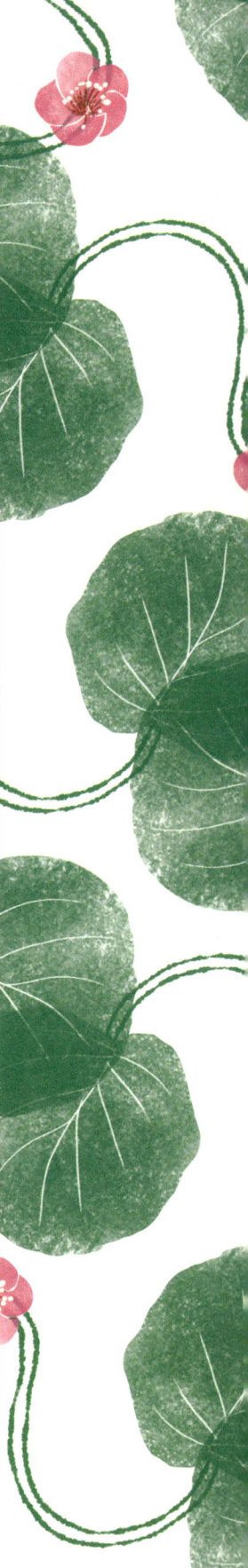

CONTENTS

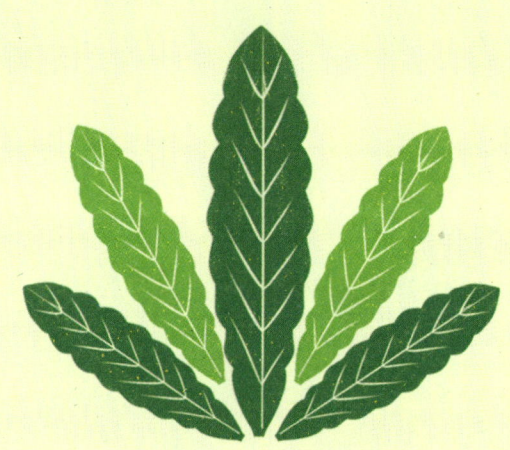

achakṣn

ELEPHANT'S FOOT

Elephantopus scaber Linn

ACHAKSN *Garo*

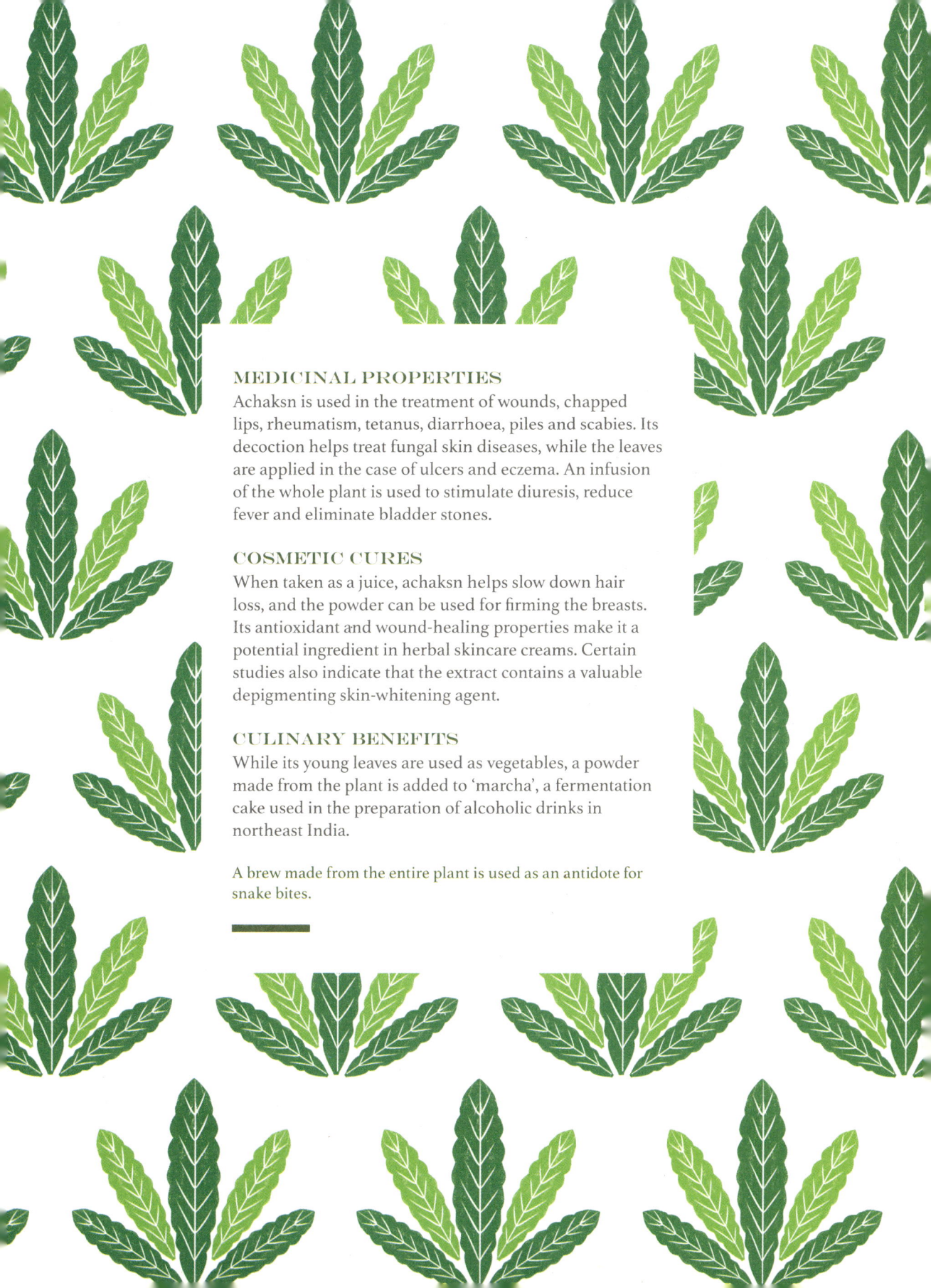

MEDICINAL PROPERTIES

Achaksn is used in the treatment of wounds, chapped lips, rheumatism, tetanus, diarrhoea, piles and scabies. Its decoction helps treat fungal skin diseases, while the leaves are applied in the case of ulcers and eczema. An infusion of the whole plant is used to stimulate diuresis, reduce fever and eliminate bladder stones.

COSMETIC CURES

When taken as a juice, achaksn helps slow down hair loss, and the powder can be used for firming the breasts. Its antioxidant and wound-healing properties make it a potential ingredient in herbal skincare creams. Certain studies also indicate that the extract contains a valuable depigmenting skin-whitening agent.

CULINARY BENEFITS

While its young leaves are used as vegetables, a powder made from the plant is added to 'marcha', a fermentation cake used in the preparation of alcoholic drinks in northeast India.

A brew made from the entire plant is used as an antidote for snake bites.

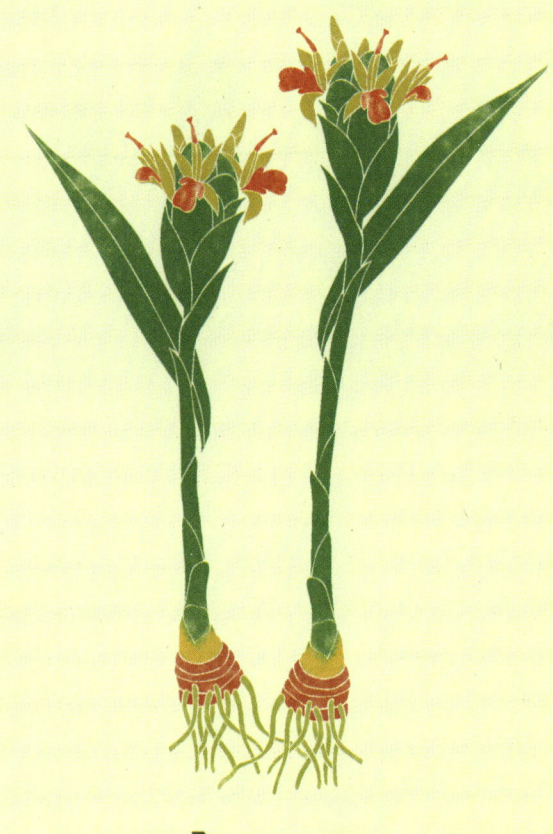

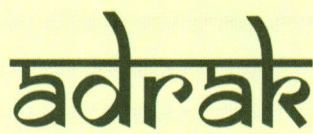

GINGER

Zingiber officinale

ADRAK *Hindi, Punjabi, Urdu* . **AADA** *Bangla* .
ADU *Gujarati* . **INGI** *Tamil*

14

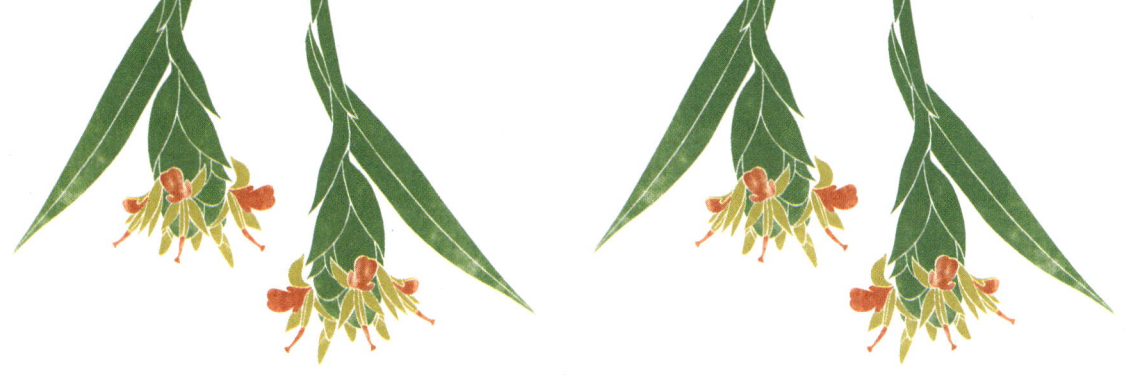

MEDICINAL PROPERTIES

Adrak has been used for thousands of years for the treatment of numerous ailments such as cold, nausea, arthritis, migraines and hypertension. The oleoresin (oily resin) from its roots contain several bioactive components, which is the primary pungent ingredient believed to exert a variety of remarkable pharmacological and physiological activities.

CULINARY BENEFITS

Adrak has now become a base spice for many culinary practices in India. It is used in numerous forms – fresh, dried, pickled, preserved, crystallized, candied and powdered. While its powdered form is used in regular cooking in Kashmir, it is used in chutneys in other parts of north India. Possibly the widest use for it is in ginger tea which is made in a variety of ways. In combination with spices like black pepper and tulasi, it makes a great decoction for colds and coughs. Ginger, steeped in hot boiling water and mixed with lemon juice and honey, is a great stress-relieving drink. To make Indian-style ginger water for cold and cough, mix ginger in a glass of water, cover with lid and keep aside for five minutes. Strain the mixture and serve ginger water immediately. Ginger tea is very popular, especially as a winter tea all across India.

Some species of ginger flowers are edible – usually raw, but also cooked. In Manipur, this is used in one of the variations of eromba, when ginger flowers are added together with vegetables that are cooked with dried fish. This adds fragrance and aroma to the popular Manipuri delicacy. In Naga cuisine, it is used extensively – in stews and teas, and is also added to vegetable and meat dishes.

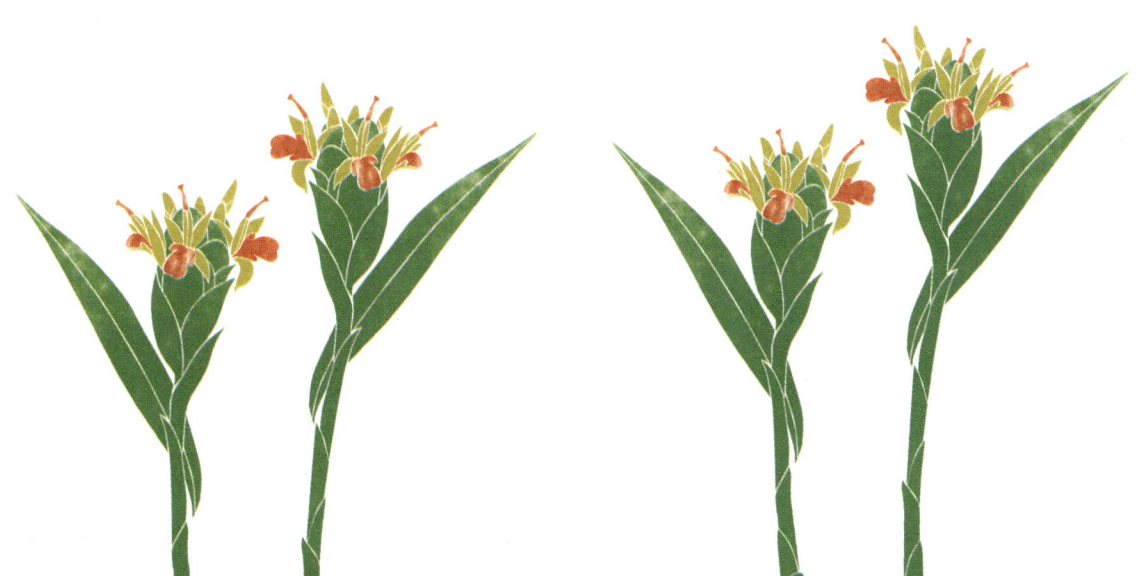

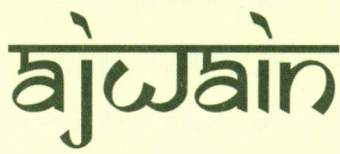

CAROM SEEDS

Trachysperpum amm

AJWAIN *Hindi* . JAMAIN *Maithili* . OMUM *Tamil* .
YAVANO *Gujarati* . JOWAN *Bangla* . AIJAVAIN *Punjabi* .
OVO *Konkani* . OAM *Tulu* . YAVANIKA *Sanskrit*

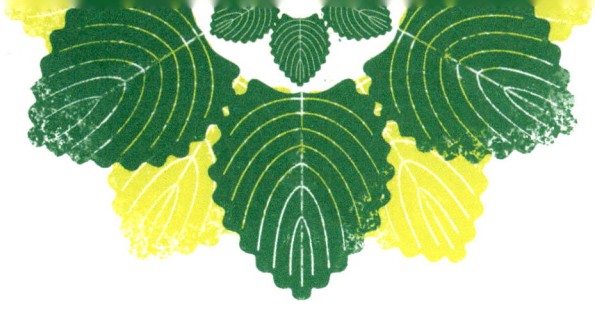
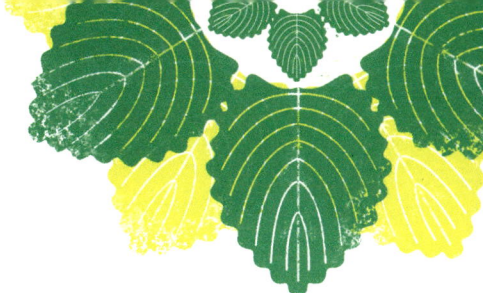

MEDICINAL PROPERTIES

Ajwain's roots are diuretic in nature and the seeds possess excellent aphrodisiac properties. The seeds made from ajwain oil contain thymol that is used in the treatment of gastrointestinal ailments and bronchial problems. Drinking ajwain water helps in weight loss by boosting metabolism, improving digestion and treating acidity. Ajwain seed oil in water also helps women post-pregnancy, as it is believed to reduce water retention and swelling.

CULINARY BENEFITS

With its characteristic aroma and pungent taste, ajwain is widely used as a spice in curries. Its seeds are used in small quantities for flavouring numerous foods, as preservatives, and the leaves are eaten like most other greens. Due to its anti-flatulence properties, it is most often added to fried foods, to balance the negative impact it can have on digestion. This approach of combining ingredients in a recipe that has opposite qualities is indicative of the overall approach and world-view of Indian cuisine – that of balance.

COSMETIC CURES

Thymol, the primary component of ajwain oil, is used to manufacture toothpaste and perfumery.

In some parts of the country, whole wheat laddoos are made with ajwain to help women recover post pregnancy.

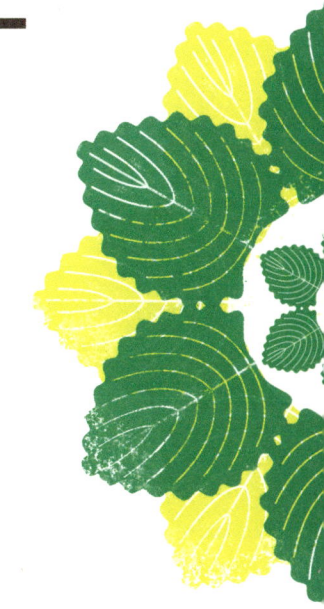

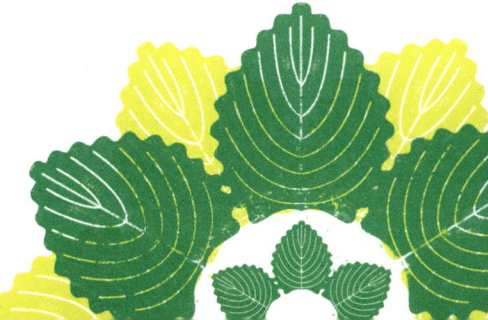

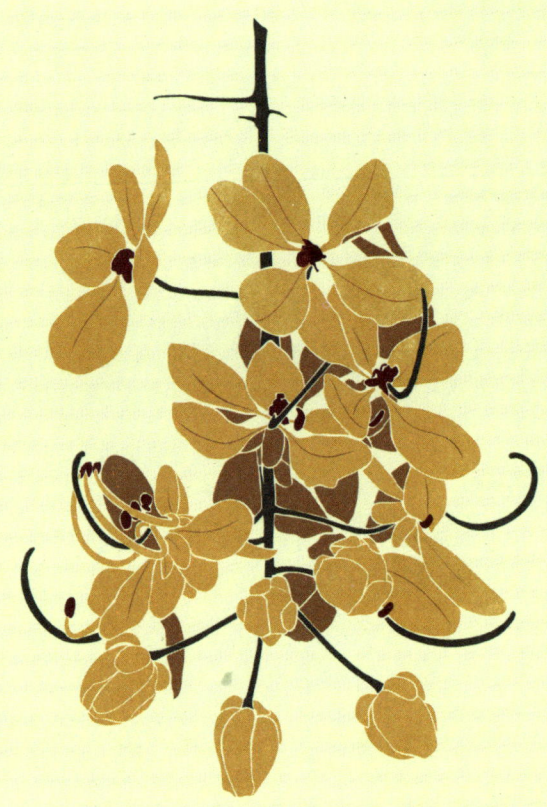

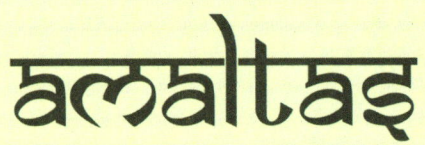

LABURNUM

Cassia fistula

AMALTAS/ SONHALI *Hindi* . GARMALA *Gujarati* .
SHAKKONNAI/KONAI/IRJVIRUTTAM *Tamil* . KONDRAKAYI,
RAELACHETTU/ARAGVADHAMU/KOELAPENNA *Telugu* .
NRIPADUMA *Sanskrit* . AMALTAAS/CHAMKAN *Urdu*

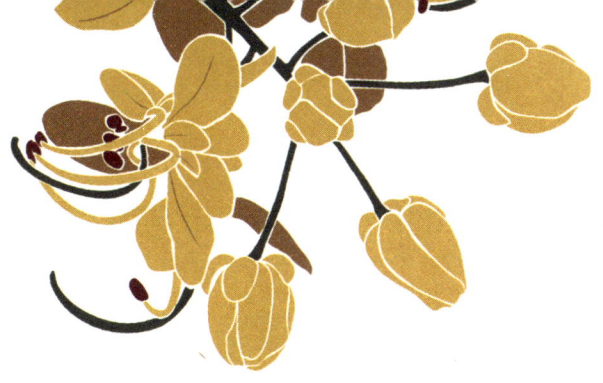

MEDICINAL PROPERTIES

Known as *Rajvraksha* in Ayurveda, amaltas is extensively used in the Unani system of medicine for various ailments in India. Taking amaltas *churna* with warm water after lunch and dinner is considered beneficial in managing blood sugar levels. It also helps in weight management by improving body metabolism and removing toxins from the body, by increasing urine production.

The flowering plant is also useful due to its antipyretic (reducing fever) and antitussive (cough-relieving) properties. Consuming amaltas fruit pulp paste along with warm water helps to manage constipation due to its laxative property. When applied externally around the navel area, the paste tends to give relief from abdominal pain due to flatulence, especially in children.

CULINARY BENEFITS

The amaltas flower can be brewed to make excellent tea. It can also be churned into a chutney, jam or preserve, when cooked with sugar or salt. One can also use it to make salads, and when mixed with chilli, kaffir lime and peanuts, it works really well as a condiment. The flower is also used with staples such as *sarson ka saag* and amaltas ki roti.

COSMETIC CURES

The pods are a detoxifier and keep the skin healthy. The paste or juice of amaltas leaves reduces itchiness and irritation in various skin problems due to its *madhur* (sweet) and *ropan* (healing) properties. As a result, amaltas gives a soothing effect when used regularly.

Applying amaltas leaf's paste along with honey or cow's milk helps one get relief from pain and inflammation, along with managing skin infections due to its antibacterial and antifungal properties.

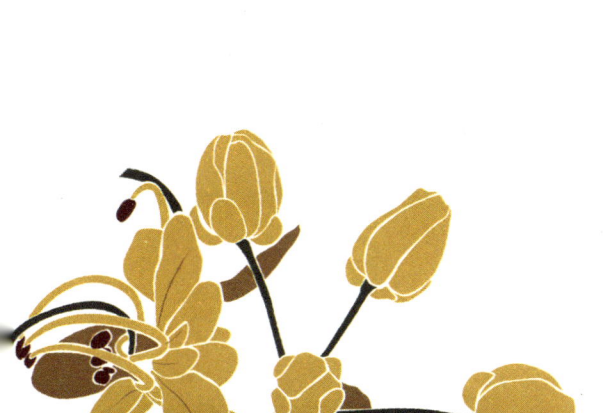

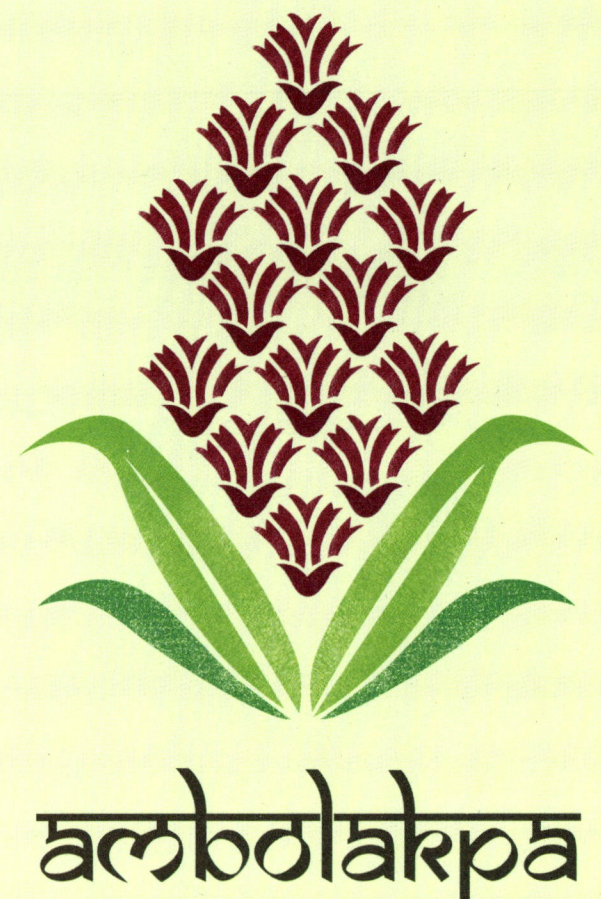

ambolakpa

HIMALAYAN MARSH ORCHID

Soo. Orchidaceae (B.388)

AMBOLAKPA *Ladakhi* . **HATAJARI** *Kumaoni* . **SALEM PANJA** *Kashmiri* .
SALAP *Urdu* . **PANCH AONLE** *Nepali*

MEDICINAL PROPERTIES

Due to its astringent quality, ambolakpa's root extract is used to cure diarrhoea, urine and kidney problems. The roots are collected, shade dried and powdered along with leaves of *Azadirachta indica*, *Ficus religiosa*, seeds of *Punica granatum* (pomegranate), fruits of *Terminalia chebula* (haritaki) and *Emblica officinalis* (amla), roots of *Aconitum heterophyllum* (atish) and mineral salts, and then made into tablets. Two to three tablets taken twice a day with hot water help treat fever.

Ambolakpa is also made into an expectorant that provides Salep, a type of flour. This is used as a nerve tonic and even as an aphrodisiac. The vaidyas of Uttarakhand often make a paste of the roots and administer it to cure diarrhoea.

Its tuber roots are considered to be energy boosters due to them containing starch, sugar, mucilage and albumen. Local practitioners in the Himalayan regions (Amchis) hence use its roots to prepare health tonics.

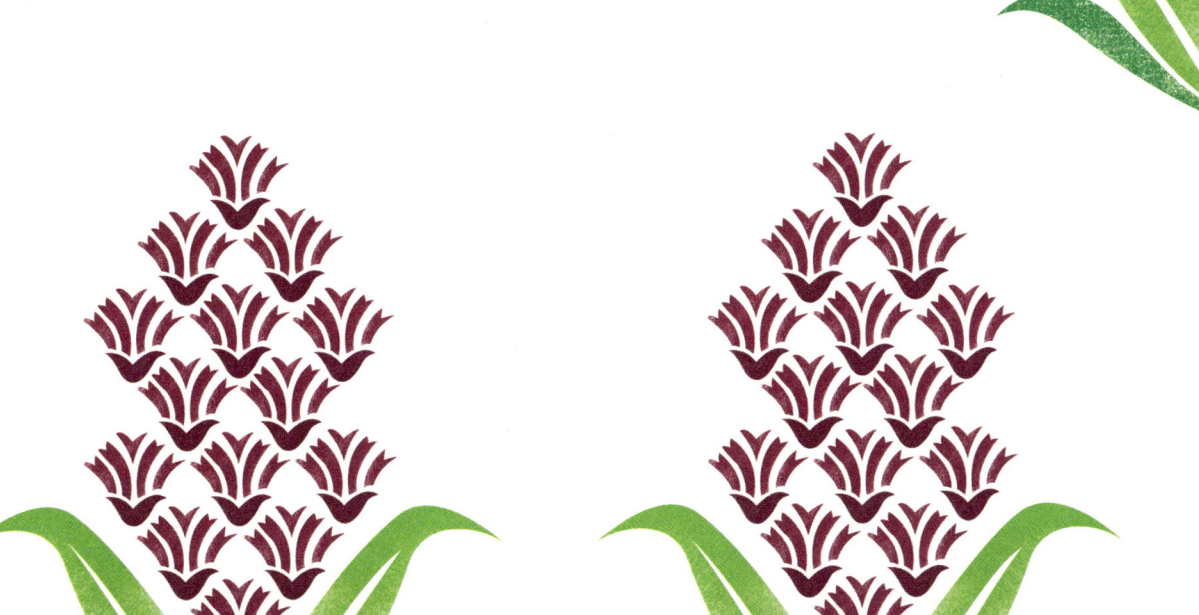

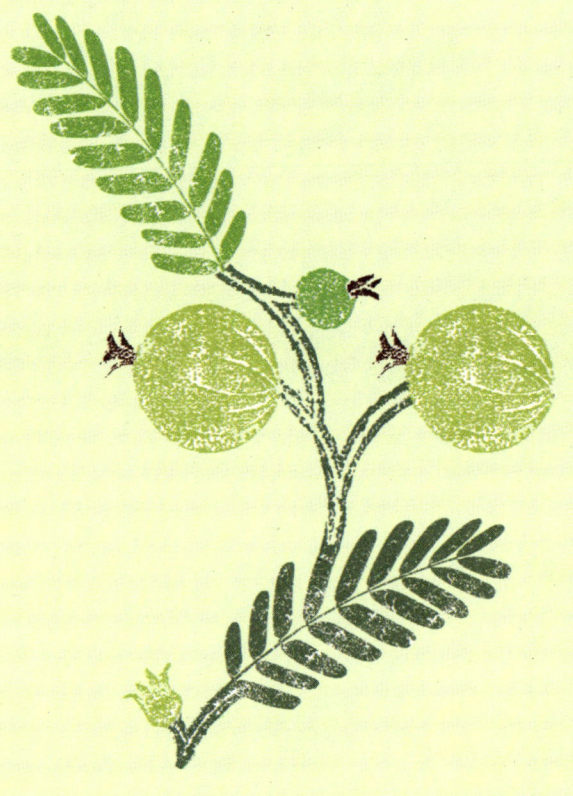

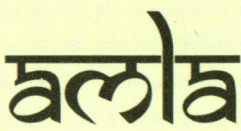

amla

INDIAN GOOSEBERRY
Phyllanthus emblica

AMLA *Hindi* . NELLIKAI *Tamil* . NELLIKKA *Malayalam* . USIRI/
USIRIKAYI *Telugu* . NELLIKAI *Kannada* . AMLAKI/AMLA *Bangla* .
AMBALA/AMLA *Gujarati* . AVALO *Konkani* . AWALAH *Marathi* .
ANLA *Oriya* . NELLI *(Tulu)*

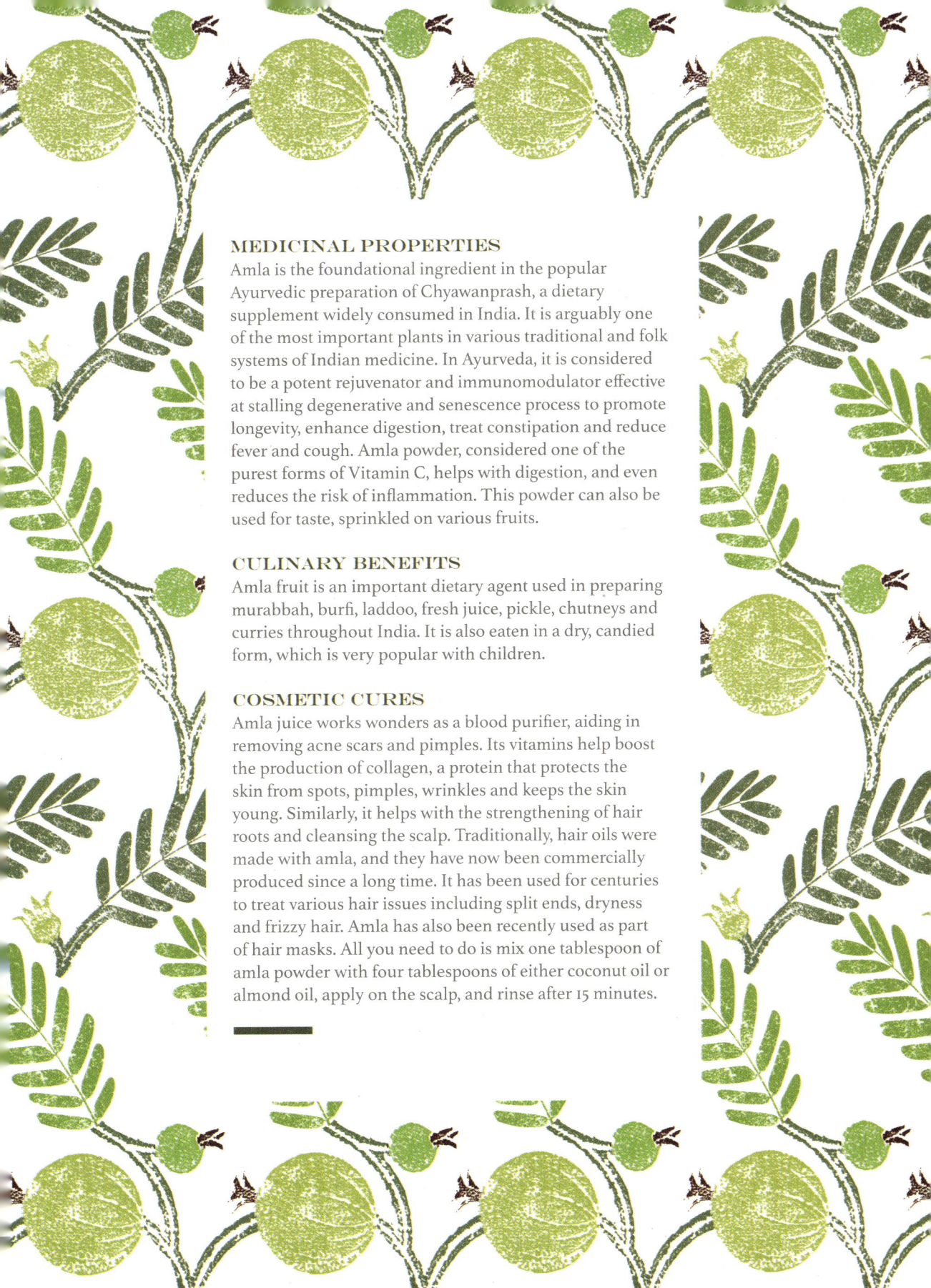

MEDICINAL PROPERTIES

Amla is the foundational ingredient in the popular Ayurvedic preparation of Chyawanprash, a dietary supplement widely consumed in India. It is arguably one of the most important plants in various traditional and folk systems of Indian medicine. In Ayurveda, it is considered to be a potent rejuvenator and immunomodulator effective at stalling degenerative and senescence process to promote longevity, enhance digestion, treat constipation and reduce fever and cough. Amla powder, considered one of the purest forms of Vitamin C, helps with digestion, and even reduces the risk of inflammation. This powder can also be used for taste, sprinkled on various fruits.

CULINARY BENEFITS

Amla fruit is an important dietary agent used in preparing murabbah, burfi, laddoo, fresh juice, pickle, chutneys and curries throughout India. It is also eaten in a dry, candied form, which is very popular with children.

COSMETIC CURES

Amla juice works wonders as a blood purifier, aiding in removing acne scars and pimples. Its vitamins help boost the production of collagen, a protein that protects the skin from spots, pimples, wrinkles and keeps the skin young. Similarly, it helps with the strengthening of hair roots and cleansing the scalp. Traditionally, hair oils were made with amla, and they have now been commercially produced since a long time. It has been used for centuries to treat various hair issues including split ends, dryness and frizzy hair. Amla has also been recently used as part of hair masks. All you need to do is mix one tablespoon of amla powder with four tablespoons of either coconut oil or almond oil, apply on the scalp, and rinse after 15 minutes.

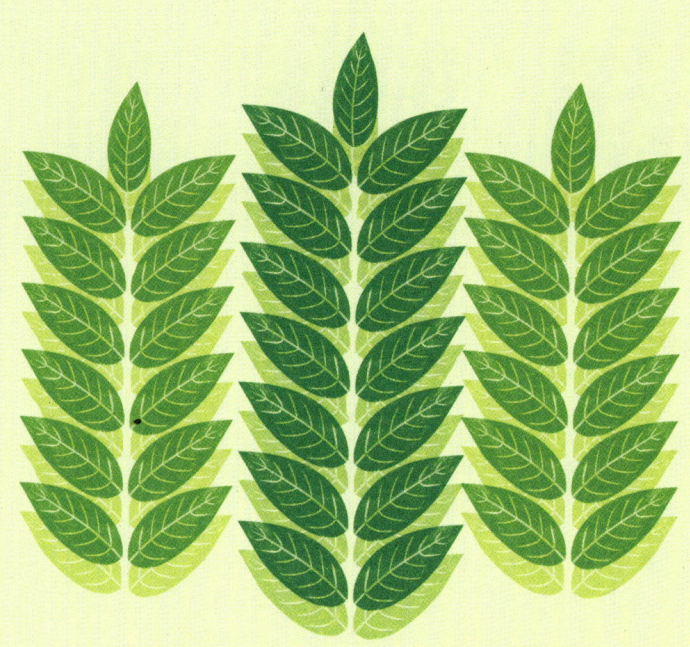

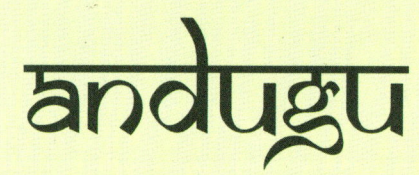

andugu

INDIAN FRANKINCENSE

Boswellia olvalifoliolata

SALAI GUGGUL *Hindi* . **KONDA SAMBRANI** *Telugu*

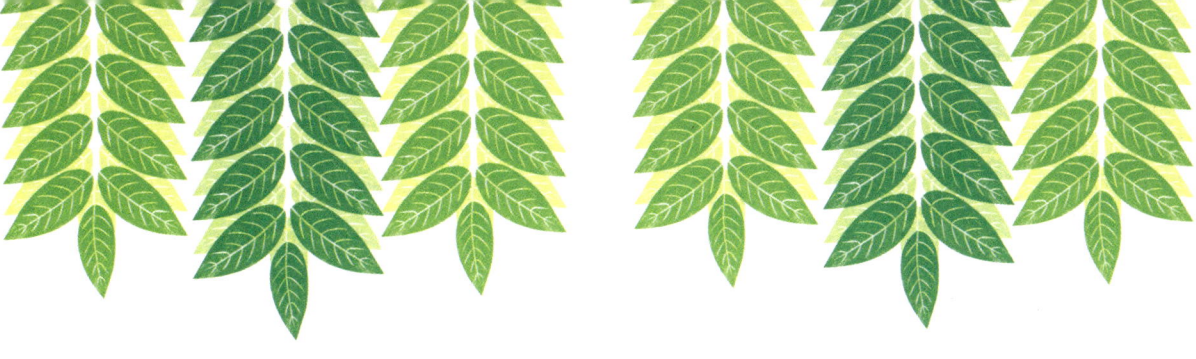

MEDICINAL PROPERTIES

Andugu acts as anti-inflammatory and is an effective painkiller. It also aids in the prevention of cartilage loss.

Tribal communities in Karnataka use the plant for arthritis, by administering one teaspoon full of its gum powder with a glass of goat milk, once daily, till recovery.

Boswellia serrata, a more commonly found but slightly different variety, can help in treating conditions such as osteoarthritis (OA), rheumatoid arthritis (RA), asthma, inflammatory bowel disease (IBD). Included here due to it being part of the same family, *Boswellia serrata* is taken orally for brain injury, joint pain, inflammatory bowel disease that affects the colon (collagenous colitis), Crohn's disease and abdominal pain. It is, additionally, used for relief from hay fever, sore throat and headaches. It is also used as a stimulant, to increase urine flow, and for stimulating menstrual flow.

Andugu is niche and uncommon, and not known to have any culinary or cosmetic uses. It is often confused with the more common *Boswellia serrata*, which is also known as Indian Frankincense and is found in many parts of the country.

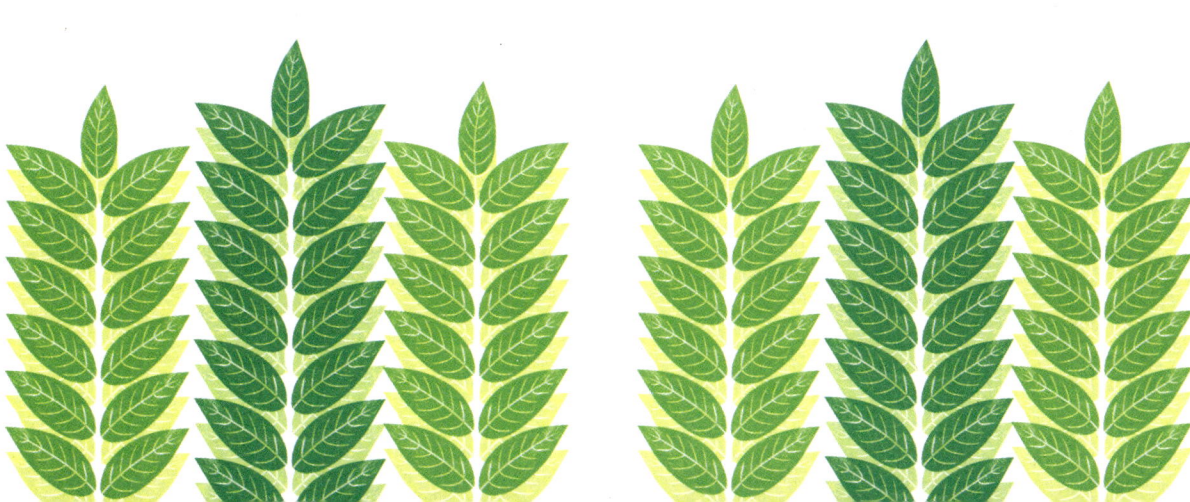

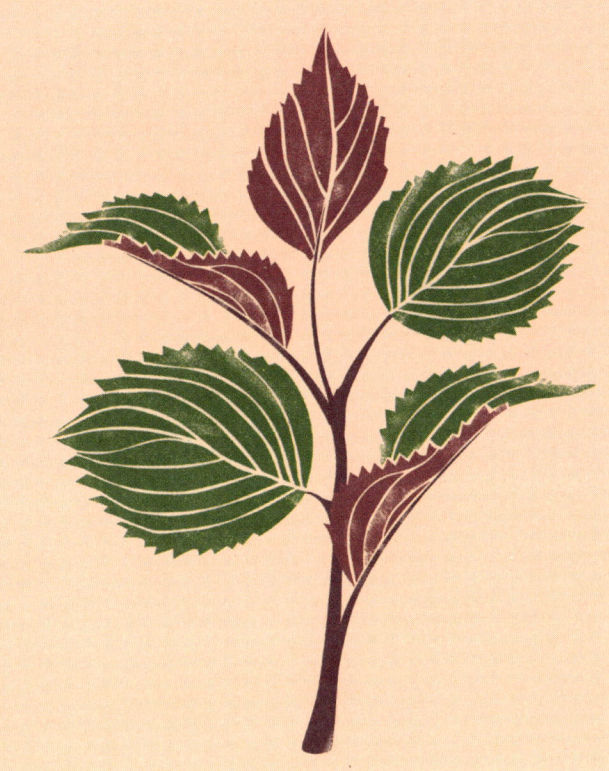

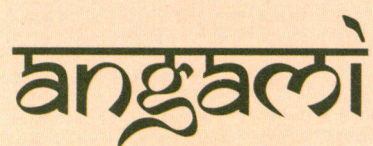

COMMON PERILLA

Britton (Lamiaceae)

ANGAMI *Assamese*

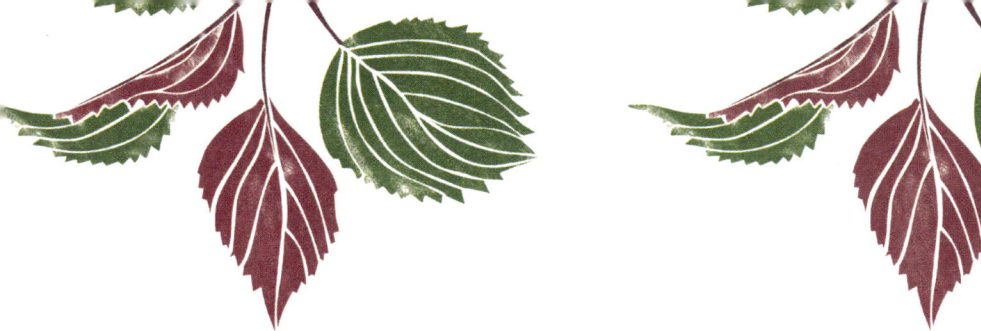

MEDICINAL PROPERTIES

Apart from aiding in the treatment of asthma, angami is also used in the case of nausea, sunstroke and reducing muscle spasms. Angami seeds are rich in dietary fibre and minerals such as calcium, iron, niacin, protein and thiamine. Angami leaves are also rich in vitamins A, C and riboflavin.

CULINARY BENEFITS

Angami has great culinary value and is primarily cultivated for preparing condiments. Oils extracted from its seeds are used as edible oil in Kumaon and northeast India. The seeds are also roasted and ground with salt, chillies and tomatoes to make a savoury side dish or chutney. The plant's young shoots and leaves are eaten cooked and added for additional flavour in various curries.

COSMETIC CURES

The extract of angami leaves contains several antioxidant, anti-inflammatory, anti-allergic and antimicrobial properties which are used as the active compound in the preparation of anti-aging skincare and moisturizing products.

Apart from its medicinal, culinary and cosmetic uses, angami is also used industrially in the manufacturing of paints, varnishes, linoleum, printing ink and for dyeing purposes.

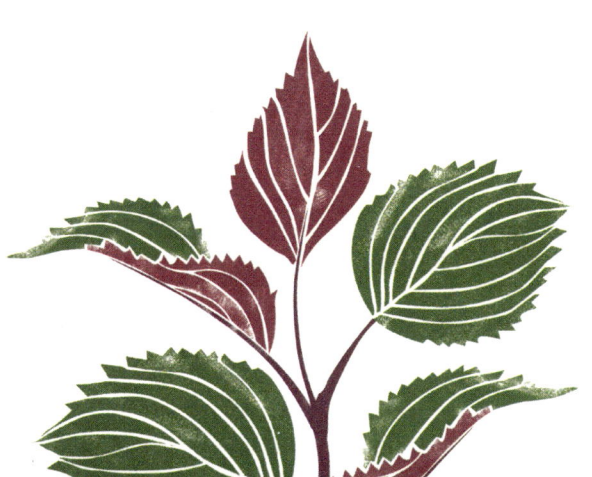

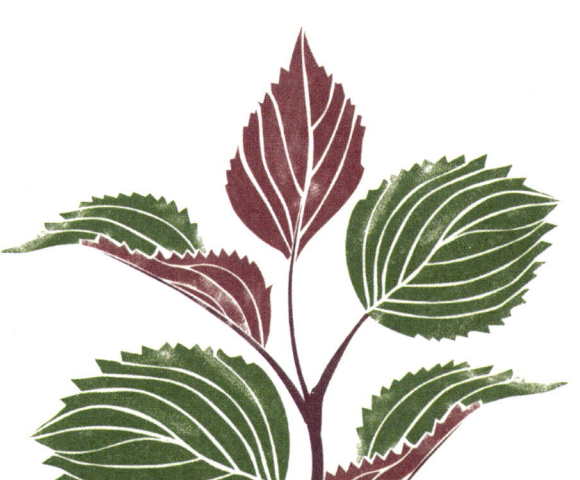

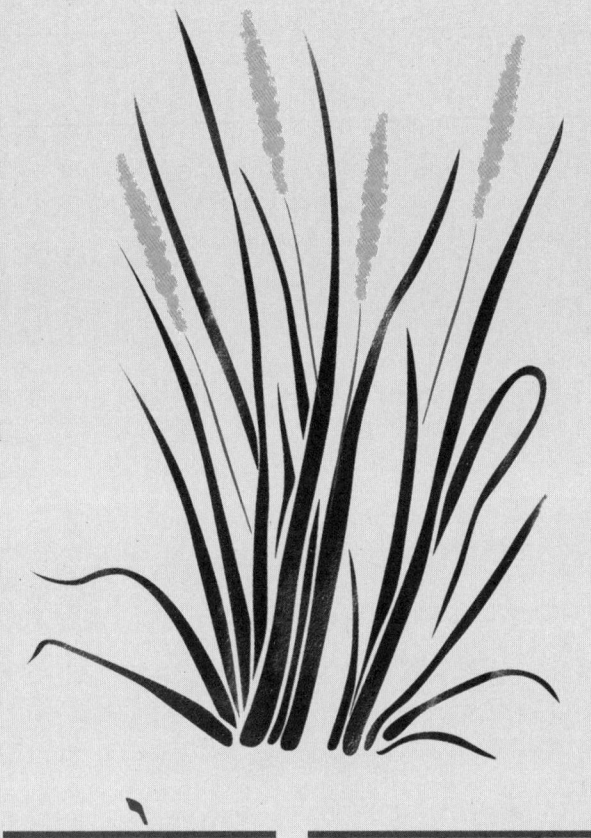

anjan grass

AFRICAN FOXTAIL GRASS
Cenchrus ciliaris

ANJAN GRASS/DHAMAN/BAIBA/KUSA/DHAMANIO *Hindi* .
KOLUKOTTAI *Tamil* . **KUSA** *Telugu*

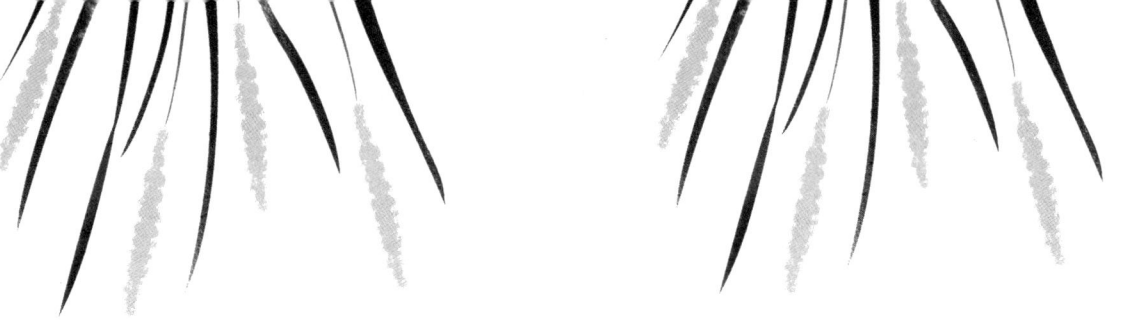

Anjan grass is a leafy prostrate and rhizomatous grass of the tropics. Planted in marginal lands and slopes to increase soil fertility and to reduce soil erosion, anjan grass is also the main source for paper production in many regions of India. It is also used in integrated pest management strategy as a pull crop, mainly in maize- and sorghum-producing areas of the country.

MEDICINAL PROPERTIES

Anjan grass' roots is an ingredient of traditional aphrodisiac prescriptions, and its seeds have diuretic properties. The seeds are pounded and eaten raw, made into porridge, or mixed and cooked with other foods. They are occasionally also mixed with pearl millet to make bread, or with sugar and ghee and given to children for nourishment.

What makes anjan grass more special is that it is relished by all livestock. It is an excellent type of maintenance quality fodder. When harvested at an early stage, anjan grass contains good proportions of crude protein with a suitable ratio of calcium and phosphorus. Even when fully ripe, the grass provides very good hay as it retains its nutritive value. Furthermore, depending on the rainfall, the yield varies greatly and in arid tract with less than 300 mm rainfall, a well-established pasture produces a yeild of 90-110 tonnes per hectare.

Anjan grass can withstand drought and is a good soil binder. Hence, it is used as a cover crop on bunds for soil and water conservation.

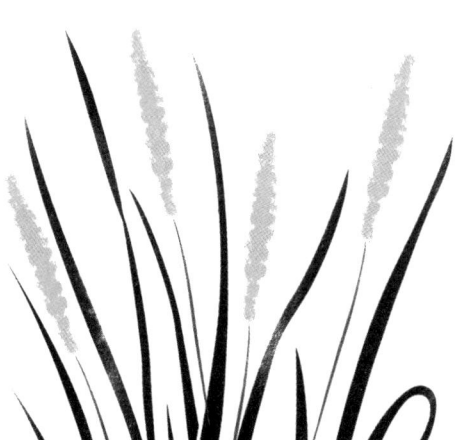

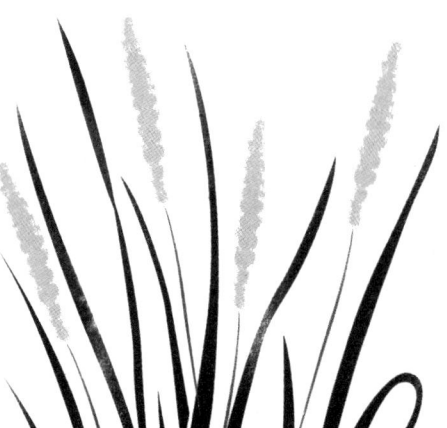

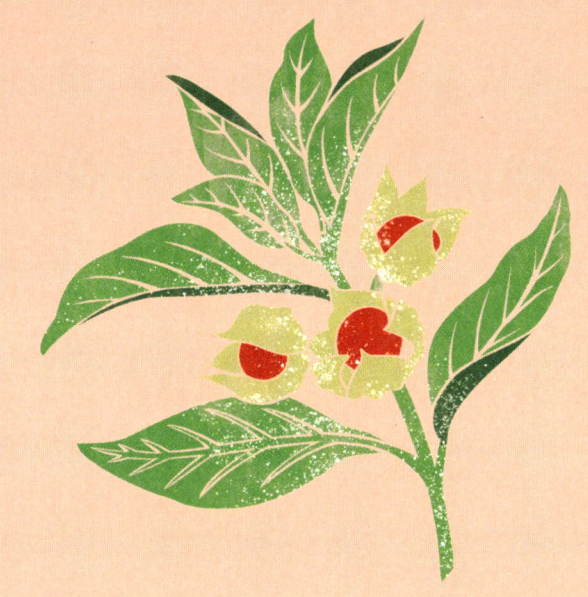

ashwagandha

INDIAN WINTER CHERRY

Withania somnifera

ASHWAGANDHA *Sanskrit, Hindi, Bangla, Assamese .* **AMUKKURAM** *Malayalam .* **HIREMADDINA GIDA** *Kannada*

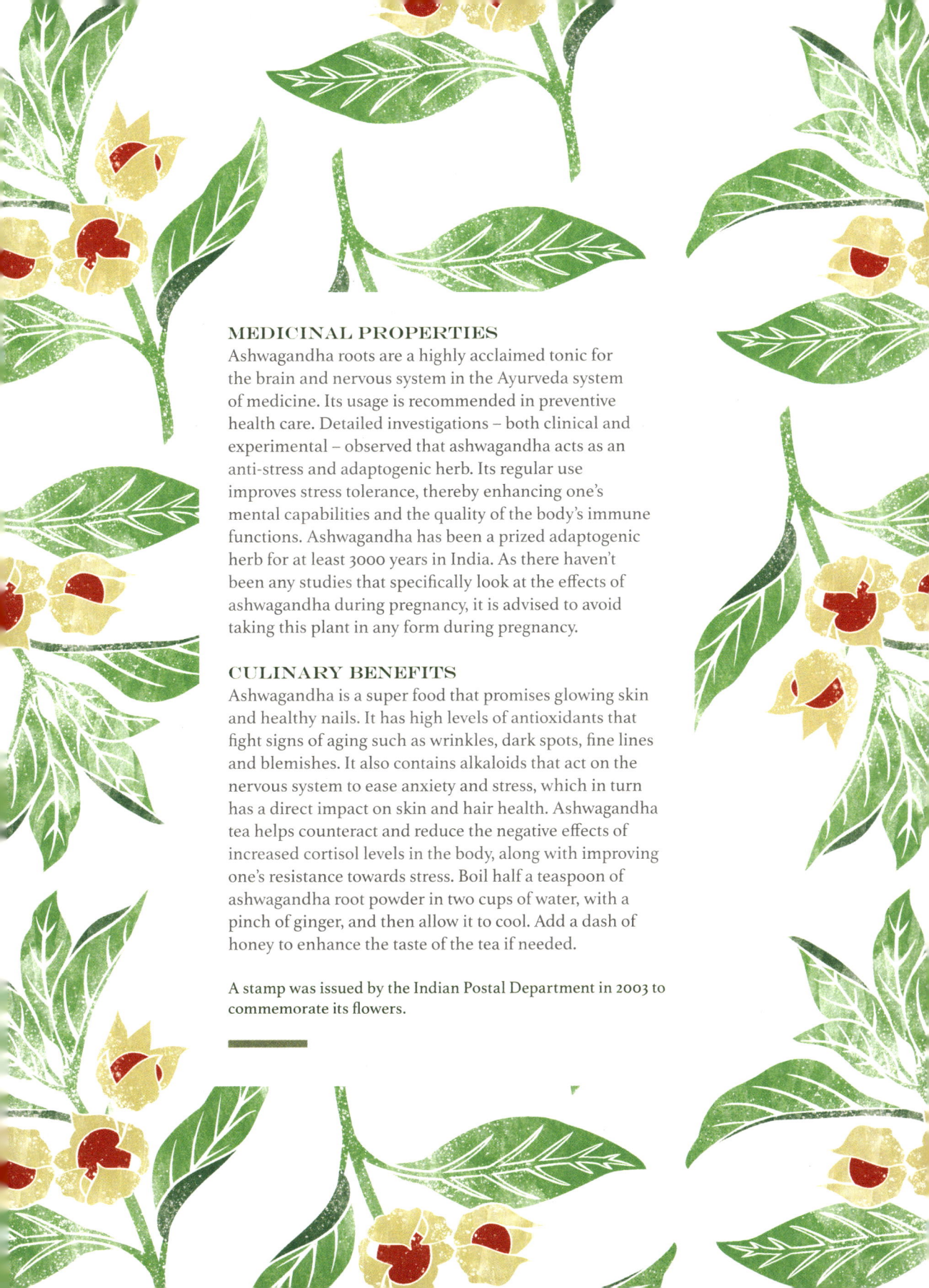

MEDICINAL PROPERTIES

Ashwagandha roots are a highly acclaimed tonic for the brain and nervous system in the Ayurveda system of medicine. Its usage is recommended in preventive health care. Detailed investigations – both clinical and experimental – observed that ashwagandha acts as an anti-stress and adaptogenic herb. Its regular use improves stress tolerance, thereby enhancing one's mental capabilities and the quality of the body's immune functions. Ashwagandha has been a prized adaptogenic herb for at least 3000 years in India. As there haven't been any studies that specifically look at the effects of ashwagandha during pregnancy, it is advised to avoid taking this plant in any form during pregnancy.

CULINARY BENEFITS

Ashwagandha is a super food that promises glowing skin and healthy nails. It has high levels of antioxidants that fight signs of aging such as wrinkles, dark spots, fine lines and blemishes. It also contains alkaloids that act on the nervous system to ease anxiety and stress, which in turn has a direct impact on skin and hair health. Ashwagandha tea helps counteract and reduce the negative effects of increased cortisol levels in the body, along with improving one's resistance towards stress. Boil half a teaspoon of ashwagandha root powder in two cups of water, with a pinch of ginger, and then allow it to cool. Add a dash of honey to enhance the taste of the tea if needed.

A stamp was issued by the Indian Postal Department in 2003 to commemorate its flowers.

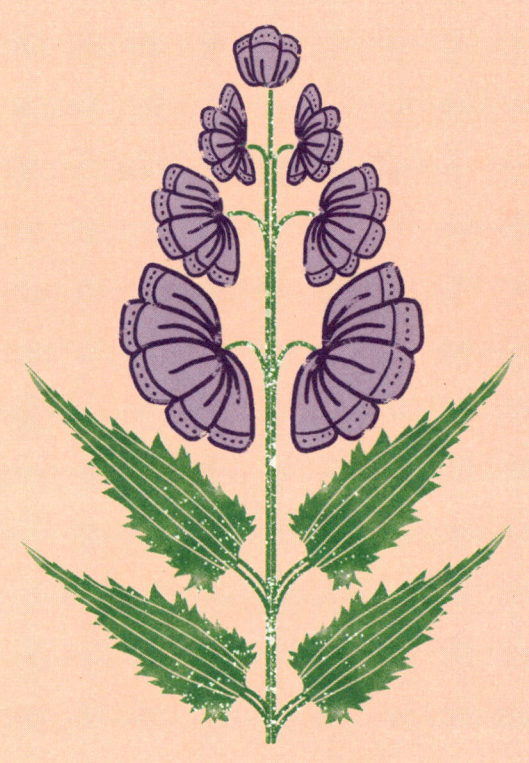

atिष

INDIAN ATEES
Aconitum heterophyllum

ATIS *Hindi* . AATAICH *Bangla* . ATBHAKHNI *Gujarati* .
ATIVISHA *Kannada* . ATIVISAM *Malayalam* .
ATIVIDYAM *Tamil* . ATI VISA *Telugu*

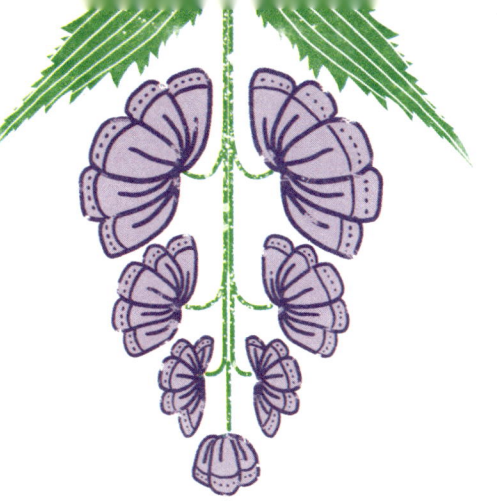
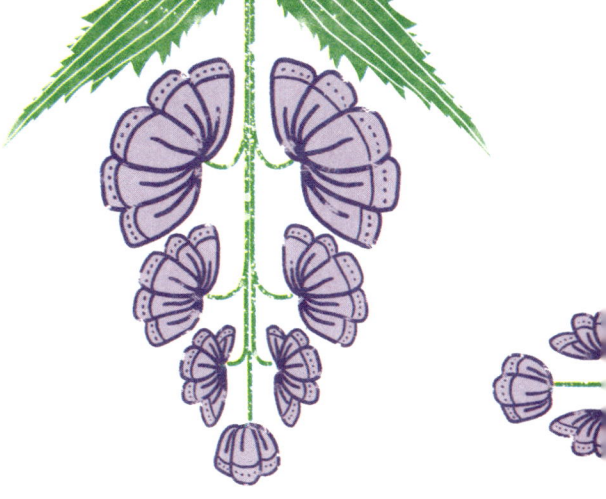

MEDICINAL PROPERTIES

Atis is part of a poisonous species used in Indian Ayurvedic medicine and accessed for its medicinal values in treating any other poison that may have entered the body. Its names in common India languages listed on the facing page show how it is known by this very quality.

The medicinal values of the root of this herb are well-known and used. Atis is an excellent medicine for treating common diseases in children like fever, cough, cold, vomiting and diarrhoea. Atis powder, when mixed with honey, helps in treating cough and cold, along with removing the accumulated mucus. Its roots can be inhaled for managing severe headaches and migraines. It is also known to be helpful in the treatment of IBS (irritable bowel syndrome), piles and haemorrhoids, especially in cases where they have been thought to be practically incurable.

It is a very powerful medicine and is administered in very small quantities, and so it should be taken under medical supervision.

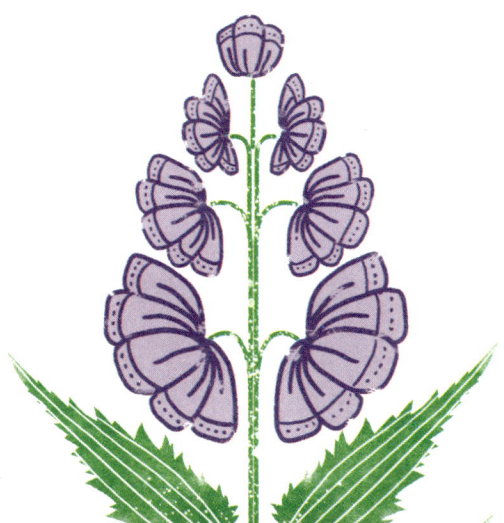
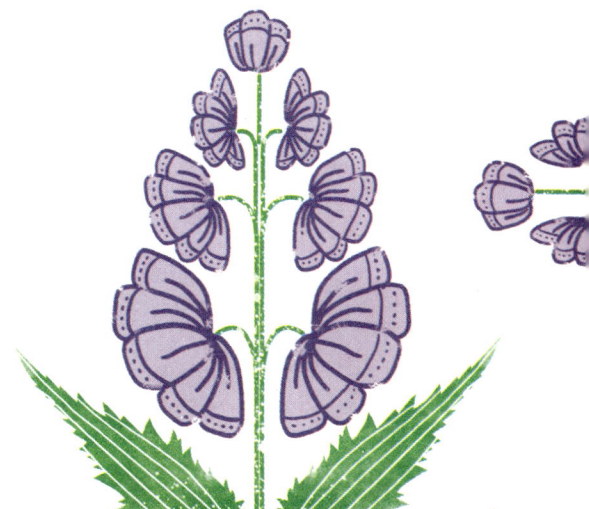

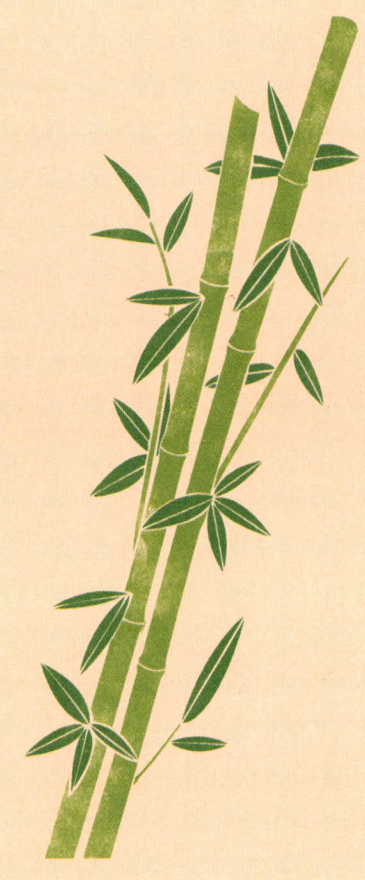

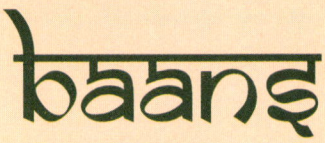

RINGAL

Chimonobambusa jaunsarensis (Gamble)

BAANS *Hindi, Nepali*

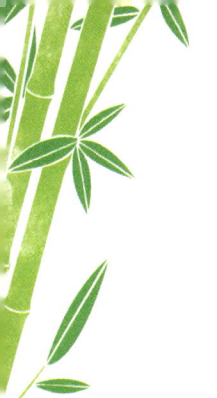
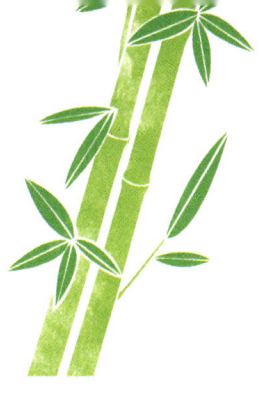
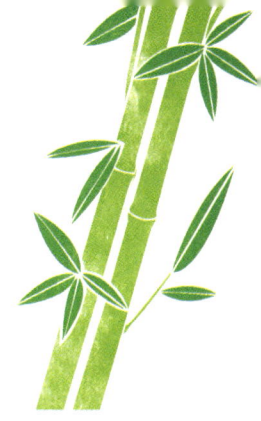

Ringal products are preferred over other bamboo products as they have greater resistance to water and therefore, survive longer in the snow-capped Himalayan region. One variety called dwarf bamboo, *Chimonobambusa jaunsarensis*, is widely preferred by the weavers (rudiyas) for its durability, quality and availability. Other varieties like that of *Thamnocalamus spathiflorus* (Dev ringal) is valued for its elastic nature, natural yellowish colour and erectness, and is used to make puja *thalis*, roofs and coverings for grass houses, hookah pipes and walking sticks, while others are used for making handicraft and agricultural items.

Ringal basketry is a popular craft in the Kumaon and Garhwal region of Uttarakhand. Some of the products made are *kandi/odagi* (a big basket used for crop residue and collection), *solta/malkhna* (a multi-purpose big netted basket), *tokari* (a round vessel for keeping chapatti, fruits and flowers), *supa* (winnower)*, changera/bisala/dabolla* (dome-shaped basket for storing grains).

MEDICINAL PROPERTIES
Ringal's medicinal value lies in the treatment of asthma, cough, paralytic complaints and other debilitating diseases.

CULINARY BENEFITS
Culinary young bamboo shoots are a delicacy in many cuisines. in several traditional cuisines of northeast India. They are an excellent source of fibre. After being rinsed and immersed in water, the shoots are cooked or fried in oil, and eaten as vegetables or combined with pork and other vegetables.

Ringal is a socioeconomically and ecologically important type of bamboo that is extensively found in the rich forests of Garhwal Himalayas. Ringal weaving is an age-old craft in the state of Uttarakhand with almost every family directly or indirectly involved. Ringal products are tough, durable and last for at least 20-25 years.

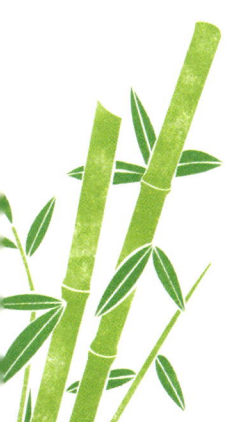
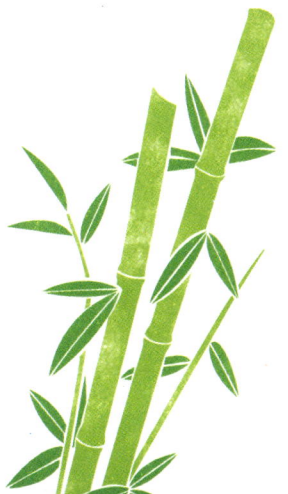
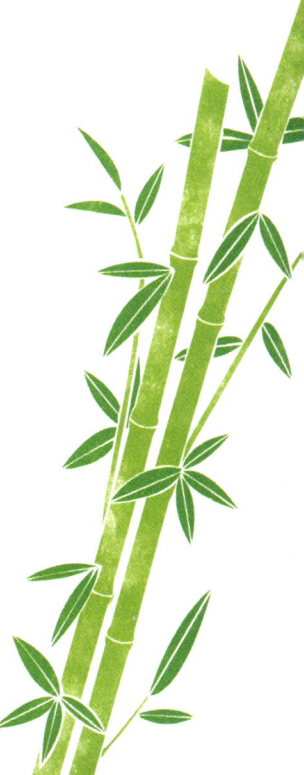

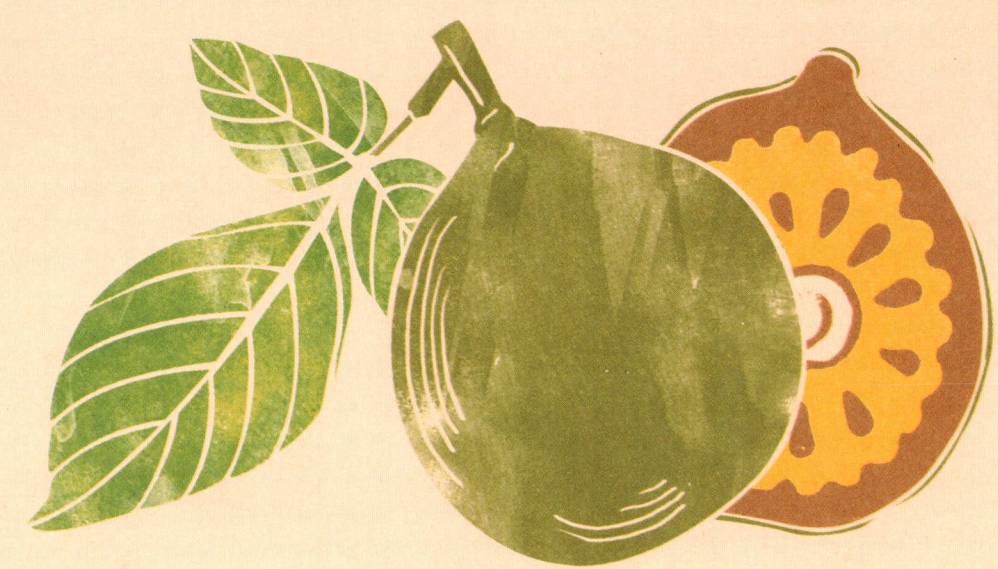

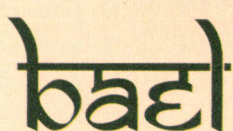

STONE APPLE
Aegle marmelos

BAEL *Hindi, Bangla, Oriya, Assamese*

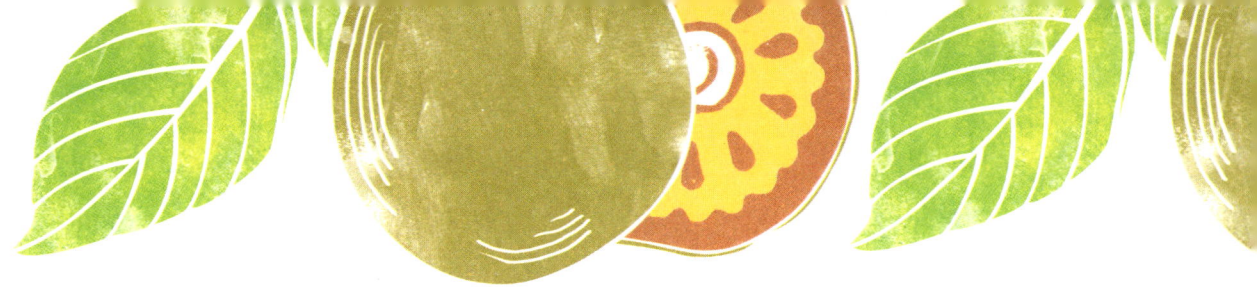

MEDICINAL PROPERTIES

When unripe, the bael is most effective remedy for diarrhoea and dysentery, while the ripe fruit is a great remedy for constipation. This fruit, along with its leaves, roots, barks and seeds are important ingredients for both Ayurveda and Unani medicinal preparations. While the burnt fruit pulp is applied on rheumatic joints, a couple of spoons of the fruit pulp is given before sleep to overcome morning sickness. Additionally, the fruit rind can be applied externally on the head to kill lice. For a stomach ache, a paste of fresh roots ground along with one black pepper, is very helpful.

CULINARY BENEFITS

The fruit of the bael has cooling properties. After soaking the fruit, its seeds and fibre are separated for an extremely cooling drink, prepared during hot summer months. In northern India, bael sherbet is available as a popular street drink that keeps people hydrated and plays a vital role in maintaining the body's energy supply, during the summer months. Typically, the fruits are also used to prepare a large number of by-products such as candy, panjiri, toffee and jam, which increases its shelf life.

COSMETIC CURES

Bael is often used as a substitute for soap and also as a source of essential oils and perfumes.

Bael is a sacred tree, which they dedicate to Lord Shiva by the offering of its leaves. Its three leaflets are believed to be emblematic of various threesomes: the three gunas (satva, rajas and tamas, or morality, superiority and immorality, respectively); the three Gods (Brahma, Vishnu and Mahesh); and the three lives (past, present and future). Bael is considered to be extremely auspicious and hence is grown around most temples.

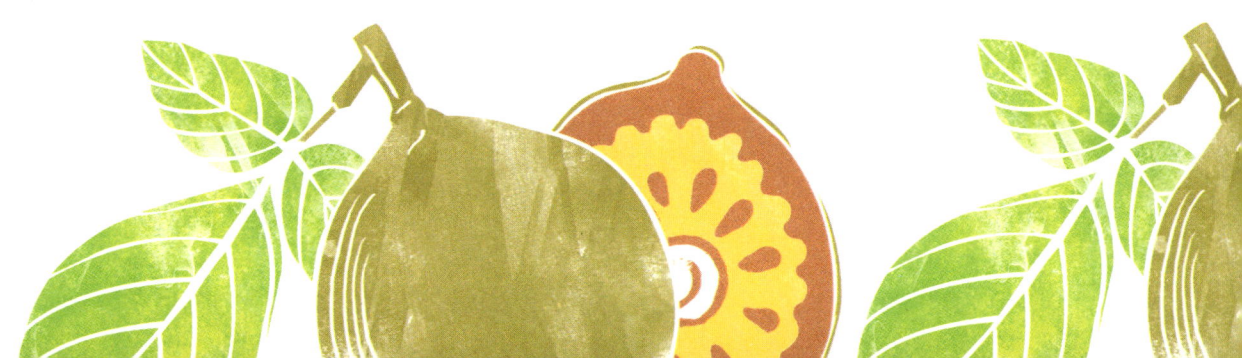

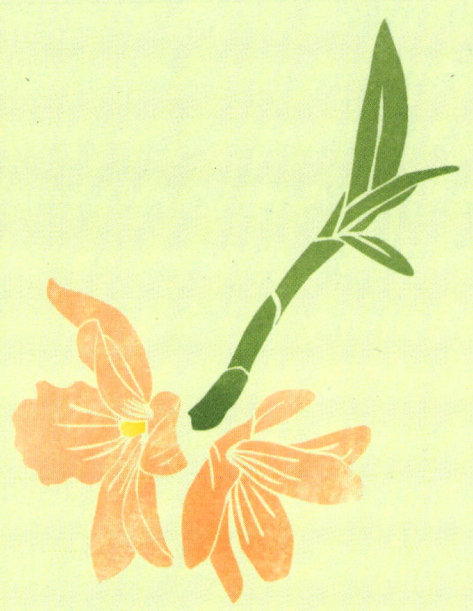

bechu

SHOE-LIPPED DENDROBIUM
Dendrobium crepidatrium Lindl

BECHU/NANGLI *Marathi*

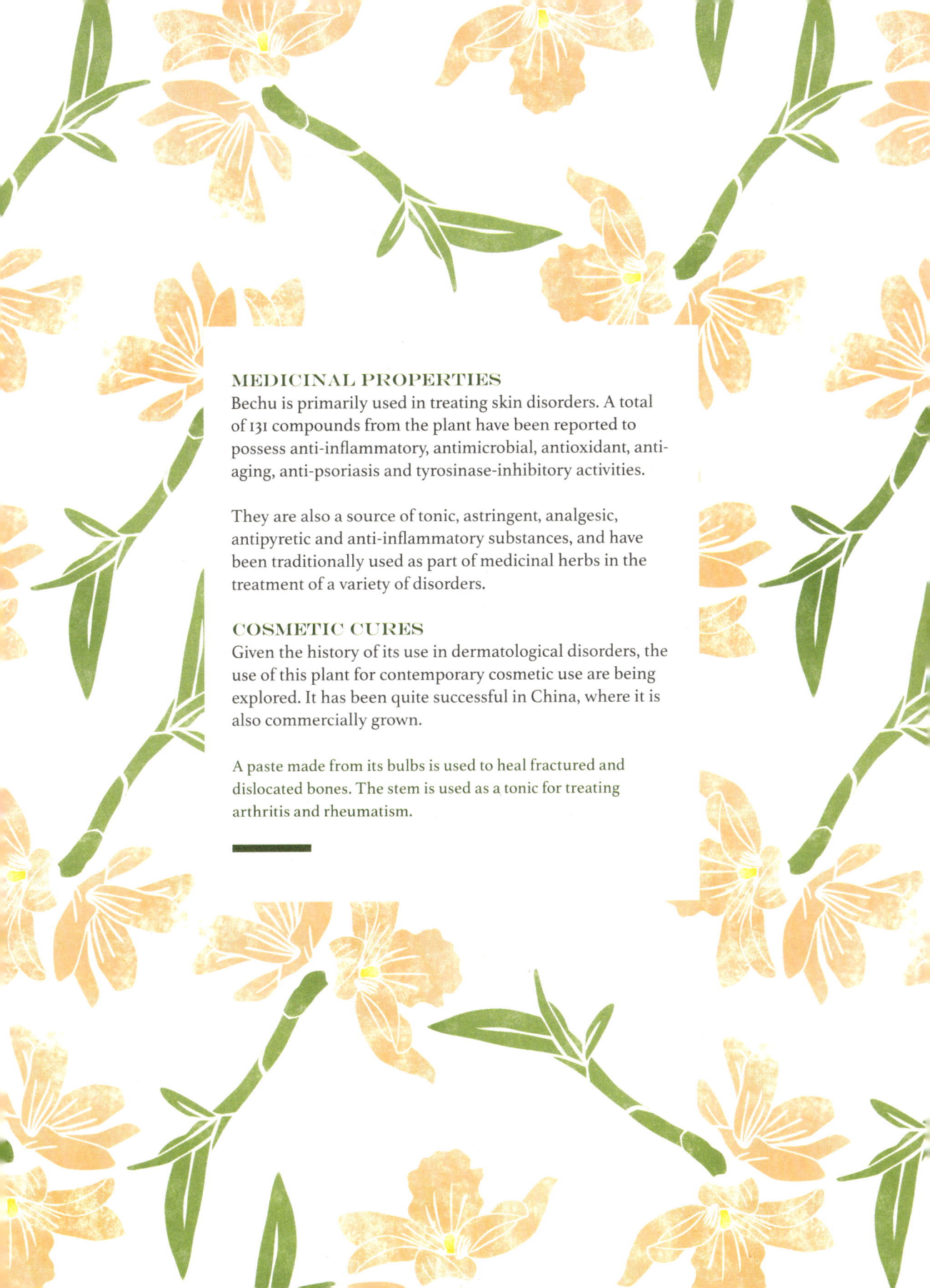

MEDICINAL PROPERTIES

Bechu is primarily used in treating skin disorders. A total of 131 compounds from the plant have been reported to possess anti-inflammatory, antimicrobial, antioxidant, anti-aging, anti-psoriasis and tyrosinase-inhibitory activities.

They are also a source of tonic, astringent, analgesic, antipyretic and anti-inflammatory substances, and have been traditionally used as part of medicinal herbs in the treatment of a variety of disorders.

COSMETIC CURES

Given the history of its use in dermatological disorders, the use of this plant for contemporary cosmetic use are being explored. It has been quite successful in China, where it is also commercially grown.

A paste made from its bulbs is used to heal fractured and dislocated bones. The stem is used as a tonic for treating arthritis and rheumatism.

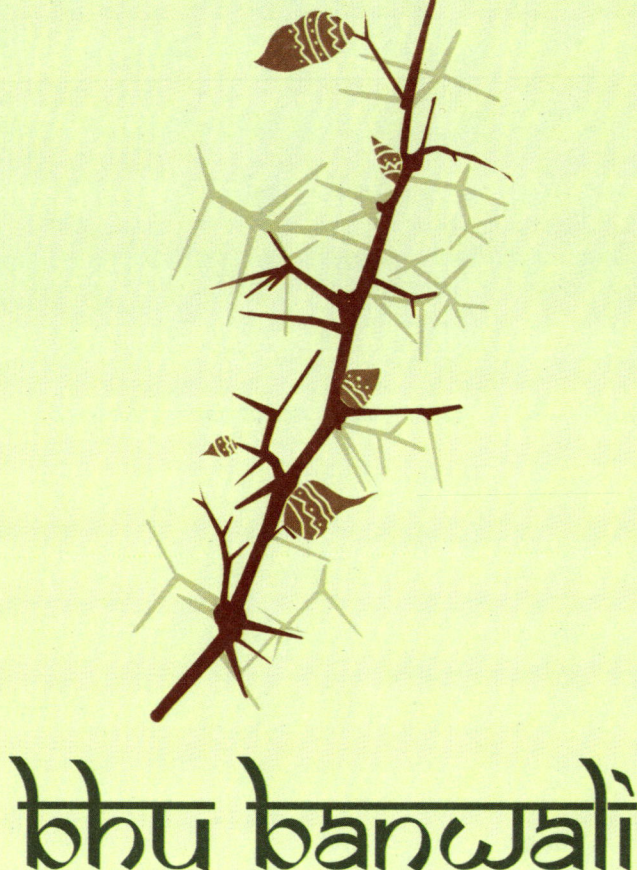

bhu banwali

DESERT ACACIA

Acacia jacquemontii

BHU BANWALI *Hindi*

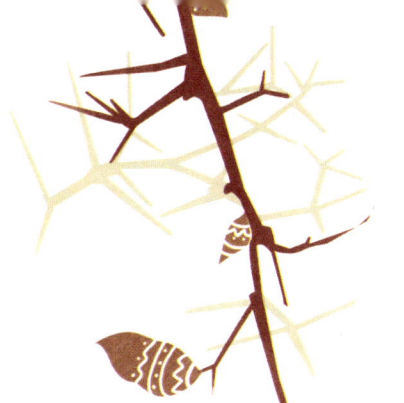
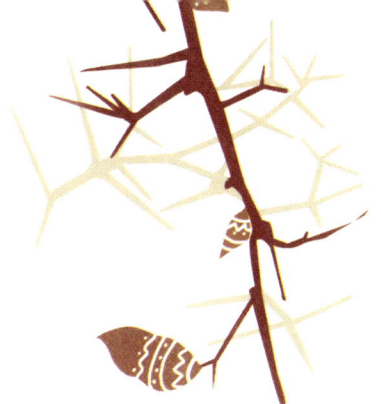

MEDICINAL PROPERTIES

Bhu banwali's bark is used in the treatment of snake bites and scorpion stings. *A. jacquemontii* produces dried gum on its stem and this gum has been extensively used by tribal communities for renal disorders. It is also added in various food preparations to serve as a health tonic, and in the treatment of asthma and mouth sores.

COSMETIC CURES

Bhu banwali is widely used in the making of toothpastes as an abrasive to clean teeth and remove stains without being too aggressive on the surface.

The leaves and pods of this plant are a good source of fodder for goats and camels. Its wood is a very useful fuel in the Indian subcontinent due to its high calorific value. The bark of the plant is used in small-sized tanneries while imparting brown or black colour to the leather. On burning, the wood gives out intense heat and is therefore preferred by gold, silver and iron smiths.

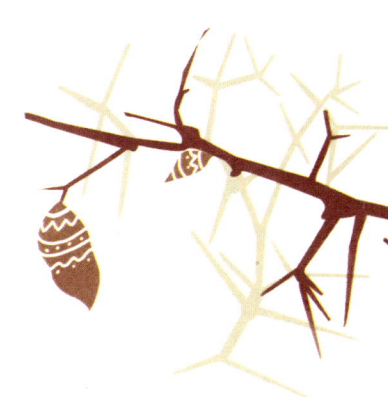

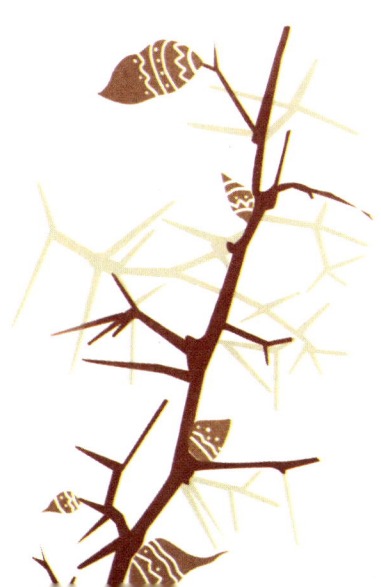
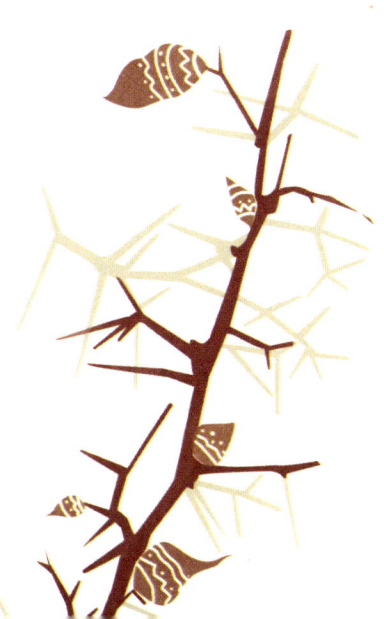

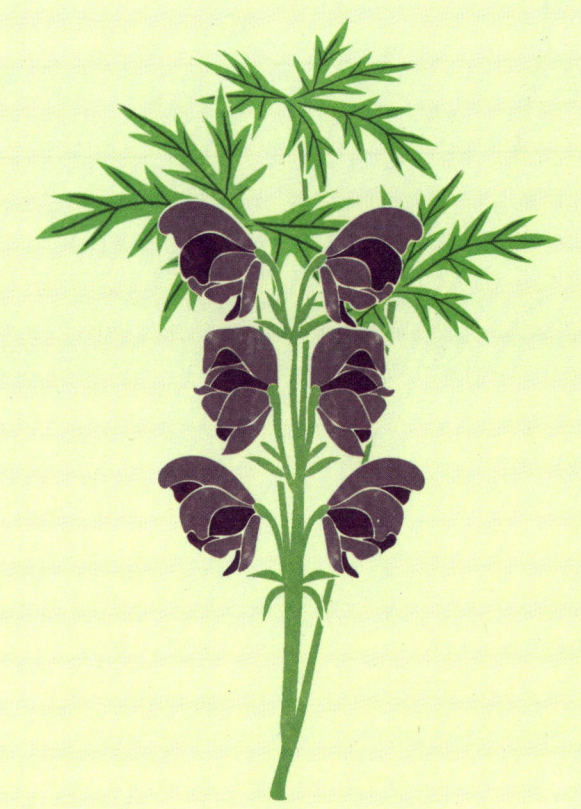

bikh/bikhma

ACONITE

Aconitum ferox Wall ex Ser (Ranunculaceae)

BIKHA/BIKHMA *Nepali*

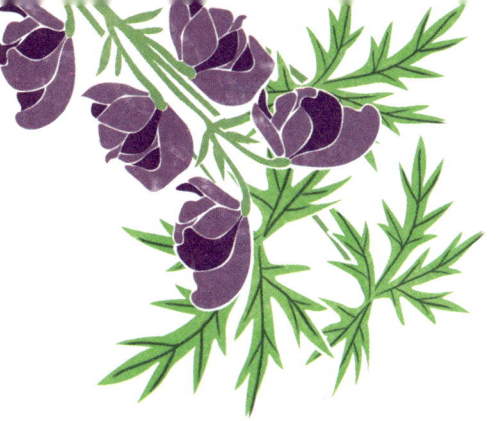
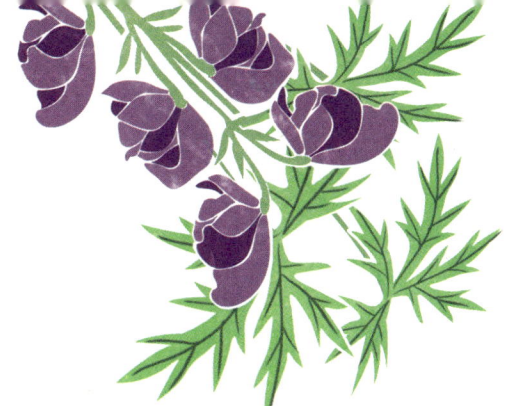

MEDICINAL PROPERTIES

Known to be very poisonous, almost lethal if had directly by humans or animals, with careful detoxification processes, this plant can be turned into a medicine.

Bikh's roots are used as an antidote for lethal poisons of local origin. The root powder is used to relieve all types of ailments such as severe body pain, diabetes, debility, asthma, ear and nose discharge, leprosy, paralysis and rheumatism. It is extremely poisonous and used against snake bites, while a local application in the form of a paste made out of its root powder helps in reducing swelling and pain. In Nepal, it is used as a folk medicine in treating leprosy and cholera.

CULINARY BENEFITS

While its young shoots and leaves are used as a vegetable, the fruits are eaten raw.

Children often use the latex of the plant for drawing tattoos.

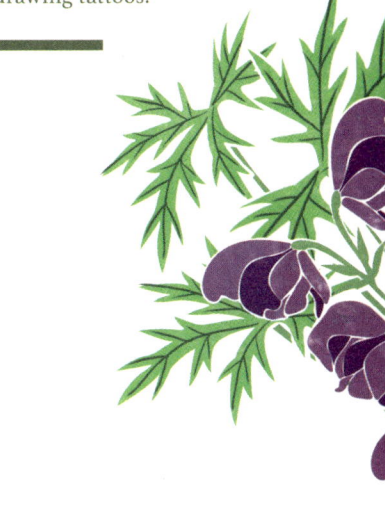

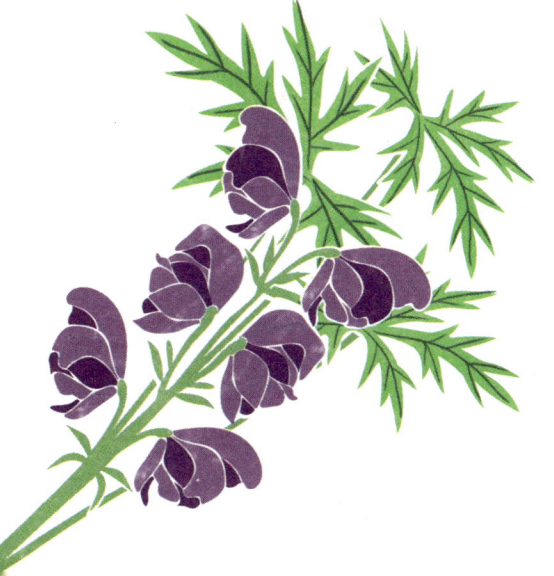
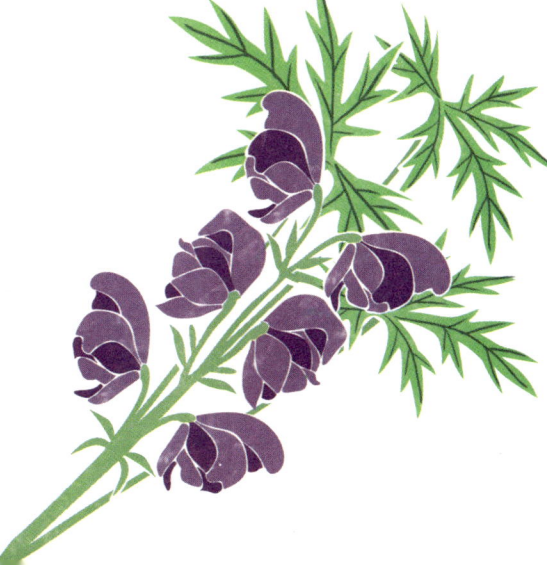

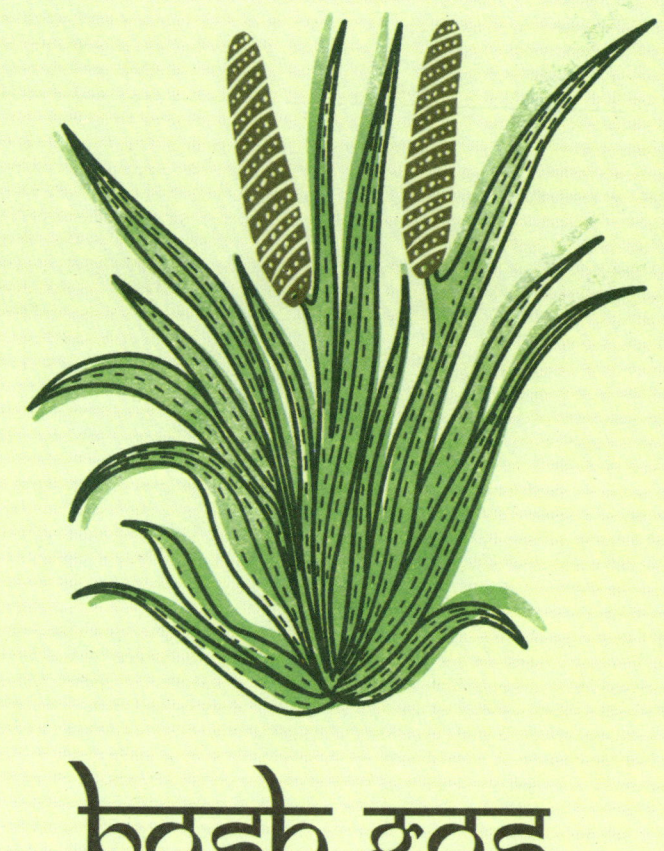

bosh gos

SWEET FLAG

Acorus calamus Linn. [Araceae]

BOSH GOS *Assamese*

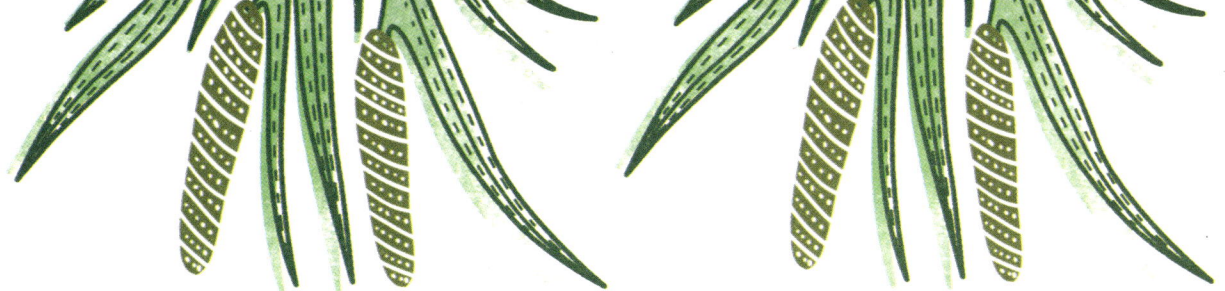

MEDICINAL PROPERTIES

When squashed and served as juice, bosh gos is often administered to patients in the treatment of diarrhoea and dysentery. The powdered roots are also used as a vermifuge. The dried roots of the plant are additionally valuable in the treatment of epilepsy, delirium, hysteria, amnesia, convulsions, dyspepsia, remittent fever, colic and snake bites. Bosh gos also acts as an emetic and in larger doses can cause violent vomiting.

CULINARY BENEFITS

Bosh gos' zesty and woody scent can supplant customary flavours like cinnamon, nutmeg and ginger. The extract is used in customary medication to alleviate headaches and migraines and other nervous system issues. It is said to reduce swelling in joints, and to calm and relax, as well as to treat vertigo and symptoms of dysentery.

COSMETIC CURES

Due to its aromatic properties, bosh gos is used in shampoos, hair conditioners, body lotions, bathing soaps, toothpastes and other personal care products. Its essential oil has a revitalizing role to play in personal care – especifically for moisturizing the skin.

The squashed root juice of this plant helps enormously in dealing with anomalies in the menstrual cycle and towards checking inordinate uterine bleeding.

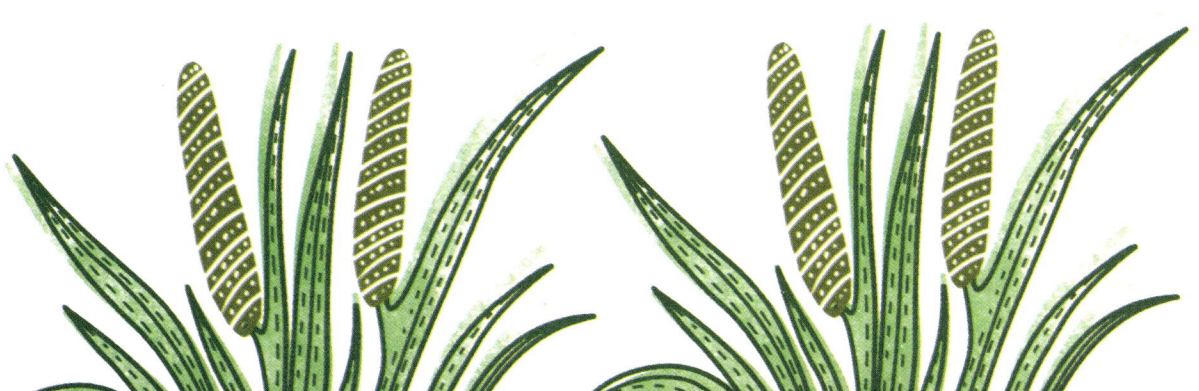

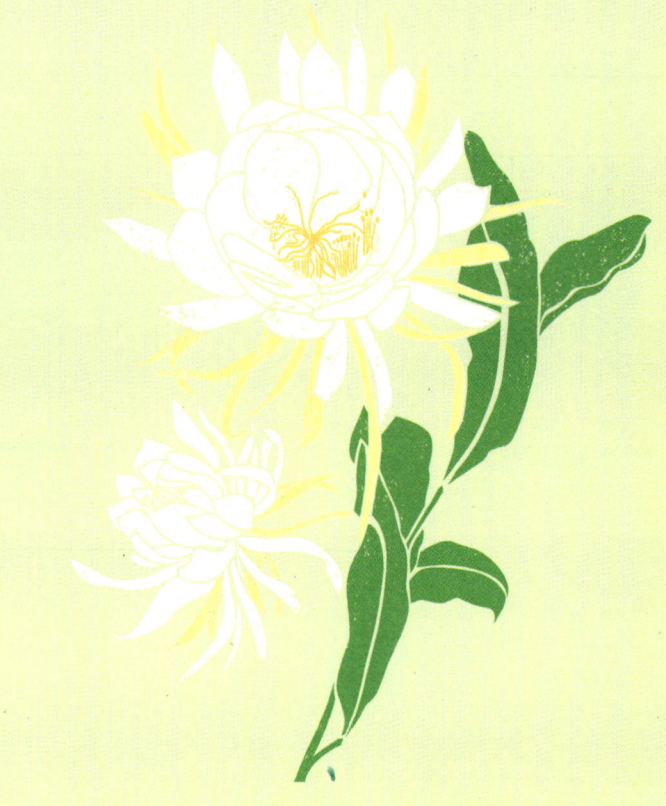

brahma kamal

SACRED SAUSSUREA

Saussurea obvallata

BRAHMA KAMAL *Hindi*

Brahma kamal, the state flower of Uttarakhand, is revered in religious purposes and known for its impressive medicinal properties. The plant, which grows above an altitude of 14,000 feet, is under imminent threat posed by over-harvesting and drastic climate change. The species – whose botanical name is *Saussurea obvallata* – is found only in the Himalayas.

MEDICINAL PROPERTIES

According to the Indian Academy of Sciences, brahma kamal clears recurrent urinary tract infections and can be used in treating fever. Considered a herb in both Tibetan and Chinese fields of medicine, its flowers, roots and leaves are often used in the treatment of bone ache, intestinal ailments, cough and cold.

CULINARY BENEFITS

Due to its bitter nature, it is an excellent liver tonic and a great appetizer. Soup made from this plant helps soothe liver inflammations and also increases blood volume in the body.

RITUAL USE

The flower is extensively used in shrines and temples in higher altitudes as offerings.

Catching the flower in bloom is a rare sight. Brahma kamal blooms in the late evening and stays for only a couple of hours. The flower remains intact throughout its life cycle. It blooms only one night in a year, exposing its star-like petals. The one who sees the blooming flower is believed to be blessed by Lord Brahma.

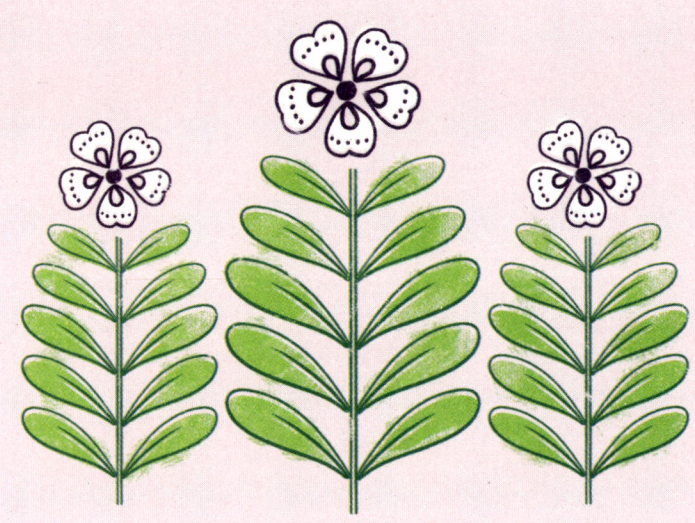

brahmi

WATER HYSSOP

Bacopa monnieri

BRAHMI *Hindi.* **BIRAMI** *Bangla* . **JALA BRAHMI** *Kannada* .
SAMBARENU *Telugu* . **NEERA BRAHMI** *Tamil*

MEDICINAL PROPERTIES
Brahmi is known for its revitalizing and nootropic activities in Ayurvedic medicine as it strengthens memory and intellect. Traditionally, brahmi was utilized in various conditions afflicting the mind and nervous system. In traditional Ayurvedic medicine, it is a *rasayana*, or a rejuvenative tonic, which promotes the revitalization of the body and tissues. Brahmi is slightly astringent and hence useful in treating diarrhoea.

CULINARY BENEFITS
Brahmi leaves are also made into a drink concentrate that can be added to either milk or water. It is believed to be cooling and energizing for the body.

COSMETIC CURES
The glycolic that is extracted from brahmi protects the skin from free radicals and attack by oxidizing agents. Hence it is used in protective day creams, skincare products, shower gels and scalp care products. It is also used in making hair oils as applying this oil strengthens hair follicles.

The term 'brahmi' originates from the Hindu god Brahma, which refers to the feminine aspect of Brahman. *Bacopa monnieri* has been so revered over the centuries that the Hindus used it in their rituals to consecrate new-born babies, believing it will open the gateways to knowledge.

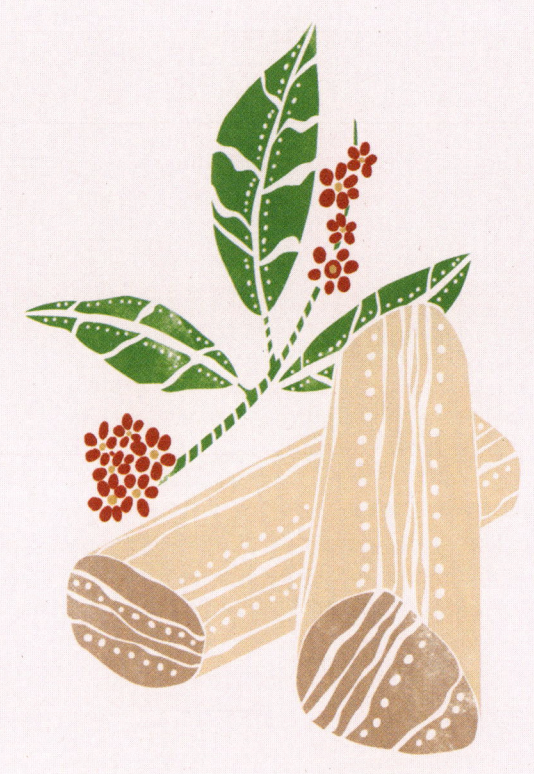

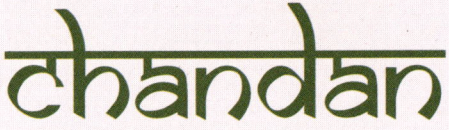

chandan

SANDALWOOD

Santalum album

CHANDAN *Hindi, Bangla,Punjabi* . CHANDANM *Tamil* . CANDANAM
Malayalam . TELLA CHANDANM *Telugu* . SUKHADA *Gujarati* .
SHRIGANDHA *Kannada*

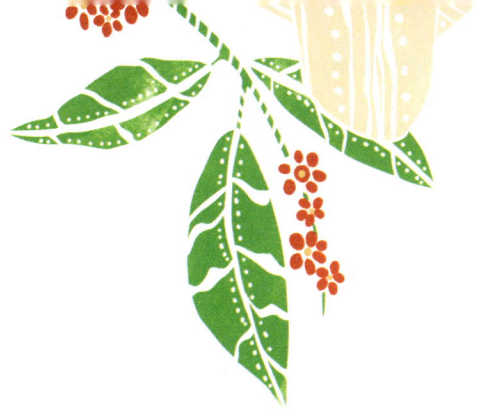
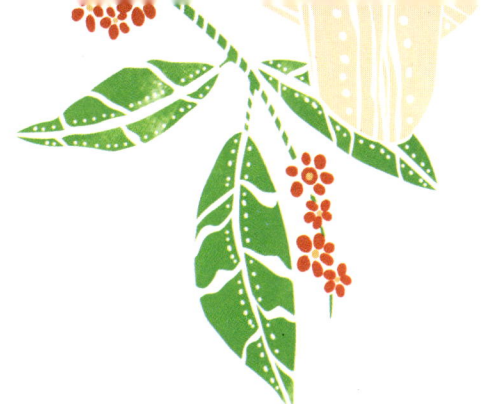

MEDICINAL PROPERTIES

Chandan oil has been used as an antiseptic and astringent, and for the treatment of headache, stomach ache and urinary disorders. In India, chandan paste is used in the treatment of inflammatory and eruptive skin diseases. The oil has also been used in the traditional Ayurvedic medicinal system as a diuretic and mild stimulant for smoothening the skin. Sandalwood oil helps manage sore throat due to its pitta balancing and sita (cold) properties. Diluting a few drops of the oil in water, and gargling once or twice a day with it helps soothe the symptoms.

COSMETIC CURES

Chandan oil aids in curing acne, blackheads, dry skin, crackling and flaking, and other skin conditions that are believed to be caused by an imbalance of pitta doshas that makes the skin prone to irritations. The goodness of chandan oil assists in restoring the damaged skin cells and maintaining its glow and radiance. Its potent astringent, antiseptic, antimicrobial, anti-aging and disinfectant properties shield the skin from harmful bacteria, virus and fungal attacks. Chandan, in powder or oil form, is popular for its cooling properties. It helps sooth inflammatory skin conditions such as eczema, dermatitis and psoriasis, as well as calm irritated skin and flatten breakouts.

RITUAL USE

One of the most important significance of chandan is in using its paste to apply on devotees' foreheads. Anointing idols with chandan tikkas is a practice in a majority of temples across India. Chandan is also used during marriage ceremonies wherein the bride and groom are anointed with a chandan and haldi paste.

Known as chandan in India, sandalwood has been used in several religious practices for centuries in the form of carvings, and is applied to the body for purification purposes and its cooling properties.

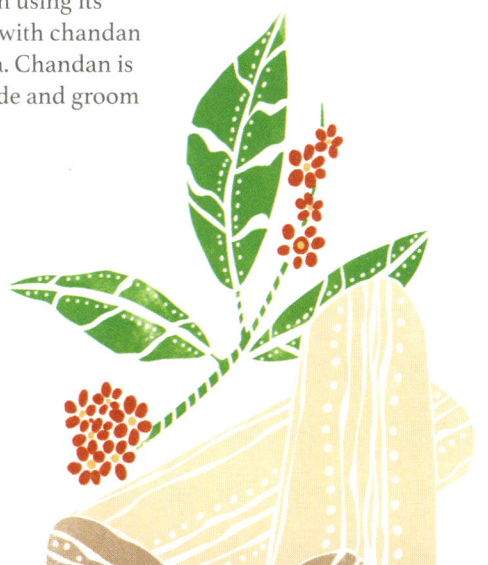

chhawntan

INDIAN NETTLE

Acalypha Indica L. (Euohorbiaceae)

CHHAWNTAN *Mizo*

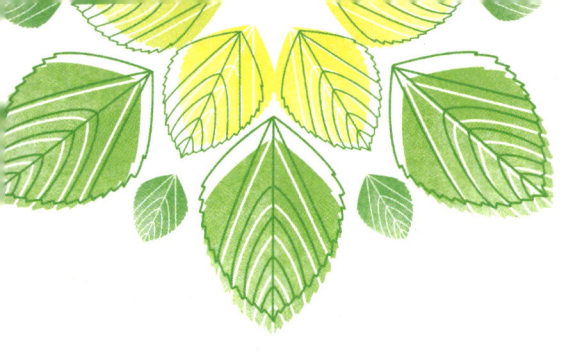
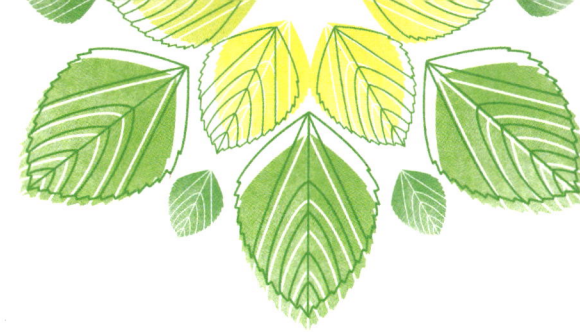

MEDICINAL PROPERTIES

The powder and paste of chhawntan leaves are applied externally in burns, scabies and centipede bites. They are also used in treating bedsores and maggot-infested wounds. Fresh juice of the leaves is applied with oil, salt or lime to treat rheumatoid arthritis. The leaves are likewise utilized as a safe and speedy purgative, and also to cure tooth and ear ache. The powdered leaf, when mixed with salt, can be applied externally to maggot-infested wounds, skin parasites and other skin issues.

CULINARY BENEFITS

Chhawntan is often cultivated for its edible roots and leaves, which are cooked as a vegetable.

COSMETIC CURES

A cosmetic use of chhawntan is in the production of anti-acne cream. In its powdered form, it is available in the market as a face mask and for hair removal.

Though chhawntan possesses diuretic, carminative, expectorant and emetic properties, it also causes gastrointestinal disturbance. It is often used in early cases of ringworm with lime juice.

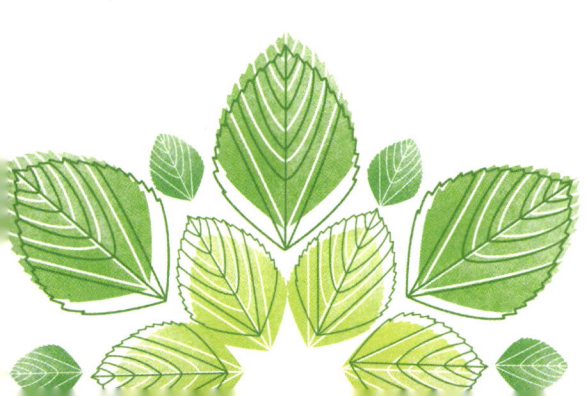
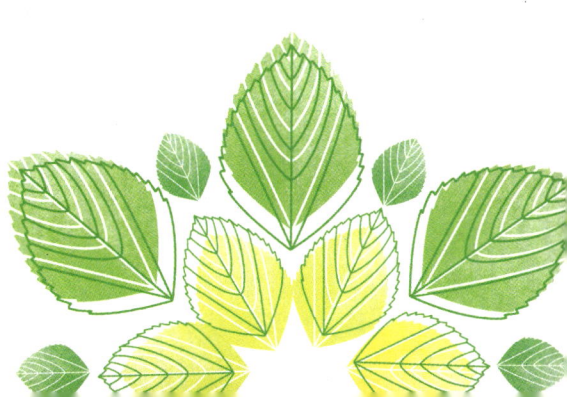

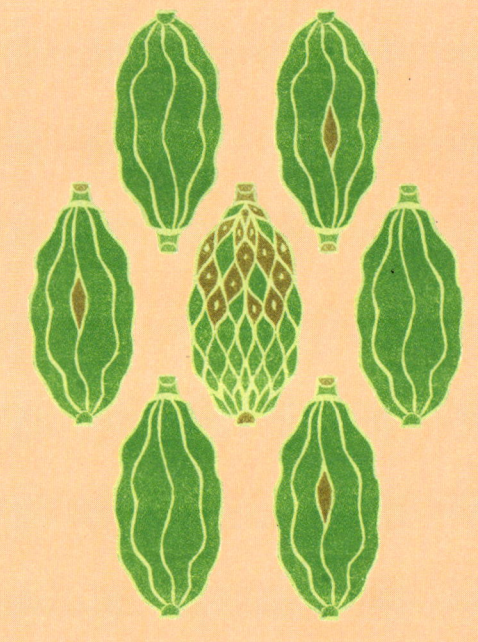

chhoti ilaichi

GREEN CARDAMOM
Eletteria cardomomum

CHHOTI ILAICHI *Hindi* . **ELAKKAI** *Tamil* . **AELAKKA** *Malayalam* .
YELAKULU *Telugu* . **YALAKKI** *Kannada* . **ILAYCHI** *Gujarati* .
ELACH *Bangla*

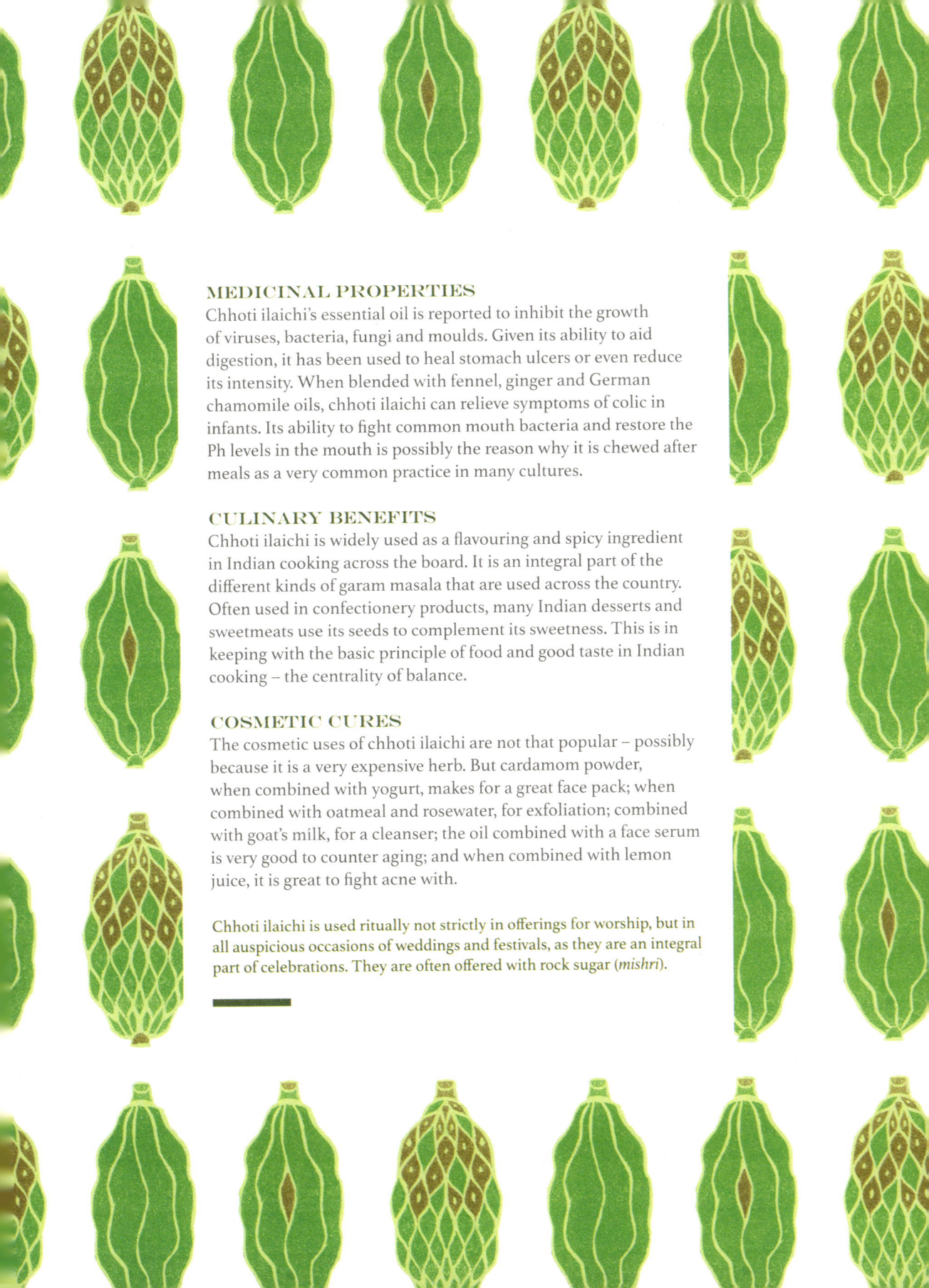

MEDICINAL PROPERTIES

Chhoti ilaichi's essential oil is reported to inhibit the growth of viruses, bacteria, fungi and moulds. Given its ability to aid digestion, it has been used to heal stomach ulcers or even reduce its intensity. When blended with fennel, ginger and German chamomile oils, chhoti ilaichi can relieve symptoms of colic in infants. Its ability to fight common mouth bacteria and restore the Ph levels in the mouth is possibly the reason why it is chewed after meals as a very common practice in many cultures.

CULINARY BENEFITS

Chhoti ilaichi is widely used as a flavouring and spicy ingredient in Indian cooking across the board. It is an integral part of the different kinds of garam masala that are used across the country. Often used in confectionery products, many Indian desserts and sweetmeats use its seeds to complement its sweetness. This is in keeping with the basic principle of food and good taste in Indian cooking – the centrality of balance.

COSMETIC CURES

The cosmetic uses of chhoti ilaichi are not that popular – possibly because it is a very expensive herb. But cardamom powder, when combined with yogurt, makes for a great face pack; when combined with oatmeal and rosewater, for exfoliation; combined with goat's milk, for a cleanser; the oil combined with a face serum is very good to counter aging; and when combined with lemon juice, it is great to fight acne with.

Chhoti ilaichi is used ritually not strictly in offerings for worship, but in all auspicious occasions of weddings and festivals, as they are an integral part of celebrations. They are often offered with rock sugar (*mishri*).

chirayata

BITTER STICK

Swertia chirayata

CHIRAYATA *Hindi* . **CHIROTA** *Bangla* . **CHIRTA** *Assamese* .
KARIYATU/KARIYATUN *Gujarati* . **NALEBEVU/CHIRATA KADDI/**
CHIRAYAT *Kannada* . **LOSE/CHIRAITA** *Kashmiri* . **NELAVEPPU/**
KIRAYATHU/NILAMAKANJIRAM *Malayalam* . **KIRAITA/**
KADUCHIRAITA *Marathi* . **CHIREITA** *Oriya* . **CHIRETTA/CHIRAITA**
Punjabi . **NILAVEMBU** *Tamil* . **NELAVEMU** *Telugu* . **CHIRAITA** *Urdu*

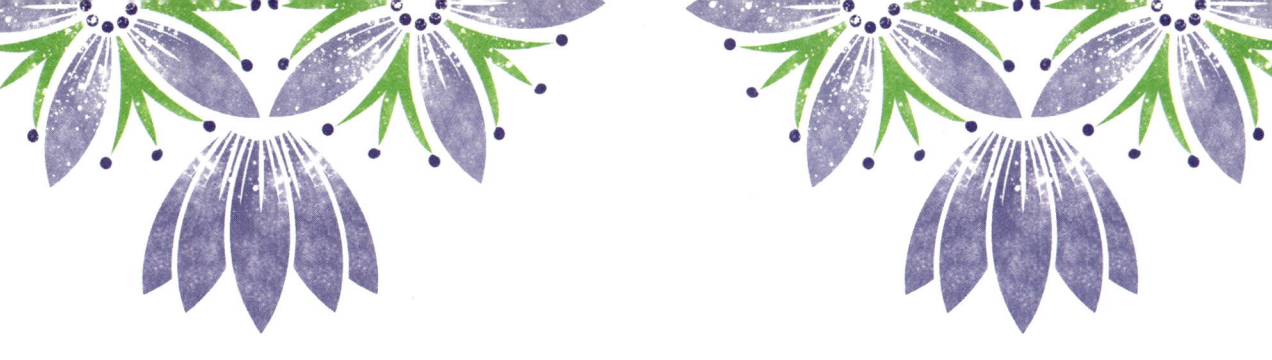

MEDICINAL PROPERTIES

Chirayata is traditionally used to treat numerous ailments such as liver disorders, malaria and diabetes, and is reported to have a wide spectrum of pharmacological properties. It is an excellent remedy for strengthening the gut and also for the treatment of dyspepsia and diarrhoea. As per Ayurveda, taking chirayata water twice a day helps manage fever due to its Jvarghana (antipyretic) property. Its powdered form, when mixed with coconut oil, helps heal wounds due to its *ropan* (healing) properties. Due to chirayata also being anti-parasitic, it helps eliminate roundworms and tapeworms from the body.

CULINARY BENEFITS

When consumed daily, chirayata can provide protection to the liver by getting rid of toxins from the body. It can also help with the generation of new liver cells. The plant is also believed to create more blood in the body, thereby helping with anaemia.

COSMETIC CURES

Chirayata is useful in managing several skin problems including acne. Applying the paste of chirayata powder along with honey reduces the redness and inflammation of the skin.

When you consume a glass of it daily – practiced in many communities and households, traditionally – it helps flush out the toxins from the body, and treats various conditions like rashes, itching, burning sensation and redness of the skin.

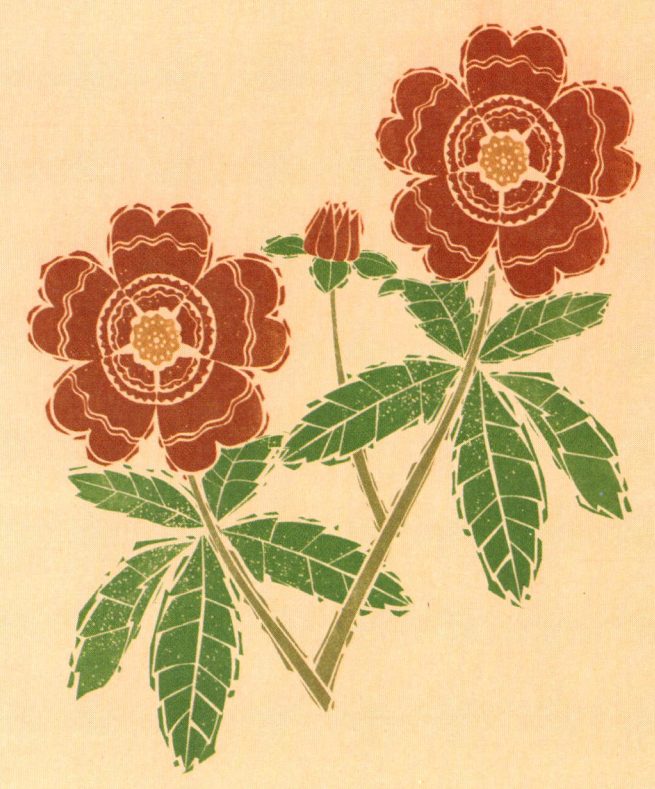

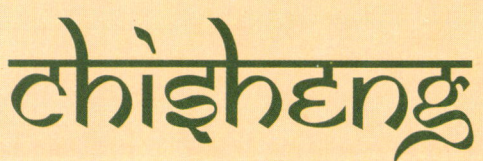

chisheng

HIMALAYAN CINQUEFOIL

Potentilla astrosanguinea Lodd, Orsaceae (B. 582)

CHISHENG *Ladakhi*

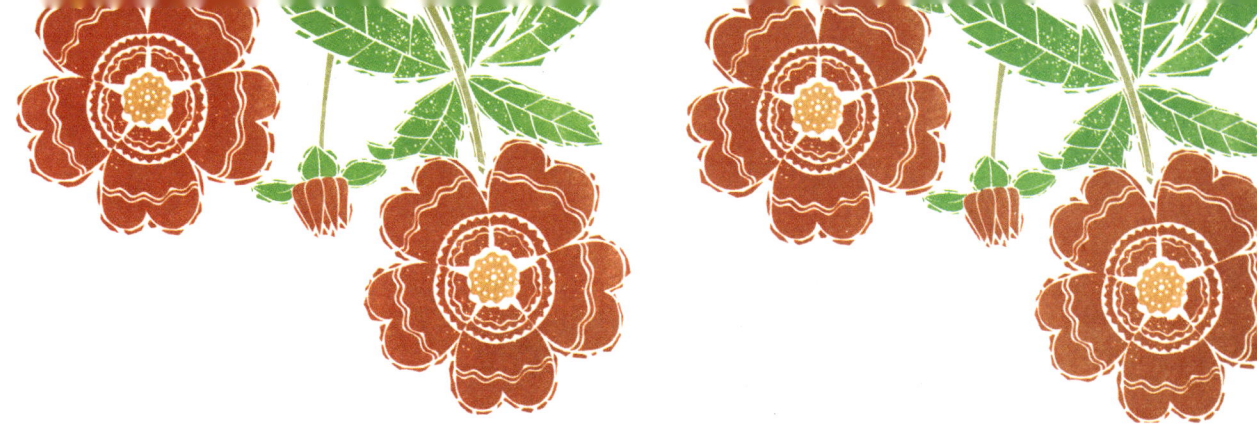

Commonly known as Himalayan cinquefoil or ruby cinquefoil, chisheng is a vigorous herbaceous perennial of the rose family whose flowers either grow isolated or in small groups.

MEDICINAL PROPERTIES

A salt tea is prepared from the whole plant after boiling it for ten minutes. Drinking one teacup three to four times a day for half a week helps in treating fever at an early stage. Different species of the plant are used in the treatment of viral infections, ulcers, fever, cough, diabetes and enterobiasis.

CULINARY BENEFITS

The leaf part of *P. astrosanguinea* has been reported to be used as herbal tea while its roots are used as food, which has a taste similar to sweet potatoes, parsnips or chestnuts.

The genus name from the Latin word *potens*, meaning powerful is in reference to the reputed medicinal properties of the plant. The specific epithet comes from the Latin word *atrosanguineus* meaning dark blood red, in reference to the flower colour. The common name of cinquefoil comes from the Latin words *qunique* meaning five and *folium* meaning leaf, in reference to the five leaflets found on the leaves of some genus plants.

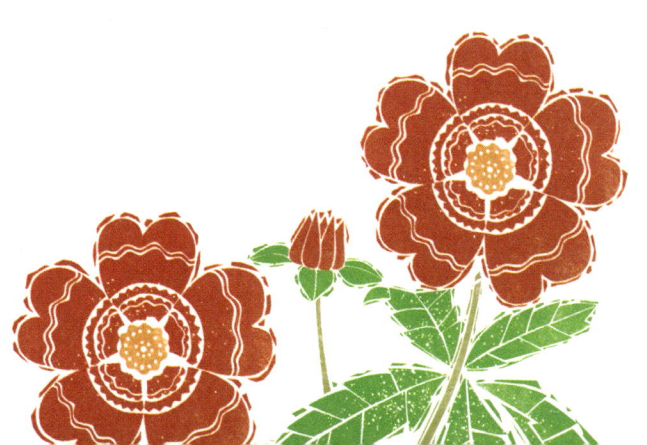

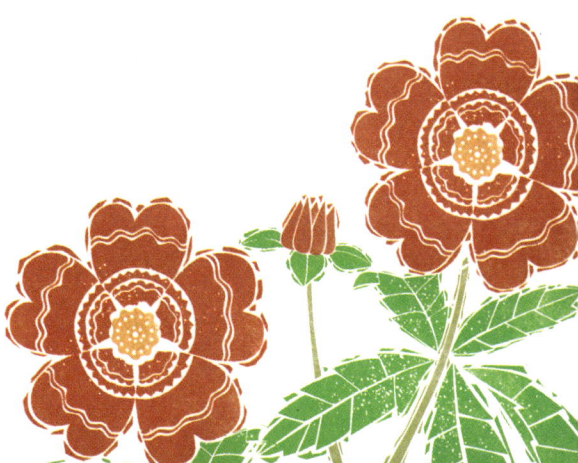

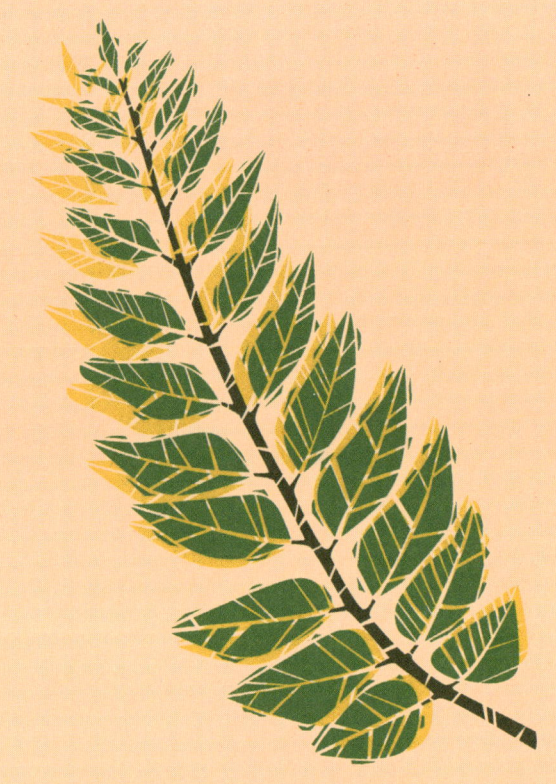

curry patta

CURRY LEAF

Murayya koenigii

CURRY PATTA/KADI PATTA/KATHNIM/MITHA NEEM/GANDHELA/
BAREANGA *Hindi* . KARIVEPPILAI/KARIVEMPU *Tamil* . KARIVEPPILA
Malayalam . KARIVEPAKU/KAREPAKU *Telugu* . KARIBEVU/BAISOPPU/
KARIBEVINA SOPPU *Kannada* . BARSANGA/KARIPHULLI *Bangla* .
MITHO LIMDO/MEETHO LIMBADO/GORANIMB/KADHILIMBDO
Gujarati . KARBAPATHI/BEVA PALO *Konkani* . KADHI PATTA/
KARHINIMB/POOSPALA/GANDLA/JHIRANG/PANDHERI KUNTHI
Marathi . BHRUSANGA PATRA/BARSAN/BASANGO/BHURAUNGA *Oriya* .
BEVUDIRAE *Tulu* . NARASINGHA *Assamese*

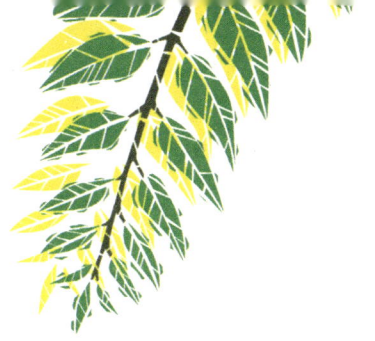
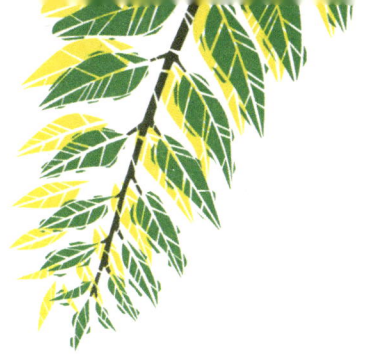

MEDICINAL PROPERTIES

Curry patta contains various antioxidant properties and has the ability to control gastrointestinal problems such as indigestion, excessive acid secretion, peptic ulcers, dysentery, diabetes and unhealthy cholesterol balance. In Ayurveda, curry leaves are considered to have antioxidant, antimicrobial, anti-inflammatory and hepatoprotective properties. A spoon of powdered curry leaves with a spoon of honey added to it, is known to relieve congestion in the chest. Curry leaf tea, best consumed on an empty stomach in the morning, is one of the best ways to maintain glowing skin due to its antioxidant properties.

CULINARY BENEFITS

Curry leaves have always been sought after for their unique flavour and usefulness in cooking, tempering being the most common use. The leaves can be dried or fried, being made into chutneys. They can also be fried crisp and used as a side to the mains in most typical Indian meals. The infusion of this herb in cooking oil adds a hint of aroma, making regular meals more flavourful and healthy.

COSMETIC CURES

It is very valuable for strengthening the hair roots. A cup of curry patta juice added to and boiled in coconut oil is considered ideal for both this, and also for preventing premature greying and fighting dandruff.

Curry leaves are a rich source of iron and folic acid. Folic acid is mainly responsible for carrying and helping the body absorb iron, and since curry patta is a rich source of both the compounds, it is your one-stop natural remedy to beat anaemia.

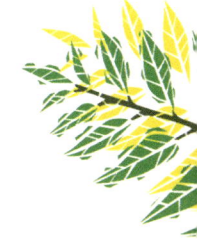
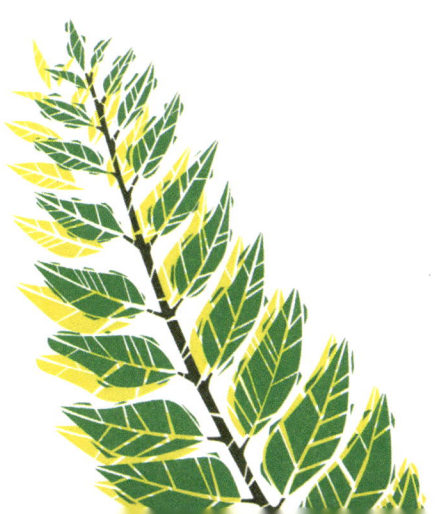
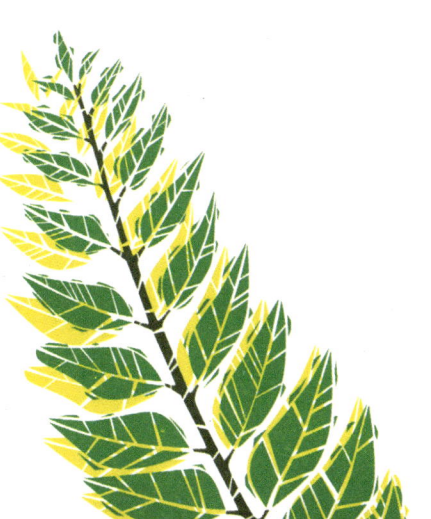

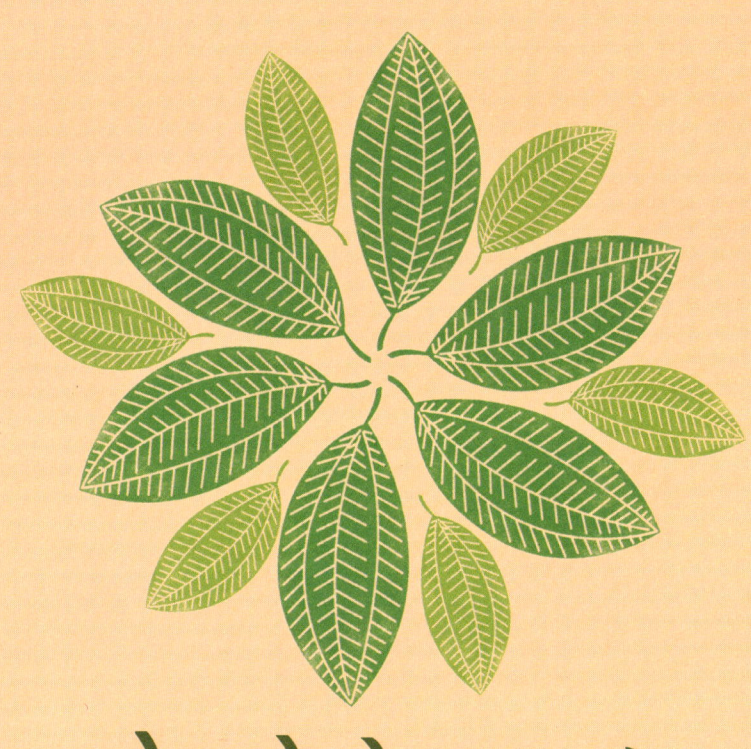

daalcheeni

CINNAMON

Cinnamomum verum

DAALCHEENI *Hindi* . DARCHINI *Urdu* . TAJA *Gujarati* .
DARCHIN *Punjabi* . LAVANGA PATTA *Telugu* .
ILAVARNGATHELY *Malayalam* . ILYANGAM *Tamil*

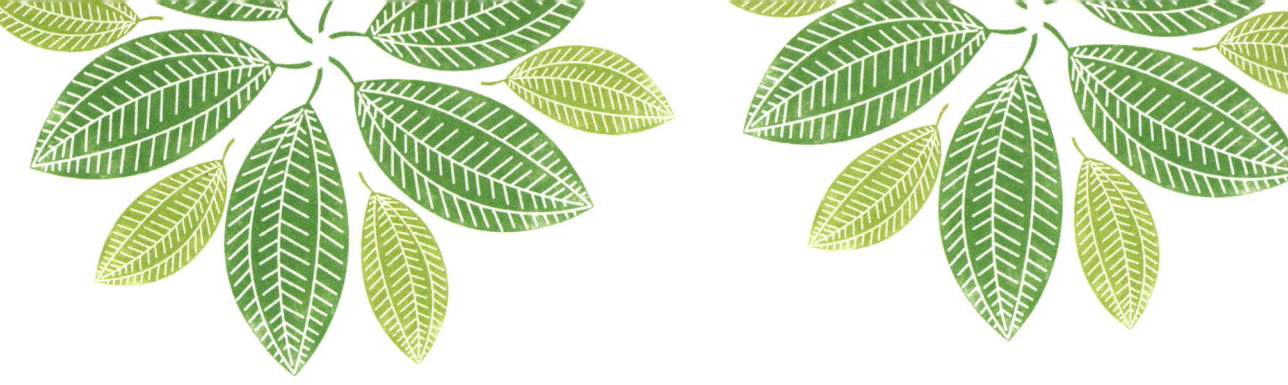

MEDICINAL PROPERTIES

Daalcheeni contains anti-fungal, antibacterial, anti-termitic, larvicidal, nematicidal and insecticidal effects. In Ayurveda, it is understood to balance the vata and pitta energies in the body and hence used as an expectorant in relieving sore throats, influenza, common cold and headaches. Taking one part powder with four parts honey, two to three times a day, helps one get relief from common cold.

Drinking a cup of warm daalcheeni water every day can briefly reduce one's pain during menstruation. In the case of rheumatoid arthritis, studies show that its regular use in small quantities does have a clear adjunct effect on the symptoms. It is also good for lowering cholesterol and strengthening cardiac muscles.

CULINARY BENEFITS

Using daalcheeni in cooking is possibly the most effective way of incorporating this spice into one's system. Widely used across cultures in India, it is a compulsory part of garam masala and is also used as a flavouring for many desserts. It has more recently been adopted in many European and American cuisines in foods like cinnamon buns and cinnamon on toast.

What is less known is that different species of daalcheeni also contribute its wood to make decorations, furniture, cabinets, and plywood. *C. javanicum* produces durable wood that is utilized in housing and construction, in general. Mosquito coils, scented joss sticks and formica are all made with the mucilage of *C. iners*.

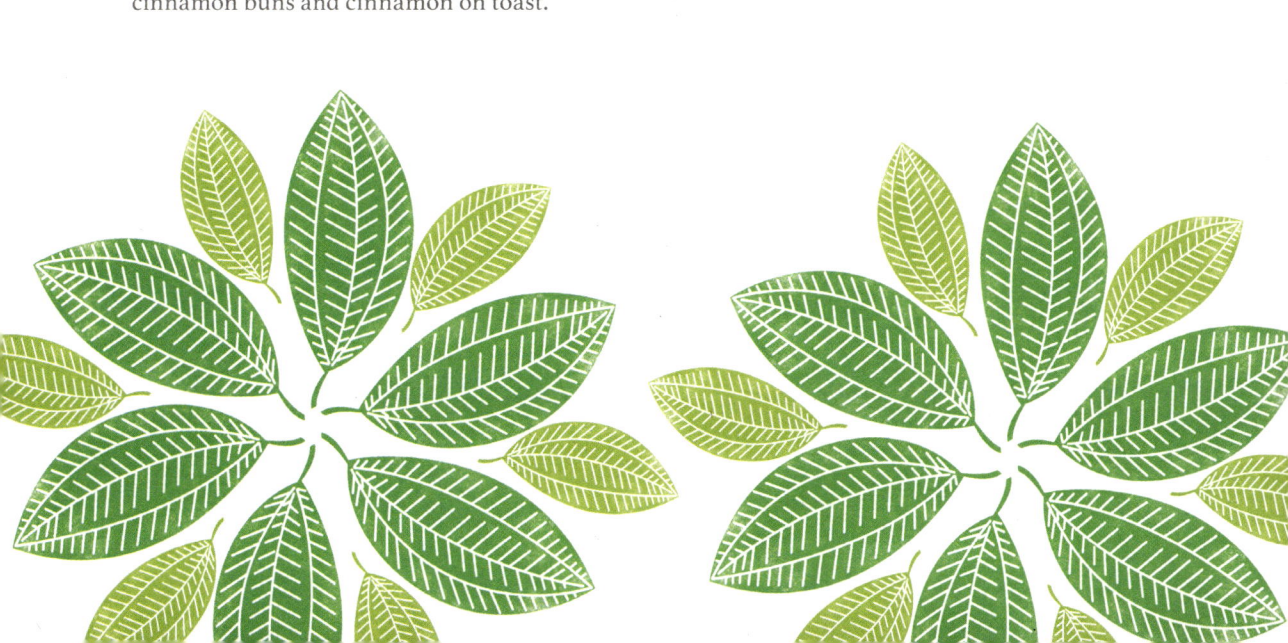

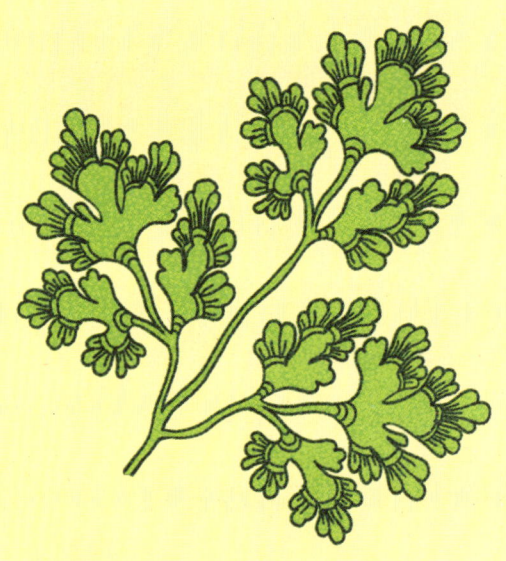

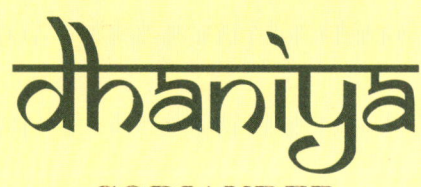

dhaniya

CORIANDER

Coriandrum sativum

DHANIYA *Hindi*

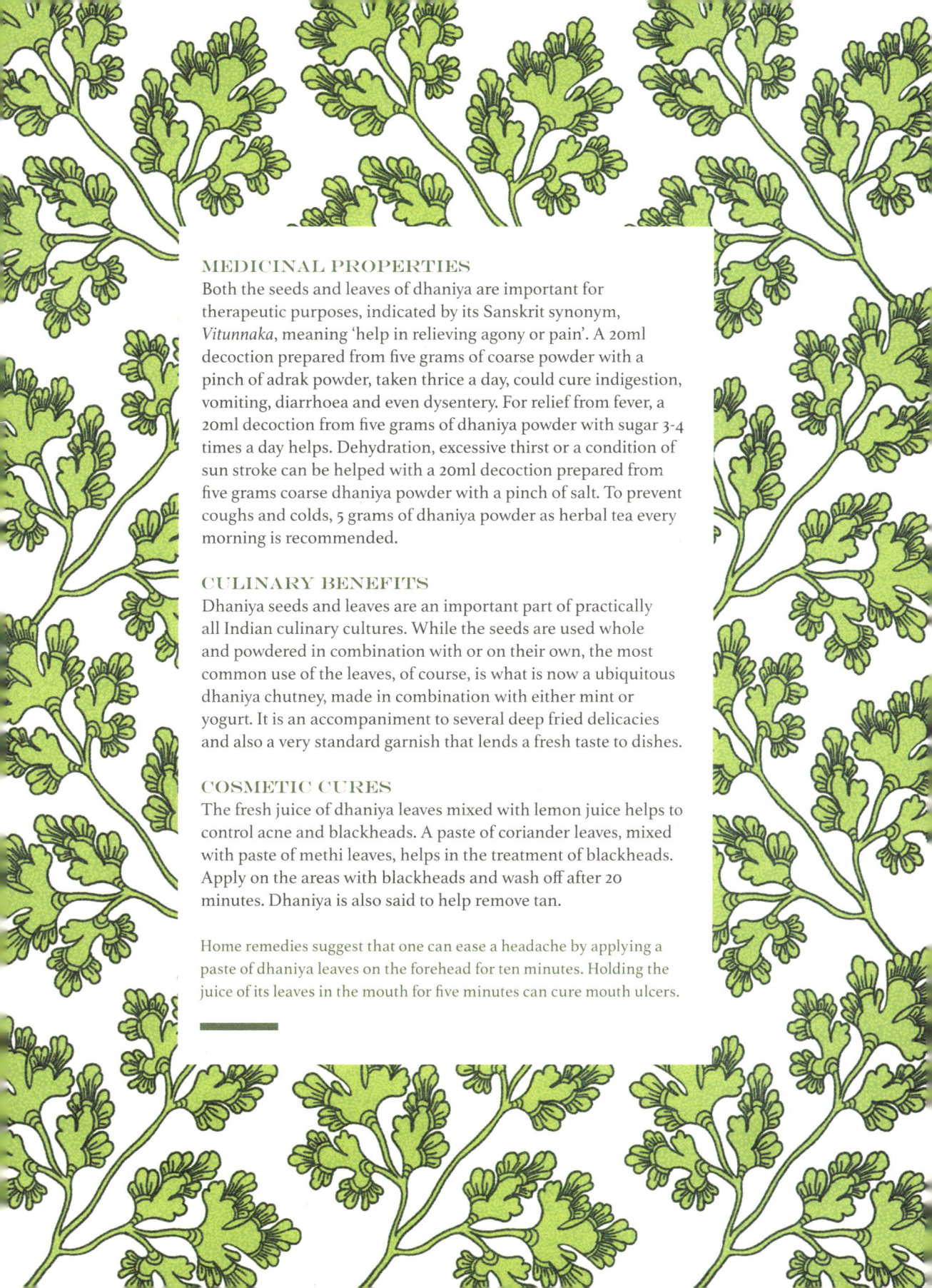

MEDICINAL PROPERTIES

Both the seeds and leaves of dhaniya are important for therapeutic purposes, indicated by its Sanskrit synonym, *Vitunnaka*, meaning 'help in relieving agony or pain'. A 20ml decoction prepared from five grams of coarse powder with a pinch of adrak powder, taken thrice a day, could cure indigestion, vomiting, diarrhoea and even dysentery. For relief from fever, a 20ml decoction from five grams of dhaniya powder with sugar 3-4 times a day helps. Dehydration, excessive thirst or a condition of sun stroke can be helped with a 20ml decoction prepared from five grams coarse dhaniya powder with a pinch of salt. To prevent coughs and colds, 5 grams of dhaniya powder as herbal tea every morning is recommended.

CULINARY BENEFITS

Dhaniya seeds and leaves are an important part of practically all Indian culinary cultures. While the seeds are used whole and powdered in combination with or on their own, the most common use of the leaves, of course, is what is now a ubiquitous dhaniya chutney, made in combination with either mint or yogurt. It is an accompaniment to several deep fried delicacies and also a very standard garnish that lends a fresh taste to dishes.

COSMETIC CURES

The fresh juice of dhaniya leaves mixed with lemon juice helps to control acne and blackheads. A paste of coriander leaves, mixed with paste of methi leaves, helps in the treatment of blackheads. Apply on the areas with blackheads and wash off after 20 minutes. Dhaniya is also said to help remove tan.

Home remedies suggest that one can ease a headache by applying a paste of dhaniya leaves on the forehead for ten minutes. Holding the juice of its leaves in the mouth for five minutes can cure mouth ulcers.

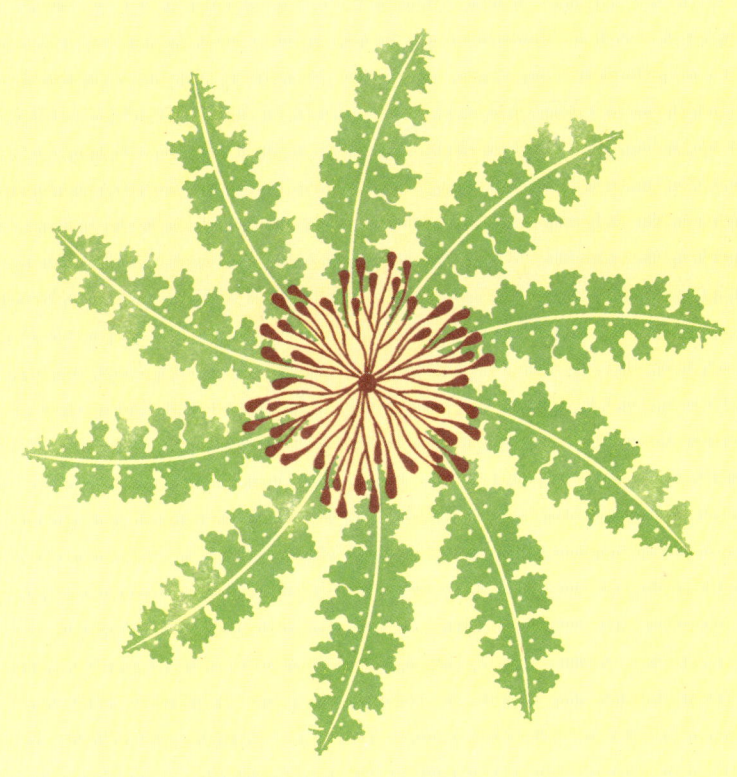

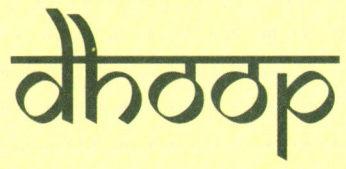

Jurinea dolomiaea Boiss

DHOOP *Hindi*

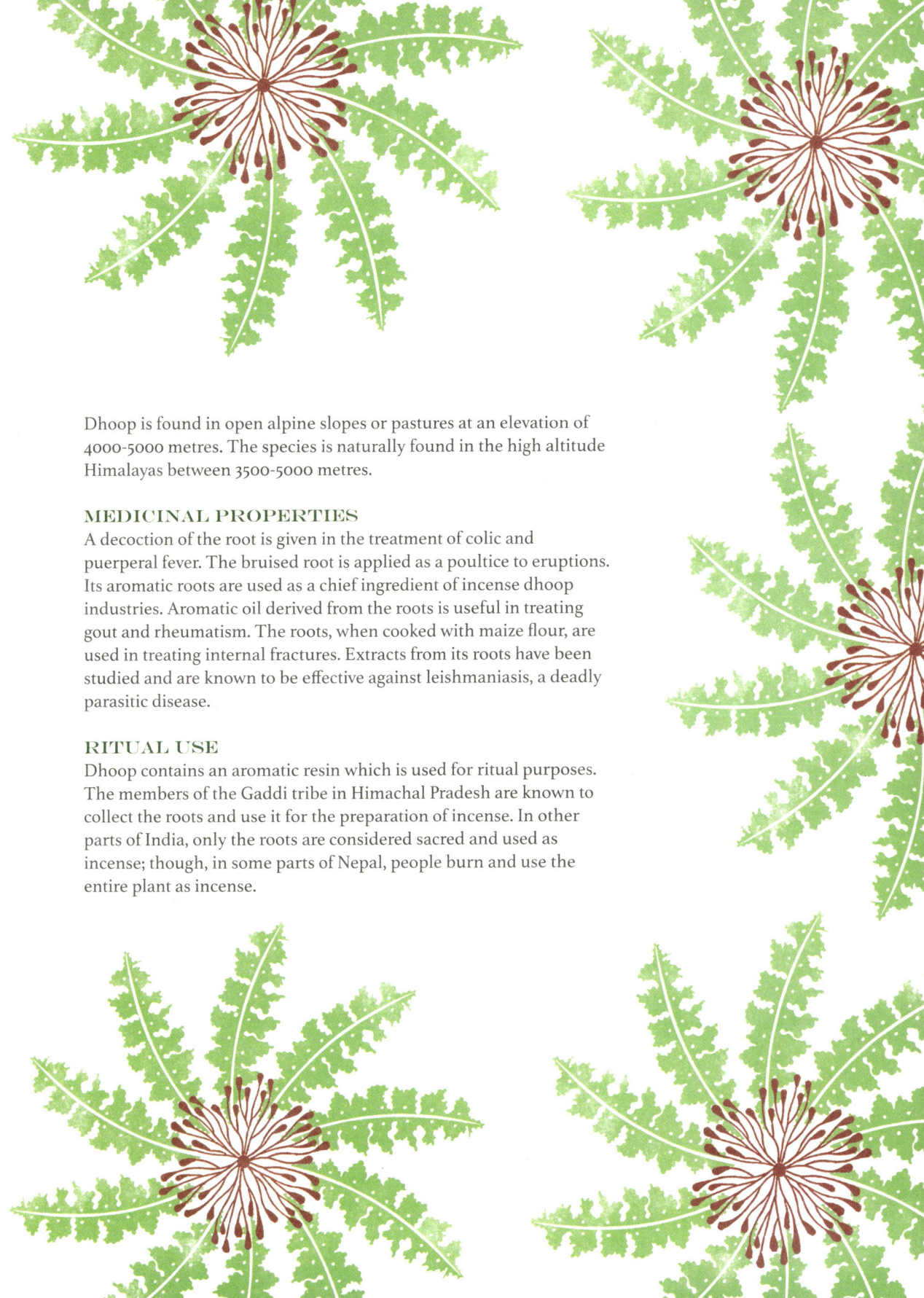

Dhoop is found in open alpine slopes or pastures at an elevation of 4000-5000 metres. The species is naturally found in the high altitude Himalayas between 3500-5000 metres.

MEDICINAL PROPERTIES

A decoction of the root is given in the treatment of colic and puerperal fever. The bruised root is applied as a poultice to eruptions. Its aromatic roots are used as a chief ingredient of incense dhoop industries. Aromatic oil derived from the roots is useful in treating gout and rheumatism. The roots, when cooked with maize flour, are used in treating internal fractures. Extracts from its roots have been studied and are known to be effective against leishmaniasis, a deadly parasitic disease.

RITUAL USE

Dhoop contains an aromatic resin which is used for ritual purposes. The members of the Gaddi tribe in Himachal Pradesh are known to collect the roots and use it for the preparation of incense. In other parts of India, only the roots are considered sacred and used as incense; though, in some parts of Nepal, people burn and use the entire plant as incense.

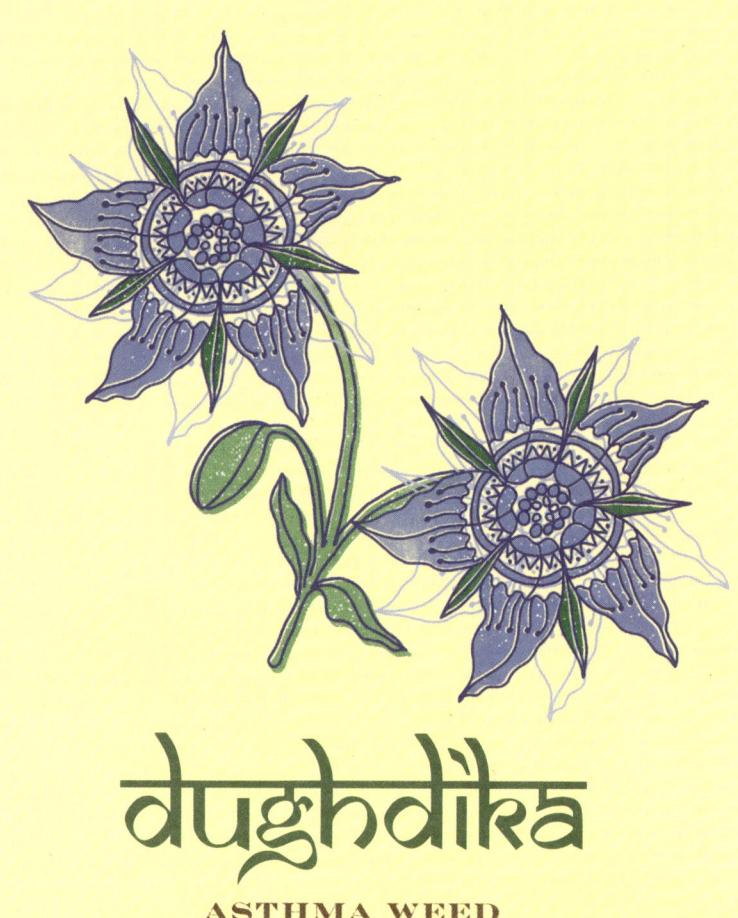

dughdika

ASTHMA WEED

Euphorbia hirta

DUGHDIKA *Sanskrit* . BARAKERU/KALAKISHRI *Bangla* .
DUDHELI *Gujarati* . NILAPALA *Malayalam* . MOTI DUDHI *Marathi* .
AMMANPACHARISI *Tamil* . NANABALA *Telugu*

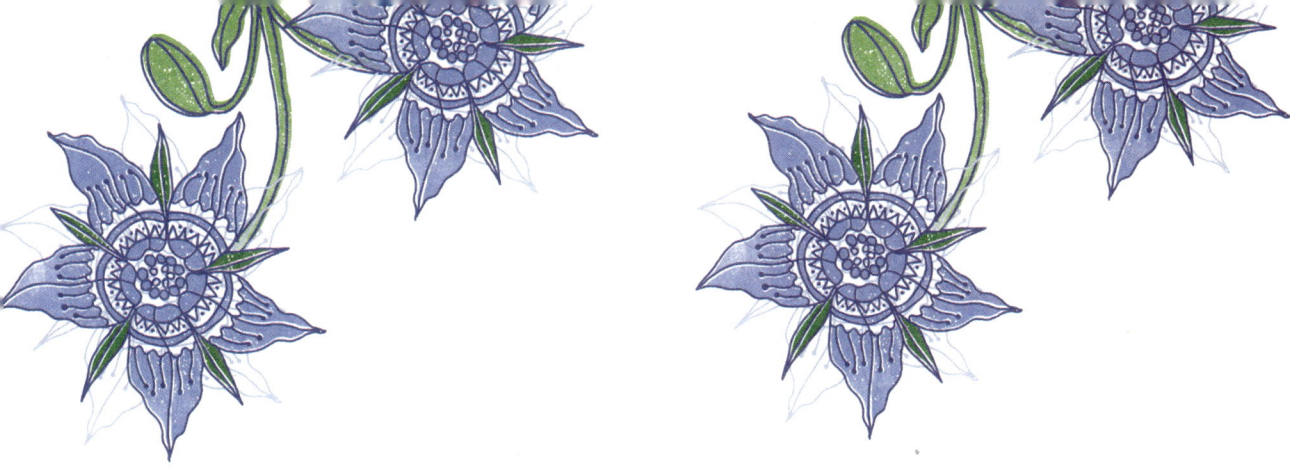

MEDICINAL PROPERTIES

Dughdika is used in a variety of different conditions – a small quantity of leaf paste with cow's milk for gonorrhoea; with warm water for intestinal worms; or the milky latex on open wounds for quick healing.

In the Ayurvedic tradition, dughdika is known as an 'asthma plant' due to its great value in treating respiratory disorders, coughs and asthma. It is also believed to be an aphrodisiac. The latex of the stem is also used on the lower lids to treat several eye infections, including conjunctivitis. The leaves, when combined with those of a couple of other plants, ground to a fine paste and added to a drink of milk and sugar, help in the treatment of jaundice.

COSMETIC CURES

As a cosmetic use, the paste of the dughdika leaves pounded with turmeric and coconut oil is very beneficial for itchy soles of feet and also otherwise for itchy skin.

The stem of dughdika produces white latex, which looks like milk, hence its name. In many parts of the country, it is used to increase lactation in women, via the addition of a few cooked leaves in the mother's diet.

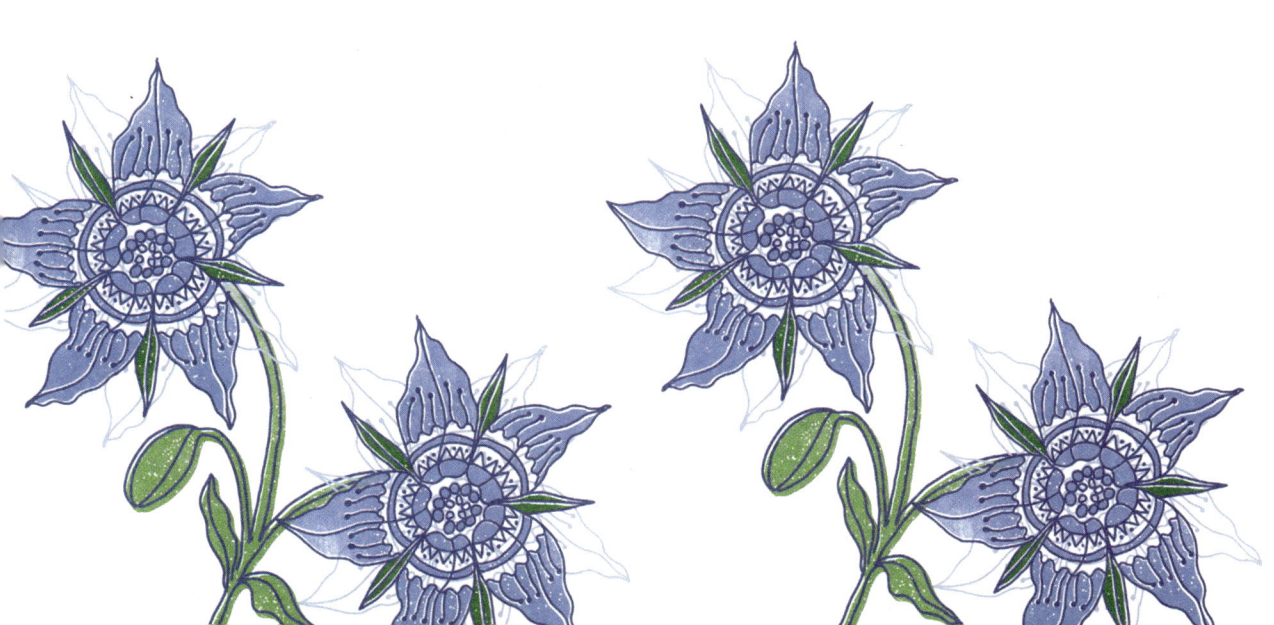

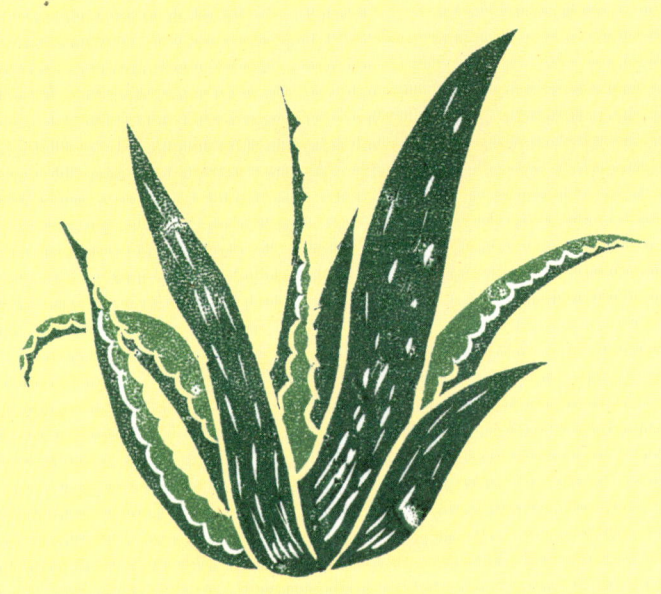

gawarpatha

ALOE VERA

Aloe barbadensis miller

GHRTA KUMARI *Sanskrit, Bangla* . **GAWARPATHA** *Hindi* .
KAORPADHA *Marathi* . **LOLISARA** *Kannada* .
KATHALAI *Tamil* . **KALABANDA** *Telugu*

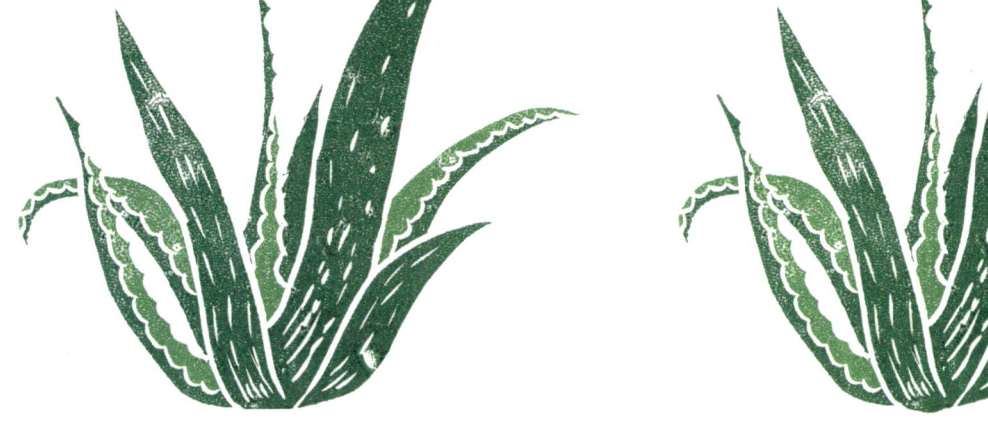

MEDICINAL PROPERTIES

The medicinal properties of gawarpatha are many. The plant consists of around six varieties of antiseptics. It can kill mold, bacteria, funguses and viruses. It can cure minor vaginal irritations and also be used for piles and fistula. Gawarpatha juice has laxative properties and drinking it can relieve most gastrointestinal disorders. Its regular use strengthens gums and improves basic health of teeth. Gawarpatha can also help in the reduction of cholesterol, triglycerides and relieve heart ailments.

CULINARY BENEFITS

Gawarpatha is an edible cactus that can be enjoyed raw, cooked, blended in drinks, soups and dips; in curries and stews, and in salads. In many parts of the country, it is cooked as everyday curry or stir fried.

COSMETIC CURES

Using gawarpatha on one's hair helps stop hair fall and makes the hair stronger. Using it on sun-burned skin helps sooth the pain, while using the gel on acne or facial warts helps lighten the colour of the skin. For instant relief from prickly heat, apply gawarpatha gel over the affected area and let it stay for fifteen minutes. Rinse well with water and repeat daily. Additionally, the natural goodness of coconut oil mixed with gawarpatha gel helps strengthen and repair the hair, along with getting rid of dandruff.

Gawarpatha's most important association for the last couple of decades has been with skincare and so it has become one of the most sought after plants for making herbal cosmetics. And this, despite the fact that its gel, which is the most crucial ingredient, is not very stable and loses its value very soon after being taken from the leaves.

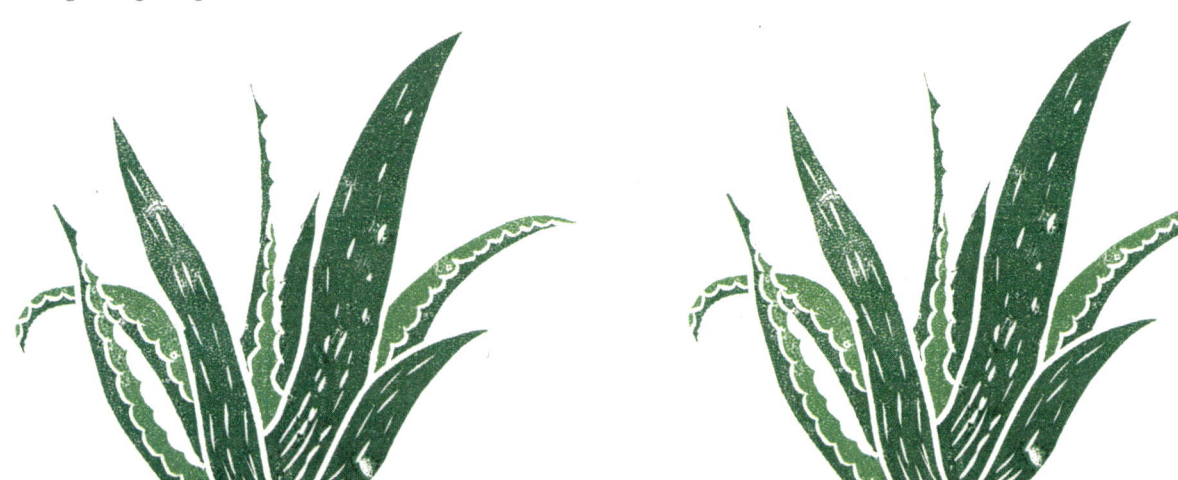

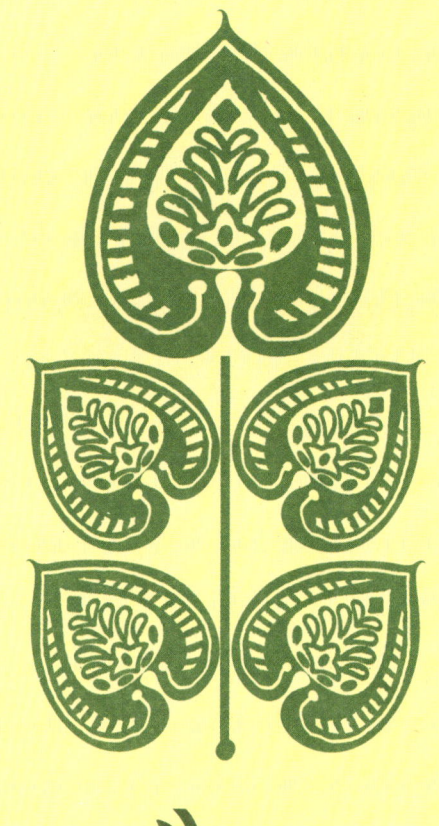

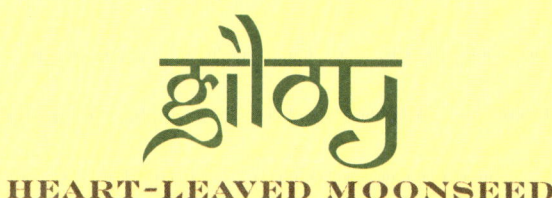

HEART-LEAVED MOONSEED

Tinospora cordifolia

GILOY/ GUDUCHI *Hindi* . GULANCHA *Bangla* . GILO *Arabic* .
GILO *Urdu* . GUDUCHI/MADHUPARNI/AMRITA/CHINNARUHA/
VATSADAANI/TANTRIKA/KUNDALINI/CHAKRALAKSHANIKA *Sanskrit* .
TIPPATIGA *Telugu* . SHINDILAKODI *Tamil* . SHINDILAKODI *Marathi* .
GALO *Gujarati*

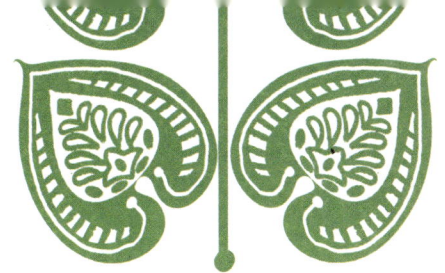
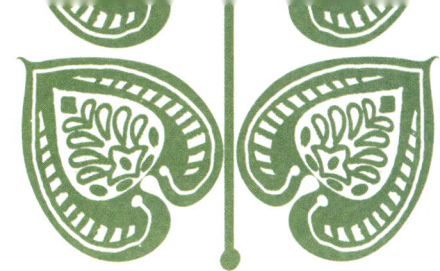

MEDICINAL PROPERTIES

Giloy's plant extracts have active compounds in the form of alkaloids, glycosides, lactones and steroids, which have immunomodulatory and physiological roles of different types, thereby demonstrating the diverse versatility of the plant. It is proven to be very fruitful for reducing mental stress and anxiety, as it relieves toxins and enhances one's memory. Applying its leaf paste on the skin helps fasten the wound healing process as it aids in collagen production and skin regeneration.

The stem is bitter, stomachic and diuretic, stimulates bile secretion, allays thirst, burning sensation and vomiting. The juice or decoction of leaves is administered orally with honey in fever and for reducing cough, cold and tonsils. Difficult to treat conditions like chest tightness, shortness of breath and wheezing due to asthma are often addressed by chewing the roots and drinking its juice. Apart from all these advantages, giloy can be applied to the eyes to strengthen one's vision. Boil giloy powder or giloy leaves in water. Once it cools down, apply it over the eyes.

It has also been shown to have a radio protective role by significantly increasing body weight, tissue weight and tubular diameter.

COSMETIC CURES

Giloy has been widely used to reduce skin dark spots, pimples and wrinkles. It also has anti-aging properties which are considered beneficial for brightening the skin.

The Banaras Hindu University in India has launched Mission Giloy in a bid to expand the plantation and use of this magical immunity-boosting herb. This mission came up particularly in continuation of the achievements of its usage during the pandemic by all practitioners across the AYUSH and local health systems.

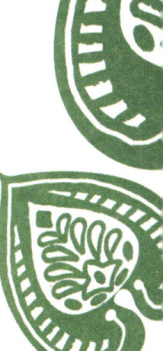

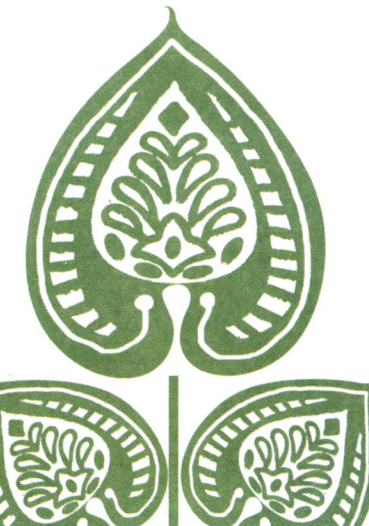

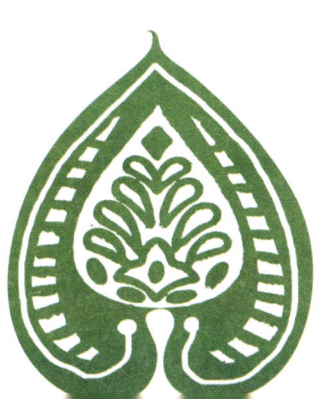

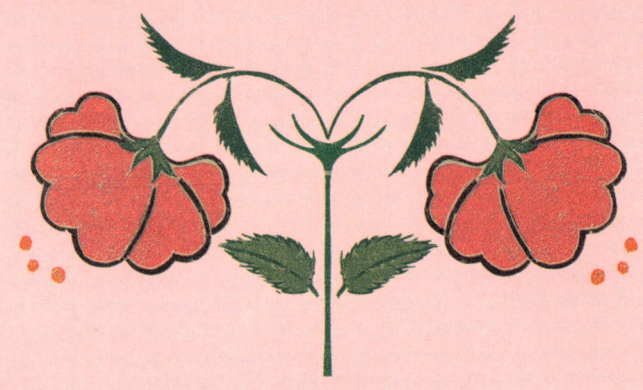

gurhal

CHINESE HIBISCUS

Hibiscus rosa-sinensis

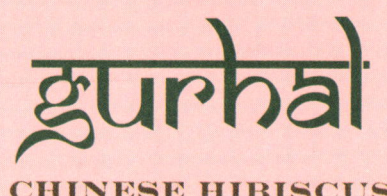

GURHAL/ JASUT/JASUM, JAVA/ODHUL/GURHAL/ARAHUL *Hindi* .
JOBA/JIWA/ORU *Bangla* . **JASAVANDA/JASSVANDI** *Marathi* . **JAPA/JAVA/**
RUDRAPUSPA/ AUNDRAPUSPA/TRISANDHYA *Sanskrit* . **JASVUA/**
JASUNT *Gujarati* . **DASAVALAA** *Kannada* . **HIMBARATHI/AYAMPARATTI/**
CHEBARATHI *Malayalam* . **MONDARO** *Oriya* . **JASUM/JAIPUSHPA/**
GURHAL *Punjabi* . **SAPATTUU/SEMPARUTTI** *Tamil*

MEDICINAL PROPERTIES

Gurhal has been found to be effective in the treatment of arterial hypertension. In folk medicine, the flowers crushed with sugar and added to fresh juice are given for controlling excessive uterine bleeding, while the flowers fried in clarified butter are also given for menorrhagia or heavy menstrual bleeding.. The flowers are made into a paste, poulticed and applied in the case of swellings, carbuncles, mumps, fever, sores and boils.

CULINARY BENEFITS

Its young leaves are sometimes used as a spinach substitute. The flowers can be had either raw or cooked – either made into a kind of pickle or used as a purple dye for colouring foods such as preserved fruits and cooked vegetables. While the root is edible and very fibrous, it is not very easy to eat. The dried flowers are also used to make a special kind of tea.

COSMETIC CURES

Dried gurhal flowers, in a powdered form, are a very good tonic for the scalp and known to prevent hair fall. A black hair dye is prepared from the petals of Japaa flowers and is extensively used for the blackening of hair.

RITUAL USE

Gurhal is ritually used in the worship of Kaali, a Hindu goddess who is the representation of the Devi. The red of the flower is believed to be evocative of that power represented in her stuck out tongue, which in everyday lore is interpreted to be her embarrassment at having stepped over Shiva in the battlefield. But the interpretation in the classical sense is that the complete cosmic power she had imbibed, which helped conquer the demons and seemed uncontrollable, was released when she opened her mouth.

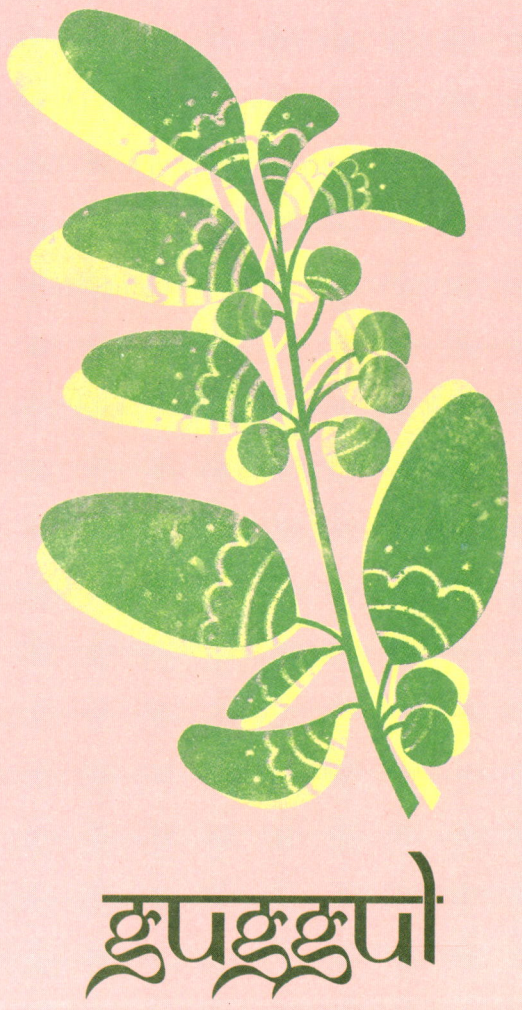

guggul

INDIAN BDELLIUM

Commiphora mukul

GUGGUL *Hindi*

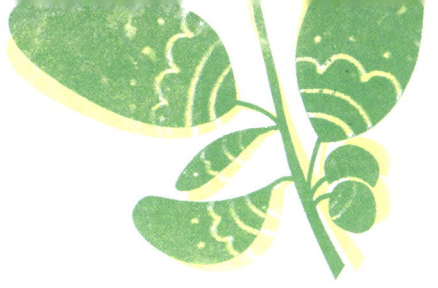
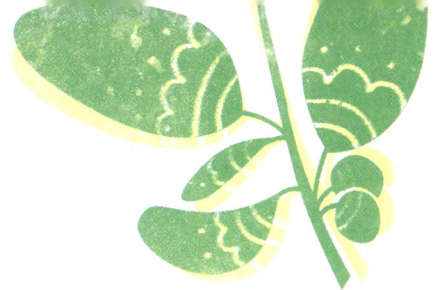

Some of its major species include *Commiphora wightii*, *Commiphora gileadensis*, *Commiphora mukul*, *Boswellia serrata* and *Boswellia sacra*. All species are a part of the *Burseraceae* family, also known as the incense family.

MEDICINAL PROPERTIES

Guggul has been used for centuries in Ayurvedic medicine. It is a holistic, plant-derived medical system to treat various health conditions such as obesity, arthritis and inflammation, due to the presence of compounds such as phenolics, alkaloids and tannins that make it a perfect natural aid to fight infections.

Sushrut Samhita describes that guggul, when taken orally, can cure liver dysfunction, intestinal worms, leucoderma, sinus and edema. It is also used as an Ayurvedic medicine for the prevention and treatment of various other diseases such as IBD (inflammatory bowel disease), acne, ulcers, arthritis and diabetes.

Guggul is often claimed to help treat obesity by promoting fat loss. One test-tube study suggests guggul may promote weight loss by inducing the breakdown of fat, thus reducing the volume of fatty tissue. Guggul supports the liver in performing its detoxifying function in a smoother manner.

Guggul sap – also referred to as guggul, gum guggul, guggula or gugulipid – is tapped from the plants in a manner similar to the way in which maple syrup is extracted from maple trees.

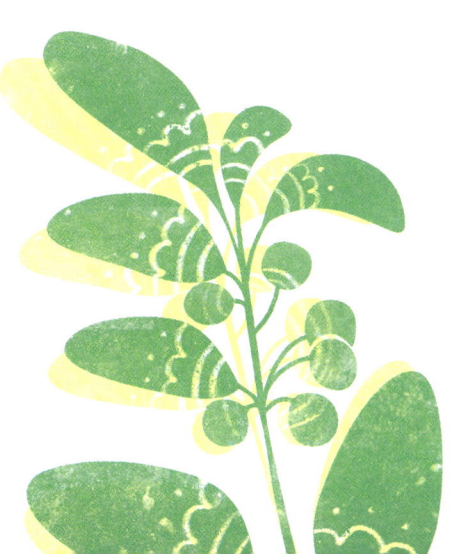
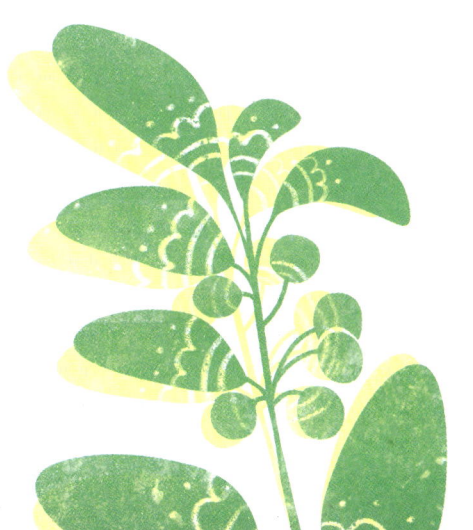

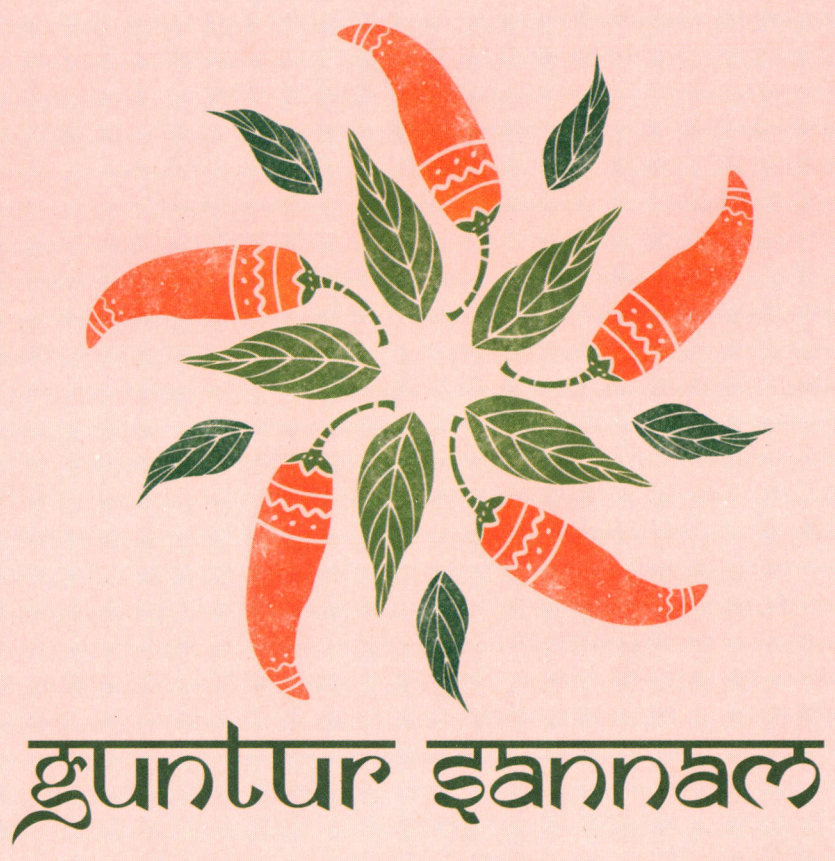

guntur sannam

RED CHILLIES
Capsicum annuum var. longum

GUNTUR SANNAM *Telugu*

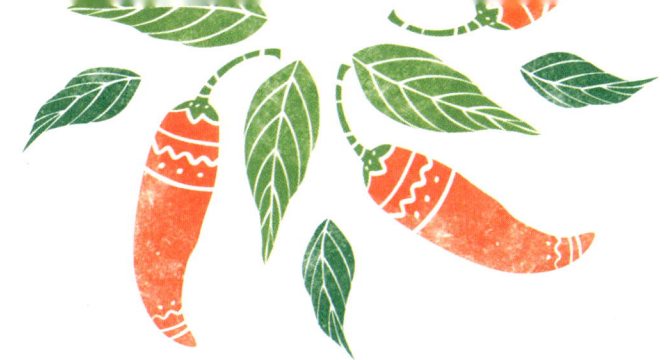

MEDICINAL PROPERTIES

Guntur chillies have several medicinal benefits. They help in clearing the mucous membrane in the stomach and in respiratory passages while also stimulating appetite. They are rich in vitamin C, contains a blend of different vitamins and phytochemicals, and an extract from them has been known to be effective against the parasite *Schistosoma mansoni* that causes schistomiasis, an infection that has affected millions of people worldwide. In fact its extracts have demonstrated antioxidant, antiviral, anti-inflammatory – all of which are being explored for further pharmacological use.

CULINARY BENEFITS

Credited for giving Andhra food its fiery edge, Guntur chillies are hot to handle yet you find yourself going back for more doses. Originating from the Guntur district of Andhra Pradesh, Guntur sannam has a thick red skin with high pungency. It is used in the preparation of various local delicacies to develop colour and flavour.

The Guntur chilli is exceptionally dark red in colour due to the rich source on capsaicin. It is said that it is this capsaicin content which is responsible for the colour of chillies. In cooking, the chilli is used as whole and thrown in during the preparation, or it is ground into a powder or a paste with other spices. No wonder when you see the dishes, they impart a rich red colour that makes them hard to resist.

With Andhra Pradesh being the largest producer of chillies in India, there are many varieties that one can explore, but the Guntur chilli seems to be a hot favourite. The locals claim that it's the distinctive flavour that it imparts to the dishes that makes it a preferred choice, if one can get past the fieriness.

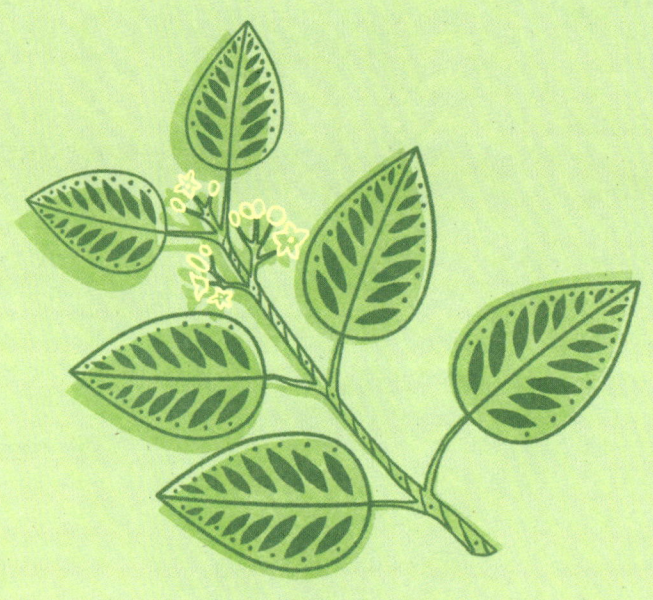

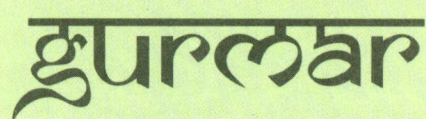

PERIPLOCA OF THE WOODS

Gymnema sylvestre

GURMAR *Kanker boli* . **KALIKARDORI/ KAVALI** *Marathi* .
MADHUNASHINI/ MESHASHRINGI *Sanskrit* .
MARDASHINGI/DHULETI *Gujarati* . **SANNAGERASEHAMBU**
Kannada . **CHERUKURINJA/ADIGAM** *Tamil* . **PODAPATRI** *Telugu*

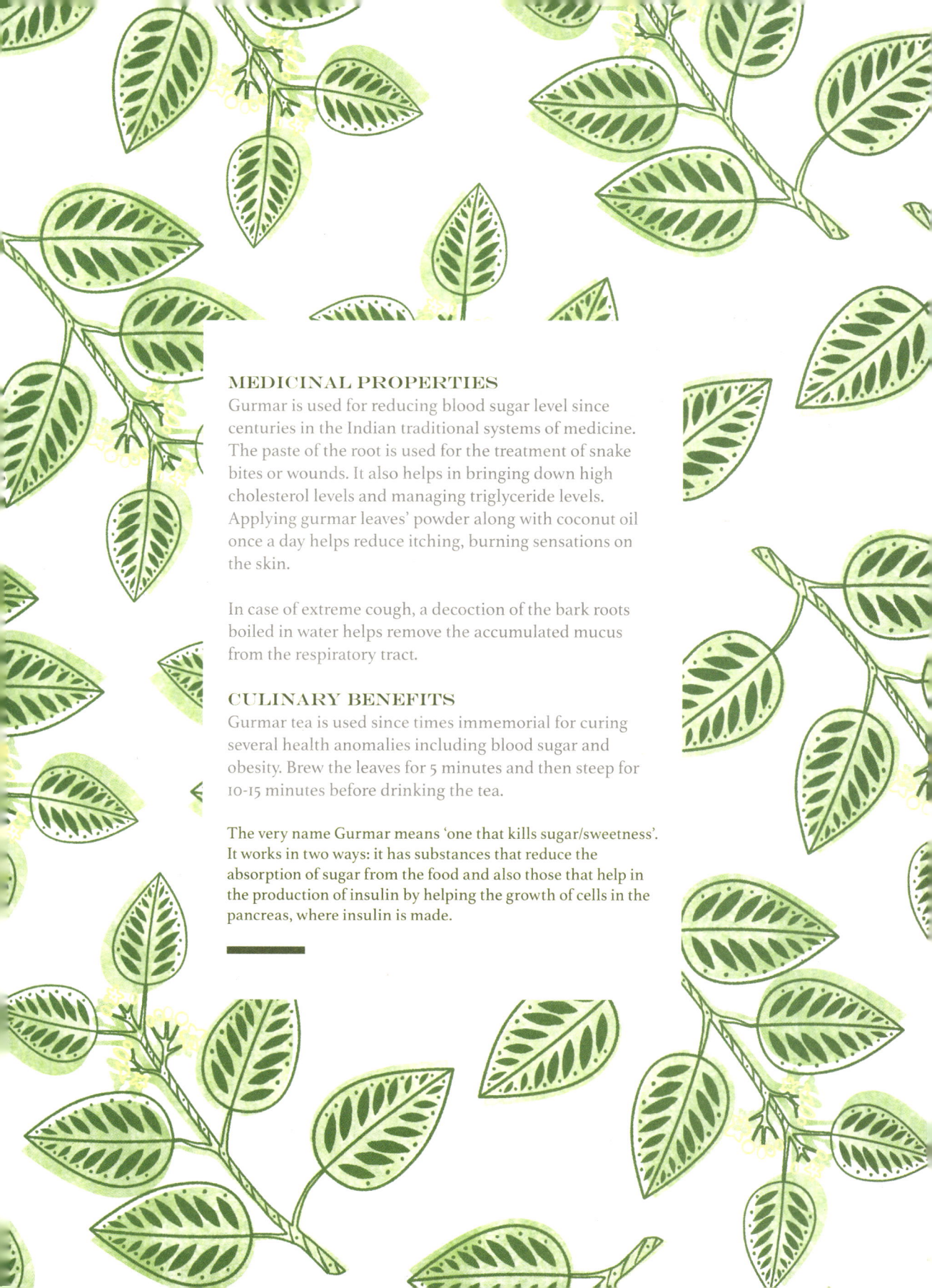

MEDICINAL PROPERTIES

Gurmar is used for reducing blood sugar level since centuries in the Indian traditional systems of medicine. The paste of the root is used for the treatment of snake bites or wounds. It also helps in bringing down high cholesterol levels and managing triglyceride levels. Applying gurmar leaves' powder along with coconut oil once a day helps reduce itching, burning sensations on the skin.

In case of extreme cough, a decoction of the bark roots boiled in water helps remove the accumulated mucus from the respiratory tract.

CULINARY BENEFITS

Gurmar tea is used since times immemorial for curing several health anomalies including blood sugar and obesity. Brew the leaves for 5 minutes and then steep for 10-15 minutes before drinking the tea.

The very name Gurmar means 'one that kills sugar/sweetness'. It works in two ways: it has substances that reduce the absorption of sugar from the food and also those that help in the production of insulin by helping the growth of cells in the pancreas, where insulin is made.

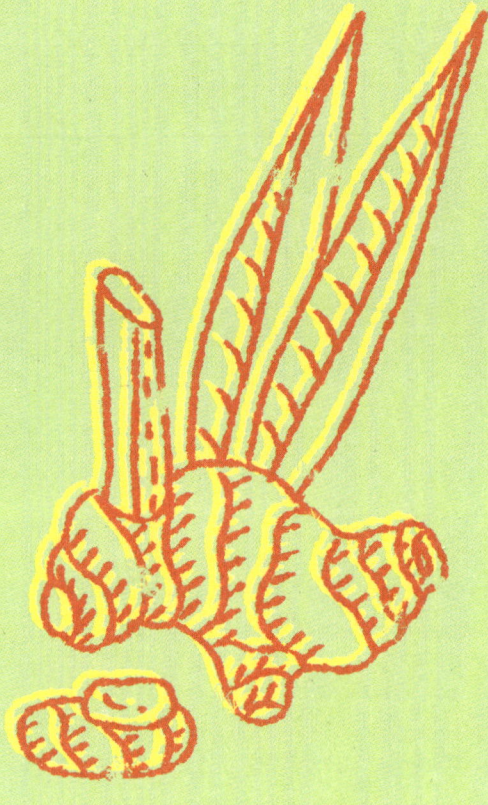

habiat

SIAMESE GINGER

Alpinia galangal

SIAMESE GINGER *English*

MEDICINAL PROPERTIES

The dried roots of habiat – called 'Greater Galangal' – are a vital medication in Ayurvedic and Unani systems of medicine. The roots are considered to be effective in treating asthma, bronchitis, hiccup, obesity, rheumatism and diabetes. The seeds contain antiulcer agents and are used in controlling diarrhoea and vomiting. It has also been proved effective when it comes to improve blood circulation in the body. It is, in addition, a rich source for iron, sodium, vitamin A and C.

CULINARY BENEFITS

The flowers are eaten raw or pickled and the roots are utilized for pickling. Its bulbs are eaten crude and can be used as a condiment, for seasoning fish and meats, especially in Thai cuisine, and also as a substitute for ginger. It has a pungent smell and strong taste reminiscent of black pepper and pine needles. White cultivars are primarily used as a spice, unlike the red cultivars which are primarily used for medicinal purposes. Habiat is also a popular addition to curries and soups.

COSMETIC CURES

The plant may possibly be an interesting alternative choice of bioactive molecules for cosmetic or cosmeceutical sectors – for example, in antioxidant skincare, anti-inflammatory cream/lotion and other botanicals due to the flavonoid phytochemical compounds found in *A. galangal*.

Habiat's roots yields an essential oil, used in perfumery as a source of Methyl Cinnamate and Cinol.

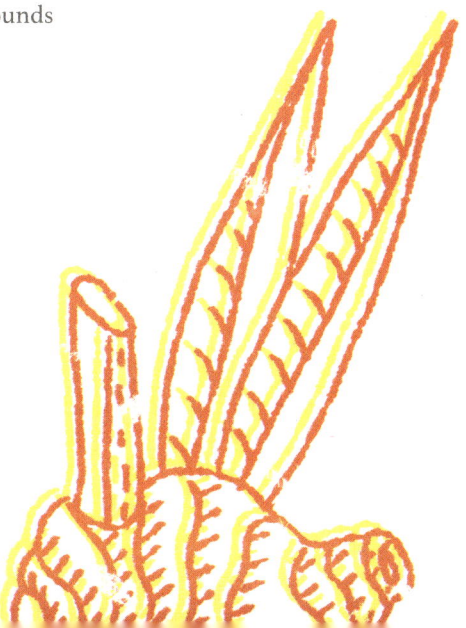

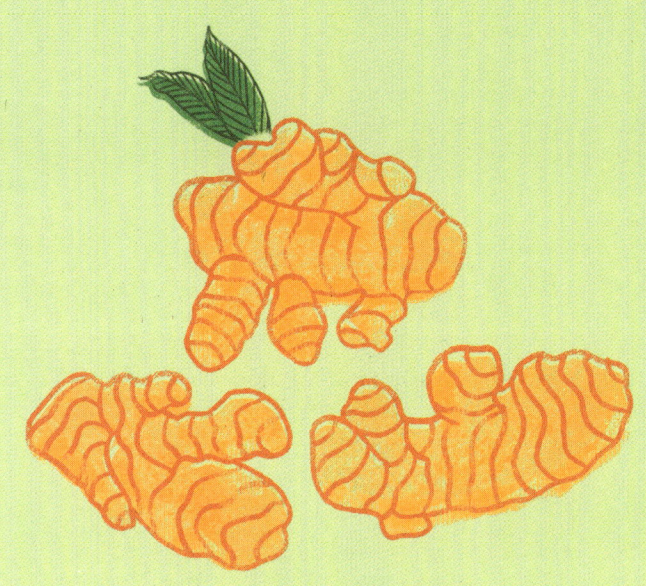

haldi

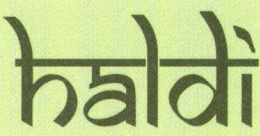

TURMERIC

Curcuma longa

HALDI *Hindi* . **ARISHINA** *Kannada* .
MANJAL/HARIDRA *Malayalam* . **PASUPU** *Telugu*

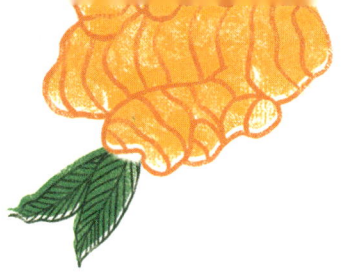
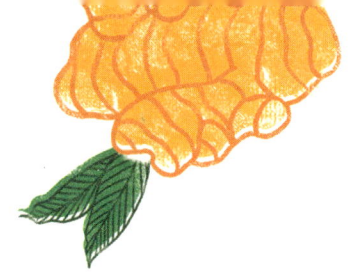

MEDICINAL PROPERTIES

Haldi is one of those herbs that are found in every Indian household and used for an unbelievably wide variety of medicinal purposes. When combined with adrak paste and applied, it helps ease strained muscles. While on the one hand it prevents skin diseases, it is also a useful application on swellings and boils due to its antibacterial properties. One of the most common antidotes for coughs and colds is haldi boiled in milk and sweetened with sugar. A teaspoon of haldi powder, when consumed early in the morning diluted in warm water, helps get rid of gastrointestinal problems thanks to curcumin, the primary compound in haldi that contains antioxidant and anti-inflammatory properties.

CULINARY BENEFITS

Haldi is used widely in foods across the country mainly because of its ability to provide protection against tropical germs. It is an essential condiment in a significant range of cuisines in India. Furthermore, our very own haldi doodh as turmeric latte has recently become a popular beverage, served in cafes globally.

COSMETIC CURES

Its essential oil lends itself to be used for basic skincare and so is now being commercially used for a range of skin products including face wash and masks. Regular use on the skin lends a glow and so it is traditionally used for brides and grooms in a special ceremony before the wedding, considered to be both cleansing and propitious. Additionally, a face pack made with honey and haldi is an easy remedy for glowing skin. Mix a teaspoon each of honey and haldi with two teaspoons of yogurt, and apply across face and neck for 10-15 minutes. Use a warm wet cloth to remove the mask.

Haldi is widely used in rituals, precisely because of its great qualities. When dried, it is powdered along with a bit of slaked lime, to be made into *kumkum*. It is also used as a dye for hand-woven cloth.

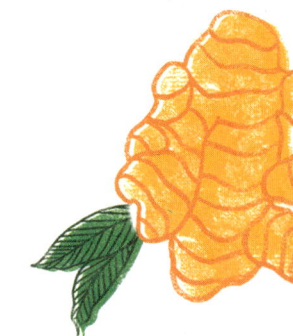

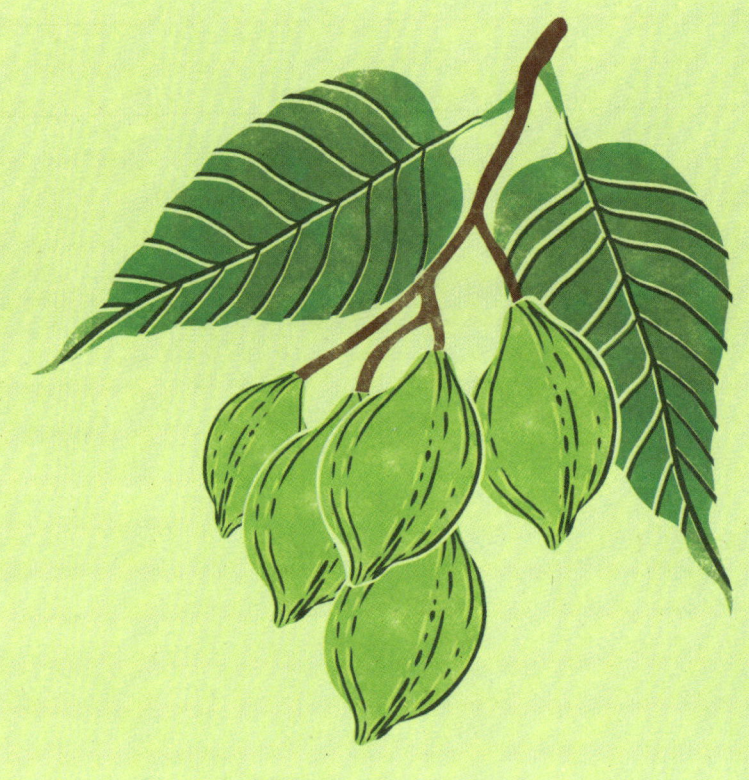

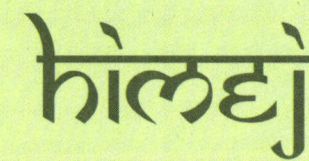

himej

CHEBULIC MYROBALAN

Terminalia chebula

HIMEJ/ HARDI/HARDE *Gujarati* . **SHILIKHA** *Assamese* . **HARITAKI** *Bangla* .
HARA *Hindi* . **ALALE** *Kannada* . **ORDO/HARDI** *Konkani* . **KATUKKA**
Malayalam . **MANALI** *Meitei* . **HIRDA** *Marathi* . **KARADHA** *Oriya* . **HALELA**
Persian . **HARITAKI** *Sanskrit* . **HAR** *Sindhi* . **KATA-K-KAY/KADUKKAI** *Tamil* .
KARAKA *Telugu* . **HAEJARAD** *Urdu*

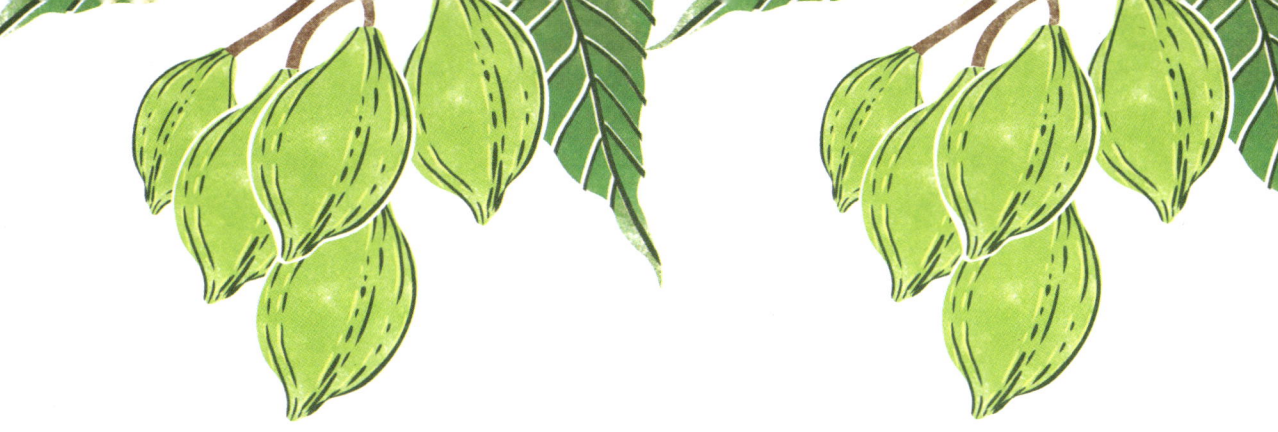

MEDICINAL PROPERTIES

Himej is highly rated for its medicinal properties and its power of healing. It is the main ingredient in the Ayurvedic formulation called Triphala which is used for kidney and liver dysfunctions. The dried fruit is also used in Ayurveda as a purported antitussive, cardiotonic, homeostatic, diuretic and laxative – while also having antioxidant, hepato-protective, anti-inflammatory, antimutagenic properties. Its decoction is used as gargle in oral ulcers and sore throat. Its powder is a good astringent dentifrice in loose gums, bleeding and ulceration in gums. It can be taken by mixing one teaspoon of the powder with lukewarm water after a meal.

Himej is often used to increase appetite and as a digestive aid, liver stimulant, gastrointestinal prokinetic agent and mild laxative. The powder of the fruits has been used in chronic diarrhoea and renal calculi, dysurea, retention of urine and skin disorders with discharges like allergies and urticaria.

Himej powder proves to be very useful for hair loss in the form of its herbal oil, which can be prepared by heating a cup of coconut oil in a pan with three pods of himej. Boil till it turns brown and the outer shell cracks. Allow it to cool and store in a jar. Himej oil also helps prevents dandruff and lice infections.

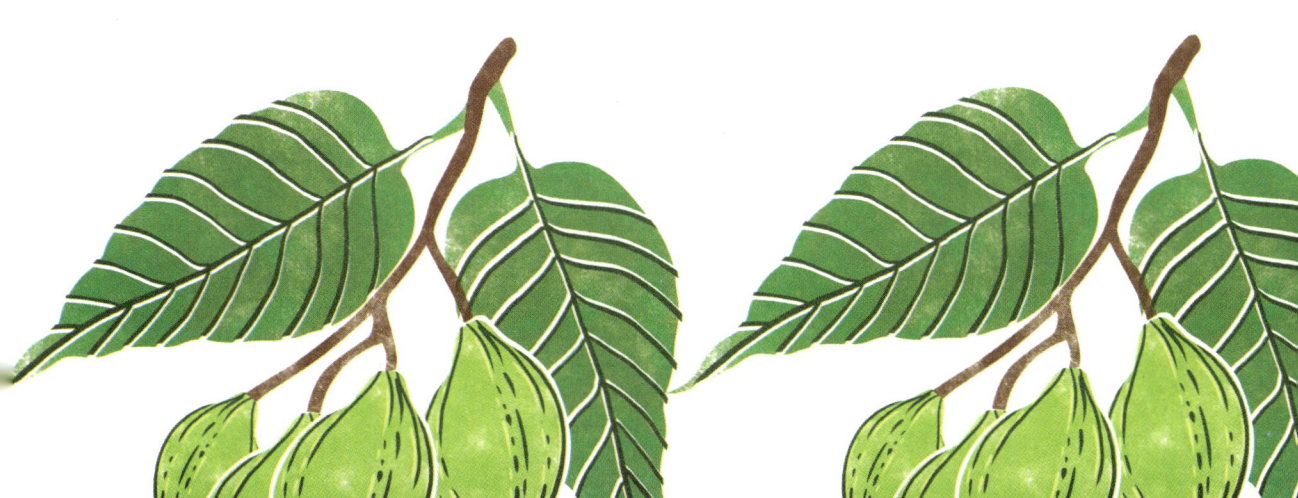

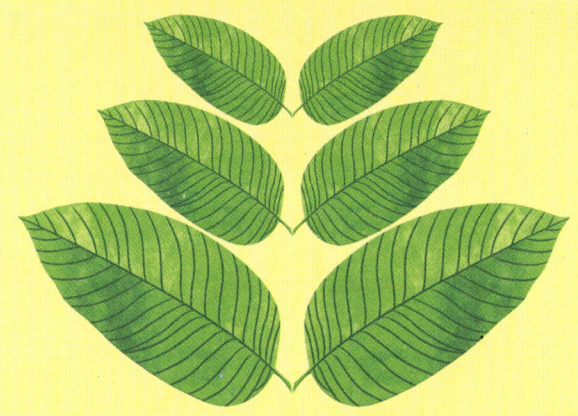

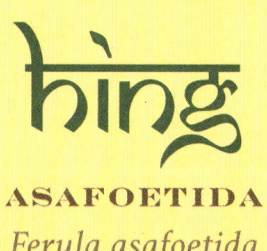

ASAFOETIDA

Ferula asafoetida

HING *Bangla, Gujarati, Hindi, Marathi, Punjabi and Urdu* .
HINGER *Kannada* . **YANG/SAP** *Kashmiri* .
PERUNGAYAM *Malayalam, Tamil* . **HENGU** *Oriya* .
AGUDAGANDHA *Sanskrit* . **INGUMO** *Telugu*

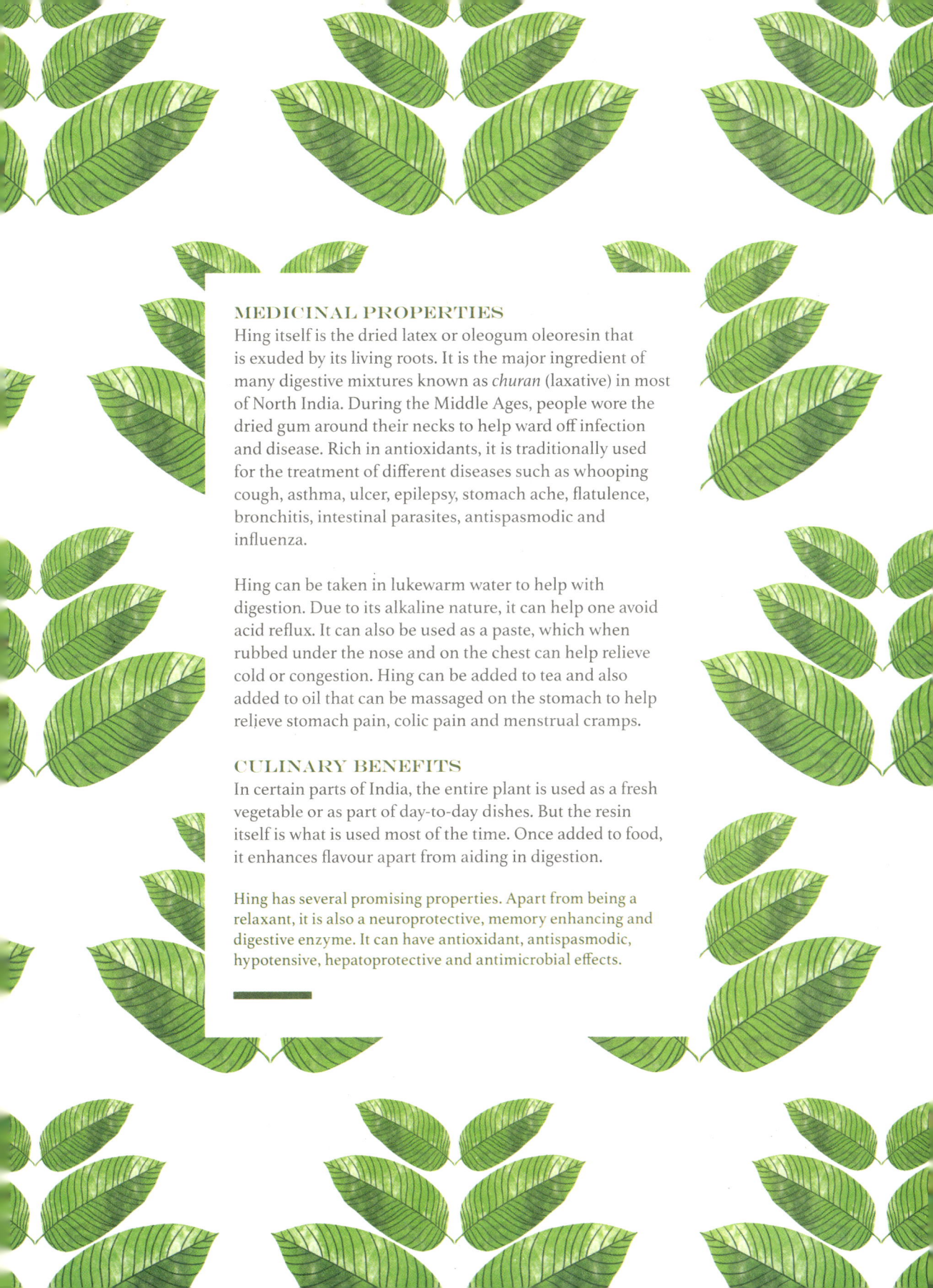

MEDICINAL PROPERTIES

Hing itself is the dried latex or oleogum oleoresin that is exuded by its living roots. It is the major ingredient of many digestive mixtures known as *churan* (laxative) in most of North India. During the Middle Ages, people wore the dried gum around their necks to help ward off infection and disease. Rich in antioxidants, it is traditionally used for the treatment of different diseases such as whooping cough, asthma, ulcer, epilepsy, stomach ache, flatulence, bronchitis, intestinal parasites, antispasmodic and influenza.

Hing can be taken in lukewarm water to help with digestion. Due to its alkaline nature, it can help one avoid acid reflux. It can also be used as a paste, which when rubbed under the nose and on the chest can help relieve cold or congestion. Hing can be added to tea and also added to oil that can be massaged on the stomach to help relieve stomach pain, colic pain and menstrual cramps.

CULINARY BENEFITS

In certain parts of India, the entire plant is used as a fresh vegetable or as part of day-to-day dishes. But the resin itself is what is used most of the time. Once added to food, it enhances flavour apart from aiding in digestion.

Hing has several promising properties. Apart from being a relaxant, it is also a neuroprotective, memory enhancing and digestive enzyme. It can have antioxidant, antispasmodic, hypotensive, hepatoprotective and antimicrobial effects.

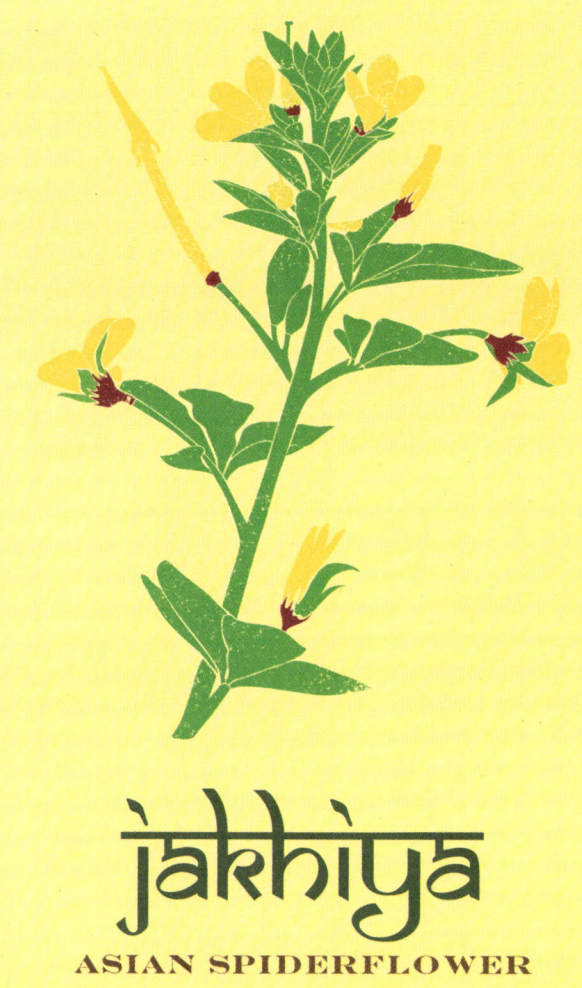

jakhiya

ASIAN SPIDERFLOWER

Cleome viscosa

JAKHIYA *Kumaoni* . BAGRA *Hindi* . HULHUL *Urdu* .
NAIVELA *Malayalam* . NAIKKADUKU *Tamil* . NAYIBELA *Kannada* .
PILITALVANI *Gujarati* . KUKKAVAMINTA *Telugu* . PIVLA TILVAN *Marathi* .
HURHURE/BAN TOREE/TORI JHAAR *Nepali*

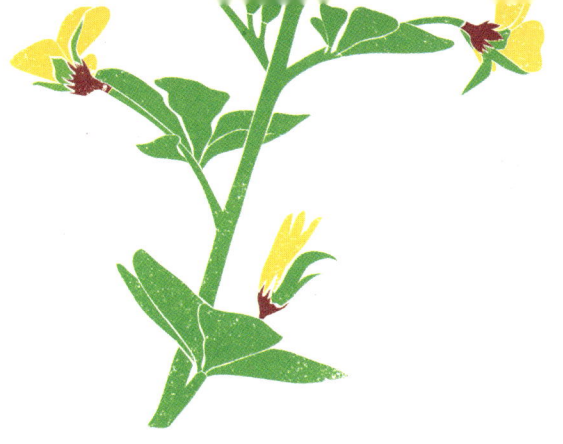
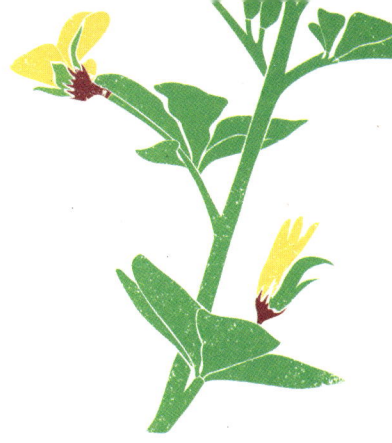

MEDICINAL PROPERTIES

Jakhiya is considered to possess cooling, stomachic, laxative, diuretic and anthelmintic properties. In both Unani and Ayurvedic medications, it is reported to be useful in the treatment of malarial fevers, skin diseases, and uterine complaints.

It is also documented to remove *kapha* (phlegm) and to cure malaria, piles, lumbago and ulcers. Interestingly, these are precisely the uses this plant is put to, by local health practitioners, though the form of their medication may be different. It is commonly used for treating fever, inflammation and bronchitis.

CULINARY BENEFITS

The seeds of the jakhiya plant are used widely by communities in both the Garhwali and Kumaoni regions of India, as a very important part of their cuisine. Due to its sharp pungent smell and crunchy taste, it is often used in the place of the more commonly used jeera or even mustard in some parts of the country. Jakhiya is regularly used in day-to-day cooking to temper pulao, dals, mooli ke parathe, and dry dishes like potatoes, spinach and other vegetables. Jakhiya has so much value in the lives of these communities there that it is often used as a gift by them.

Also known as dog mustard, Asian spider flower or tick weed, all the parts of this plant are used in a wide variety of ways.

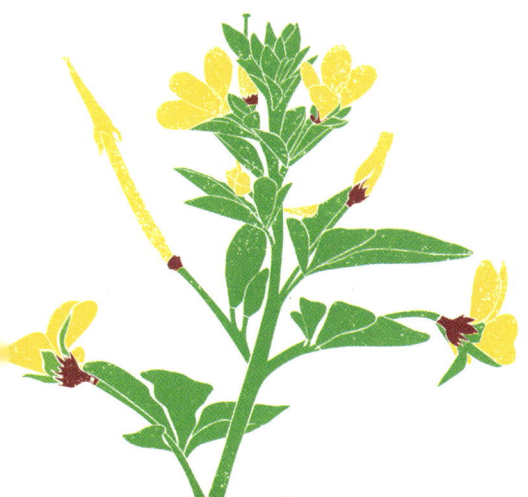
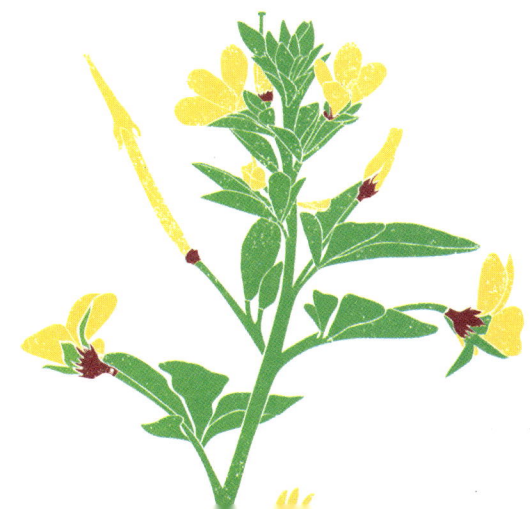

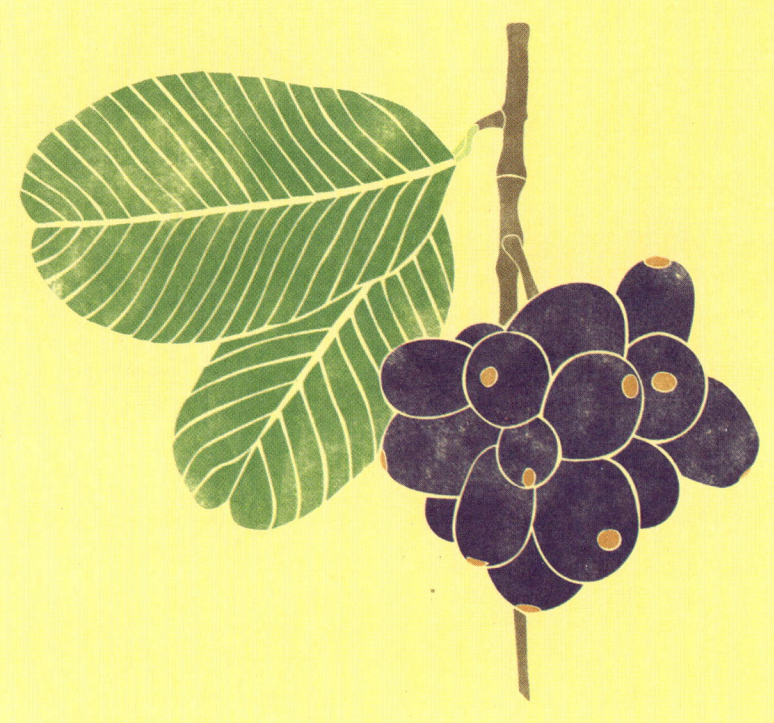

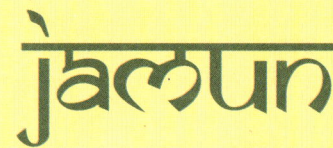

jamun

INDIAN BLACKBERRY

Syzyglum cumini

JAMUN *Hindi* . NERIL/NEERALU/NEERALA/NERALE *Kannada* .
JAM *Meitei* . PHANIR/JAAMBU/JAMUNA *Nepali* . NEREDU *Telugu* .
HMUIPUI/LHENHMUI *Mizo* . CHOMSTHATHEI *Tangkhul*

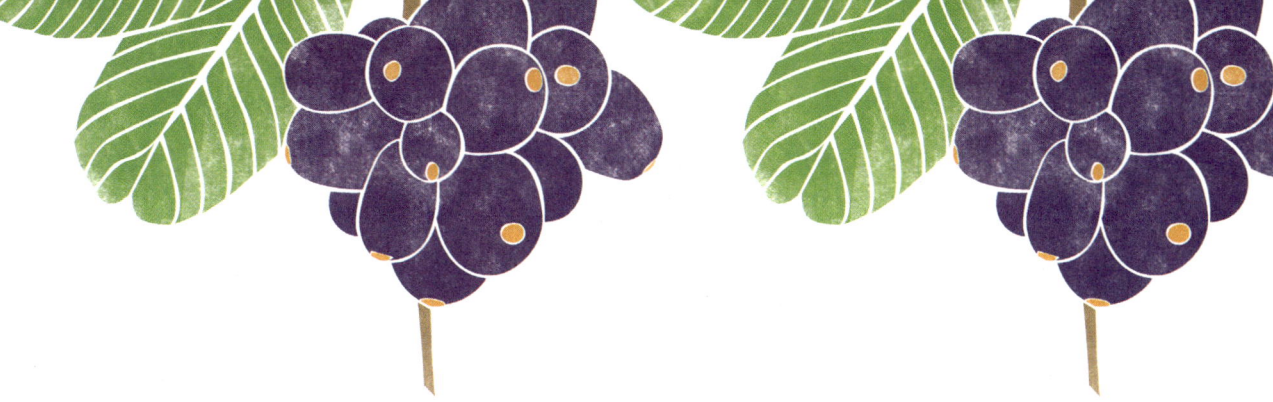

MEDICINAL PROPERTIES

Over the decades, jamun has become best known for its great value for diabetes mellitus. When its seeds are dried, powdered and administered orally thrice a day for 3-4 months, the glycoside in them helps prevent the conversion of starch into sugar. Furthermore, fresh bark juice mixed with milk is used to treat diarrhoea. It is also used in the case of sore throat, bronchitis, asthma and ulcers, along with keeping one's blood pressure in check.

The peel, pulp and seed of jamun are all good sources of antioxidants, minerals, vitamins and polyphenols.

The rich content of Vitamin C and other antioxidants in jamun that can boost the production of white blood cells. Hence they have been used to treat ailments like cough, diabetes, dysentery, inflammation, and also as a lotion for ringworm of the scalp.

CULINARY BENEFITS

The fruit is consumed by being made into tarts and jam. Good quality juice is made into sherbets, syrups and squash. When the fruit is astringent, they are often pricked and then soaked in salted water, to be enjoyed. In some parts of India, the same is made into wine.

COSMETIC CURES

The astringent properties of jamun help in preventing acne, blemishes and pimples. It also contains anti-aging properties and aids in hair growth and skin conditioning. Application of jamun seed powder on the skin can help fade off scars and blemishes. Applying a mixture of jamun powder and almond oil on the scalp helps reduce dandruff and supports healthy hair growth. Combining the powder of dried seeds with honey and using it as a face mask aids in reducing pimples and dark spots.

A serving of 100 grams jamun contains 79 mg of potassium, which makes it appropriate for a high blood pressure diet. The fruit aids in the conversion of carbohydrates to energy and regulates blood sugar levels. Because of its low glycemic index, diabetic patients can benefit from consuming jamun during the hot summer months.

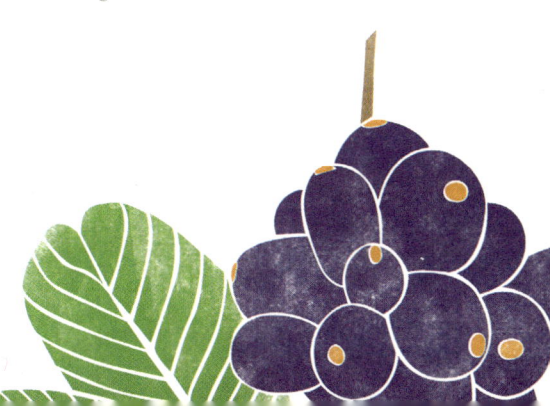

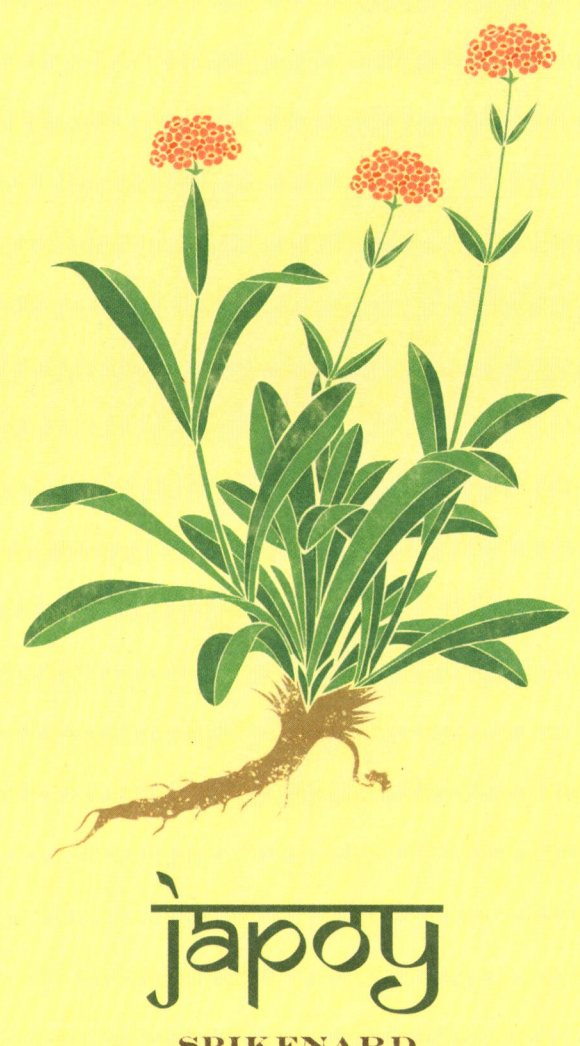

japoy

SPIKENARD

Nardostachya j atamansi DC

JAPOY *Nepali*

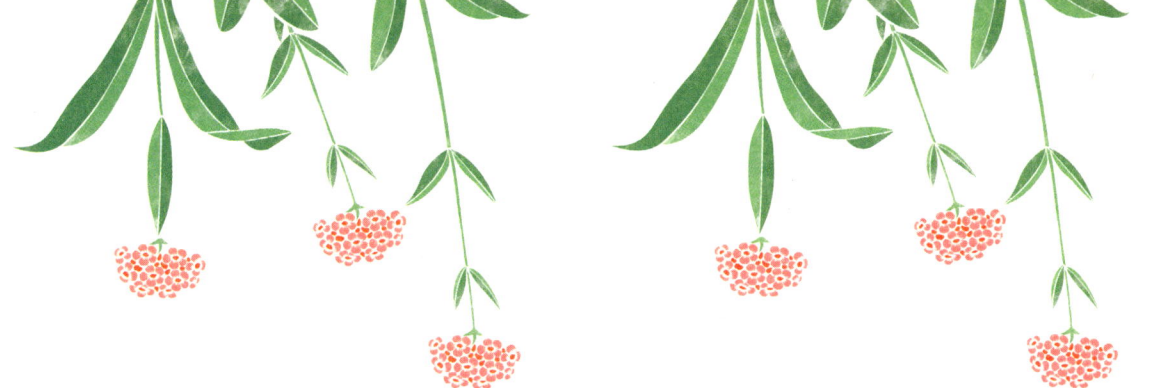

MEDICINAL PROPERTIES

The sweet-smelling root which is thin in the constitution is covered for the most part by coarse earthy coloured hair. As the mainstream valerian, it is directed as an energizer and an anti-spasmodic in cases of hysteria and epilepsy. The dried root is also used as an ingredient in the preparation of hair oil, and for hair growth.

Applying japoy on cuts and wounds helps prevent bacterial infections. It also has a calming effect on people and acts like a good sedative while helping with problems like insomnia and anxiety by providing a good night's sleep if taken in proper dosage. Along with treating hypertension, it also helps regulate blood pressure.

COSMETIC CURES

In the powdered form, japoy is used as a conditioner for hair, as it improves hair growth, decreases hair fall and cools the scalp, also making the hair delicate and plush. It is likewise utilized in the preparation of herbal antioxidant face cream. Apart from skin recuperating properties, it can be utilized as a hair mask by mixing with coconut or jojoba oil, or as a face mask by making a paste with turmeric powder and saffron.

Consuming 3-5 grams of japoy powder mixed in plain or lukewarm water after meals help prevent sleeping disorders.

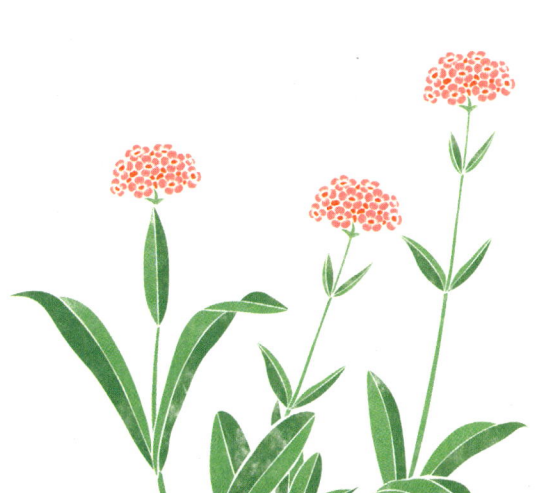

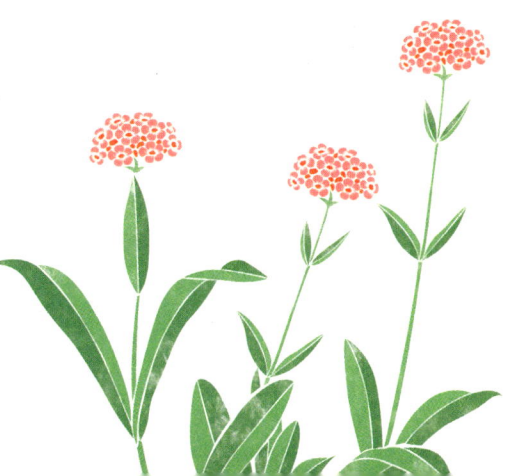

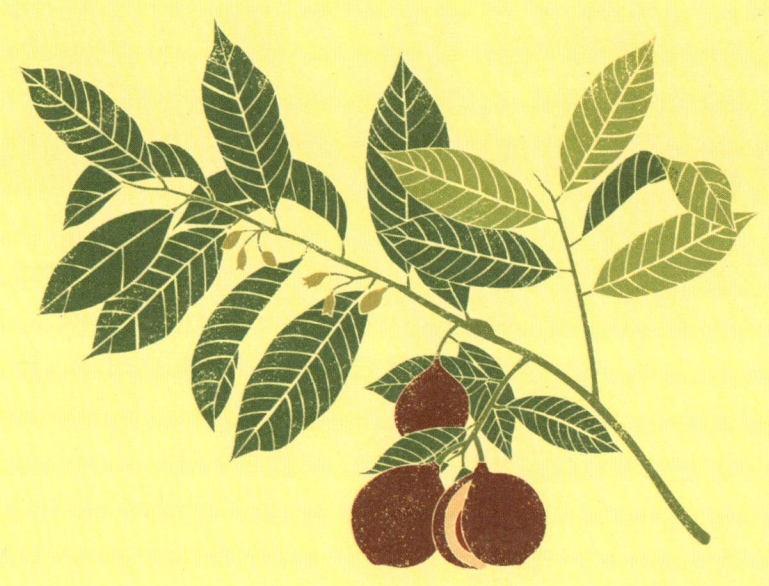

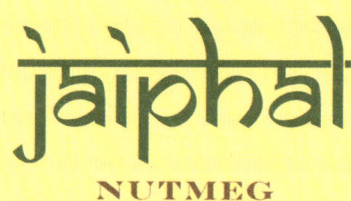

NUTMEG

Myristica fragrans

JAIPHAL *Hindi* . **JAJIKAYA/JATIPHALAMU/JAPITRI** *Telugu* .
JAVITRI *Bangla* . **ONTHI** *Bodo* . **JAJIKAYI** *Kannada* .
ZAAFAL *Kashmiri* . **JATHIKKAI** *Malayalam*

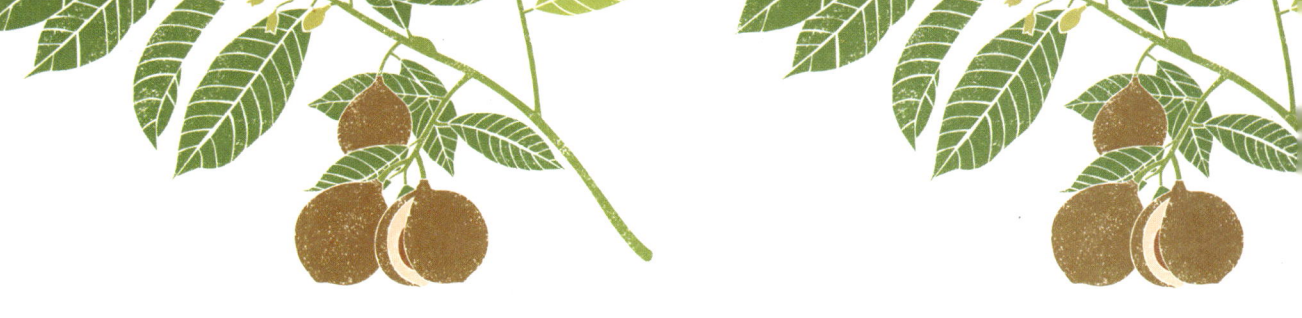

MEDICINAL PROPERTIES

Jaiphal contains many essential volatile oils such as myristicin, elemicin, eugenol and safrole whose anti-inflammatory properties make it useful for treating joint and muscle pain. Its essential oils also aid in the better secretion of digestive enzymes which promote digestion. Jaiphal is an adaptogen for the brain, which means its qualities can be used to either stimulate or be a sedative as required for the system.

CULINARY BENEFITS

In Indian cuisine, jaiphal takes the pride of place. Used often for a subtle taste in pulaos and meat curries, it also goes into the making of pickles and chutneys. It is a must for Mughlai cuisine and is sometimes also added to garam masala. Jaiphal is well-known for its warm nutty flavour, which makes it a perfect addition sweet and savoury dishes and also to flavour cakes, cookies, custards and ice-creams.

COSMETIC CURES

Due to its anti-inflammatory properties, jaiphal has the quality to decrease hyperpigmentation, balance oily skin and calm irritation. It is especially useful with sensitive and oily skins, to be used in the preparation of face masks, serums and creams. It has been used in Ayurvedic medicine to reduce acne scars, a facet that is slowly being revived today. An effective home remedy to cleanse one's skin involves adding a few teaspoons of aloe vera gel and milk to a fine paste of jaiphal powder, and applying it over the skin for ten minutes.

Jaiphal has acquired fame as part of the narrative of conquest as extraction in Amitav Ghosh's *The Nutmeg's Curse: Parables for a Planet in Crisis.*

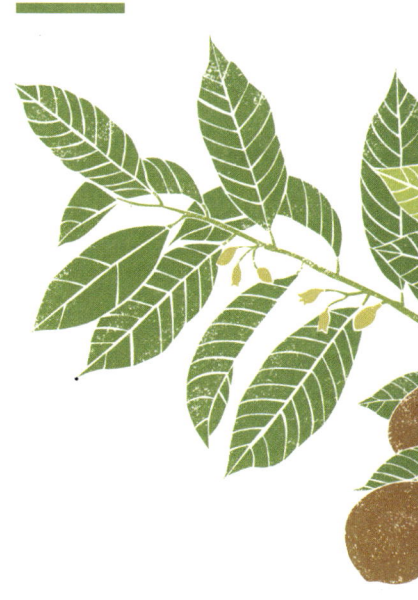

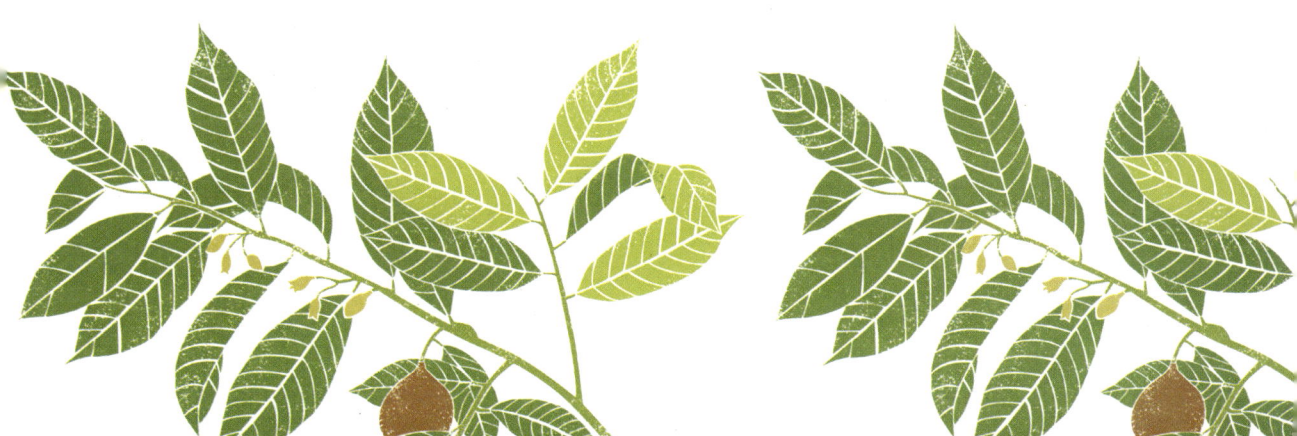

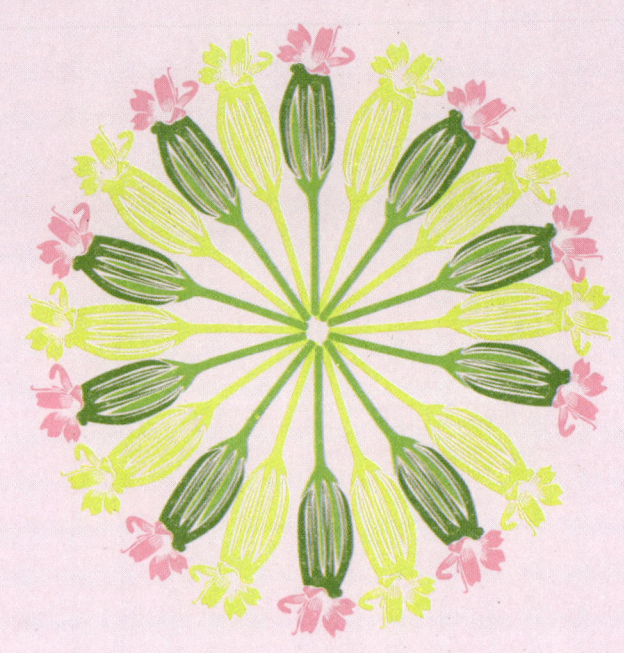

jeera

CUMIN

Cuminum cyminum

JEERA *Hindi* . **JEERE** *Bangla* . **JEERAKAM** *Tamil* .
JEERU *Gujarati*

MEDICINAL PROPERTIES

Jeera has been widely used in traditional medicine to treat a variety of diseases such as diarrhoea, dyspepsia and hypolipidemia. The literature presents ample evidence for the biological and biomedical activities of jeera, which have generally been ascribed to the action of its active constituents such as terpens, phenols and flavonoids. Jeera seeds are packed with antioxidants, anti-inflammatory properties, vitamins A and C, copper and manganese. Add one tablespoon of jeera seeds to a glass of water, with some chopped ginger, and bring to a boil. Strain and consume once cooled, two to three times a day, for relief from cold and asthma.

CULINARY BENEFITS

Jeera is an integral part of Indian cuisine because of its warm aroma, which is from the essential oils it carries. While it is the ubiquitous tempering for cuisines across the country, a roasted and powdered form is the perfect seasoning to savoury yogurt drinks or dishes across India, especially in accompaniments like raitas and drinks such as chaas.. In the powdered form, jeera is the base for many gravies, ingenuously combined with other spices in an incredible array of tastes across the country.

In north India, a jeera drink is had cold in the summer months while hot jeera water is a part and parcel of the everyday Kerala diet throughout the year, as it helps detoxify the body, remove all the toxins from it, suppress hunger hormones and even speed up one's metabolism.

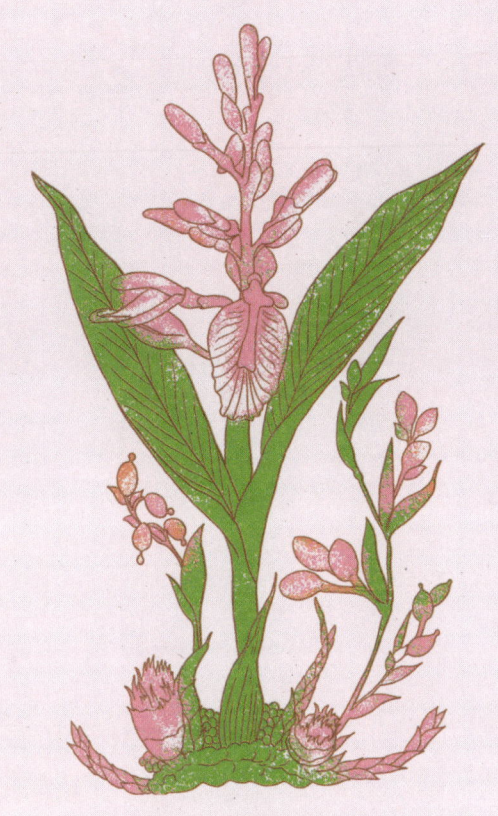

kali ilaichi

LARGE CARDAMOM

Amomum subalatum Roxb

KALI ILAICHI *Hindi* . **PERALAM** *Malayalam* .
PEDDA YALAKAYA *Telugu*

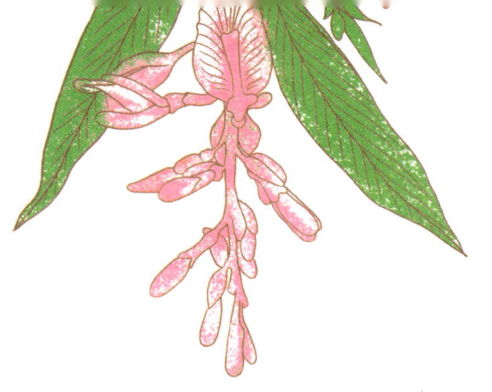
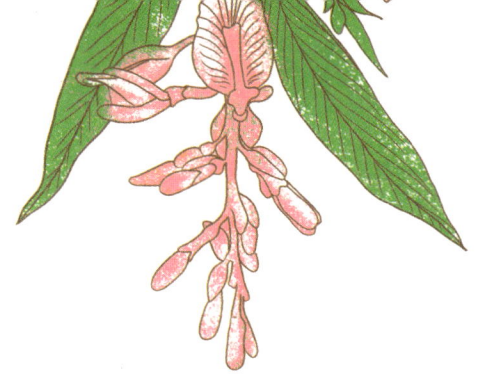

MEDICINAL PROPERTIES

There is scientific evidence to show that the antibacterial and antioxidant properties of kali ilaichi can contribute in developing immunity in the body. Eating it is supposed to normalise the flow of mucous through the respiratory tract. From this then, many diseases of the respiratory tract like whooping cough, tuberculosis and bronchitis have the potential to be treated by using kali ilaichi in new pharmacological preparations. Given its very strong aroma, it can also successfully ward off bad breath and help resolve other oral health issues. Chew a single cardamom seed to treat bad breath and gum infections.

Traditionally, kali ilaichi has been known to cure dyspepsia, anorexia, dysentery, hyperacidity, stomach ulcers and skin diseases. Kali ilaichi is also used in a preparation called 'Alui' for the treatment of malaria along with jeera. Its seeds can act as an antidote to snake bites and scorpion stings.

CULINARY BENEFITS

Widely used in Indian cooking as a flavouring in both savoury and sweet preparations, kali ilaichi is also used as a preservative to different types of coffee, liquors, confections, beverages and tobacco.

COSMETIC CURES

Its essential oils are extremely good in combating dandruff. Applying the oil all the way from the scalp to the hair strands, and massaging for 10-15 minutes gives excellent results.

Roughly one inch in length, the pods are dark brown to black in colour and have a tough, dried, wrinkly skin. It has notes of resin and camphor, as well as menthol's slightly minty aroma that provides balance to an otherwise funky flavour.

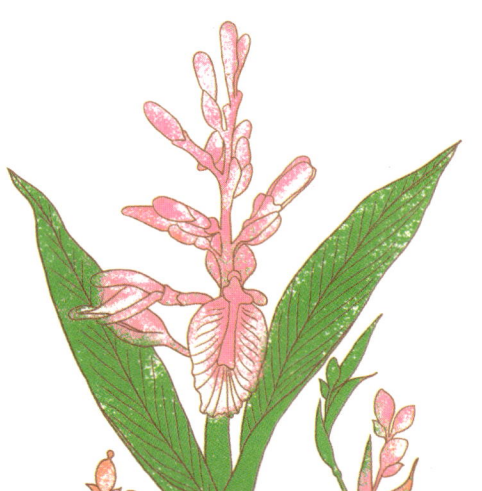
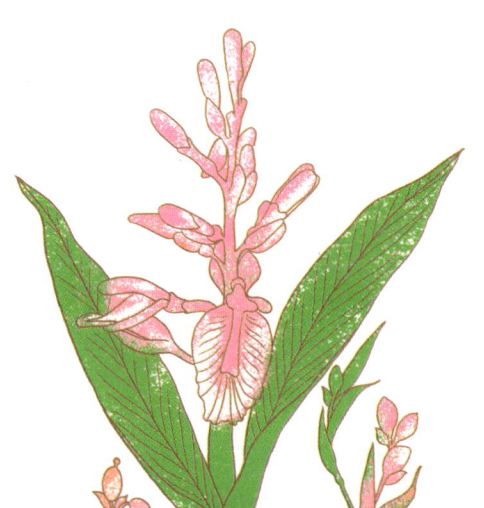

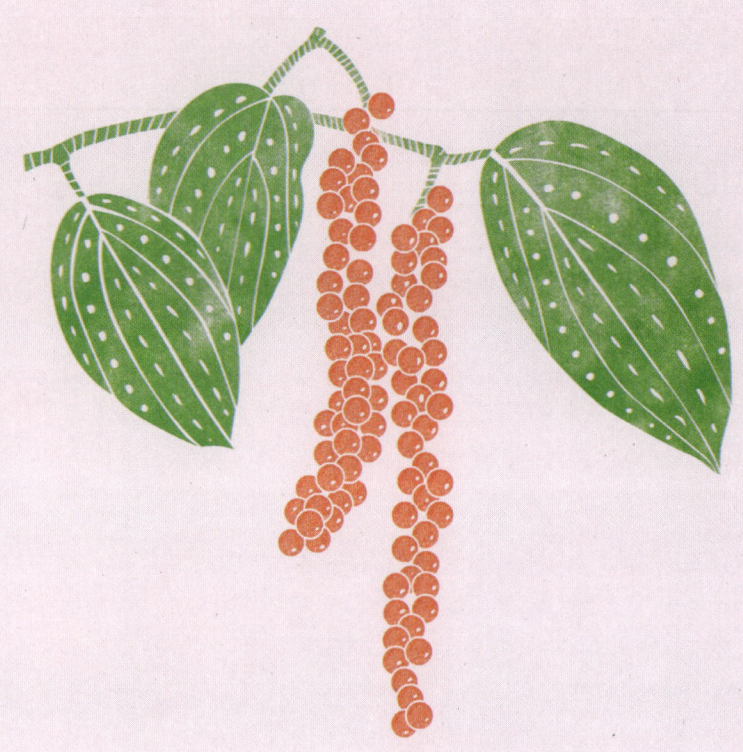

kali mirch

BLACK PEPPER

Piper nigrum

KALI MIRCH *Hindi* . GOLMIRCH *Marathi* . KURUMILAGU *Tamil* .
KURUMULAKU *Malayalam* . MIRYALATIGE *Telugu* .
KARIMENASU *Kannada* . SYAH MIRCH *Urdu* . KALO MIRCH *Gujarati* .
LALIMIRI *Marathi* . THINGMARCHA *Mizo*

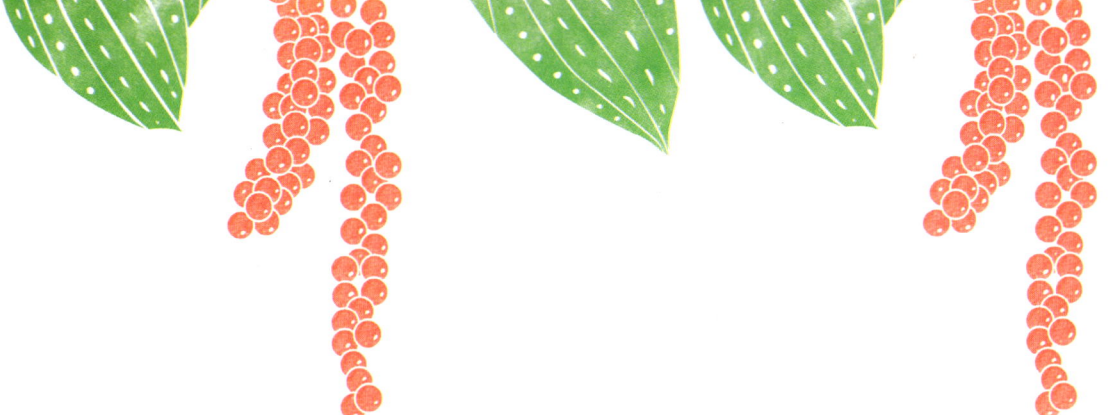

MEDICINAL PROPERTIES

Traditionally considered to be a hot, pungent herb that stimulates 'agni', or digestive fire, by supporting the secretion of fluids and circulation of blood in the gastro-intestinal tract, kali mirch's most active constituent, Piperine, has been found to support the absorption of other herbs, specifically the curcumins found in turmeric, as well as resveratrol. Kali mirch's antibacterial nature helps relieve cold and cough, especially when mixed with honey and consumed in the grounded form.

CULINARY BENEFITS

Nicknamed 'black gold' or the 'king of spice', kali mirch has been traditionally used in Indian cooking and has the potential to make food more beneficial when used in various recipes, as part of a marinade and as a table spice. In south India, kali mirch is widely used in the preparation of rasam, a spicy soup-like dish that is usually served with rice.

COSMETIC CURES

Kali mirch's antibacterial and anti-inflammatory properties help cure skin infections and acne. Traditionally used as a face scrub, it exfoliates dead skin and stimulates blood circulation causing more oxygen to flow to the face. Add coarsely ground kali mirch to your face pack and apply it for 10-15 minutes Wash your face with warm water afterwards.

In Kerala, many start their day with a cup of black coffee with a pinch of kali mirch powder. The aroma of the freshly ground spice is difficult to ignore.

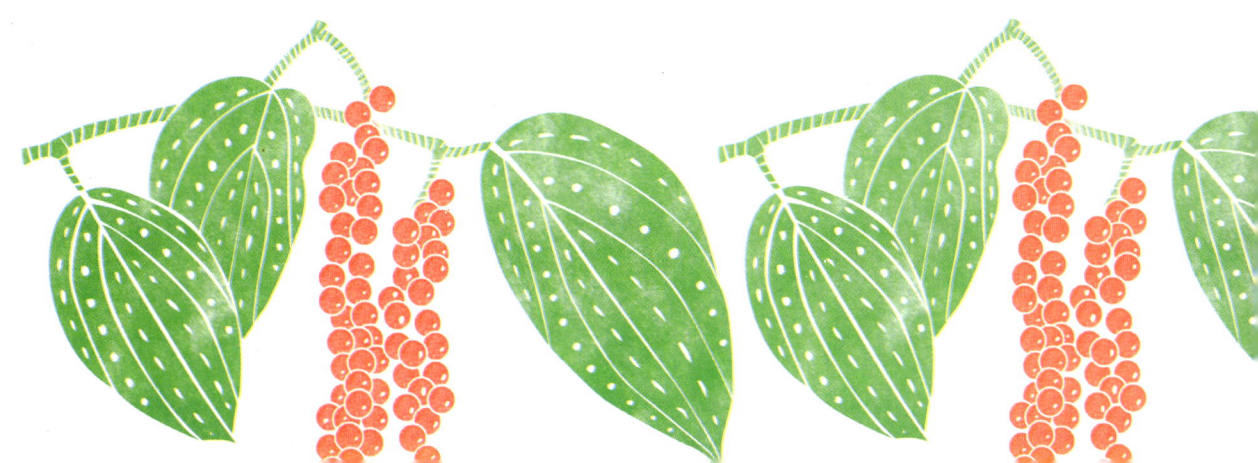

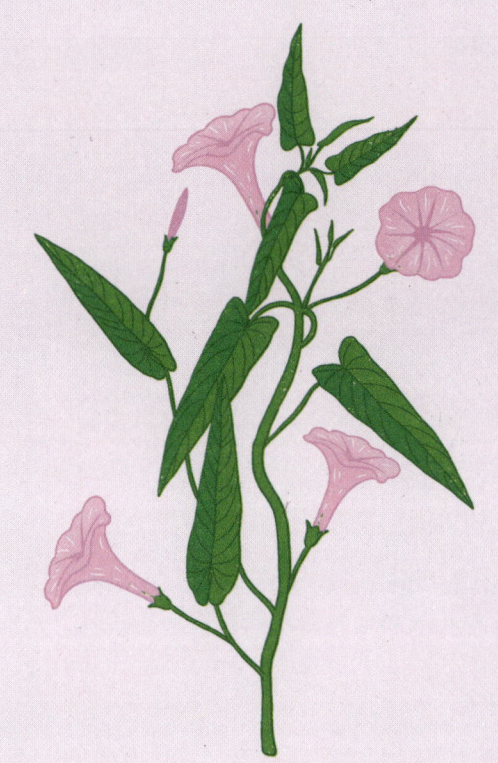

kalmi shak

WATER SPINACH

Ipomoea aquatic

KALMI SHAK *Kokborok*

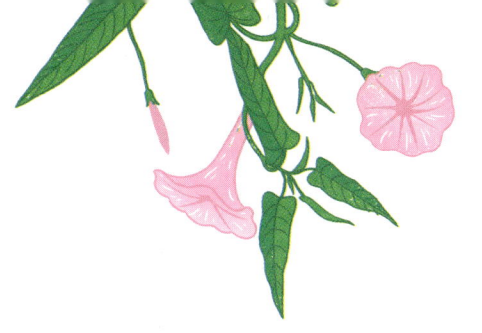
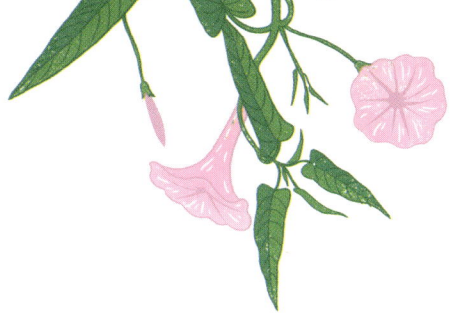

MEDICINAL PROPERTIES

Apart from essential nutrients, kalmi shak also contains a high concentration of beta-carotene, which acts as an antioxidant to reduce free radicals in the body, thus preventing cholesterol from becoming oxidized. Its leaf extracts are used against jaundice and nervous debility. Consuming kalmi shak in a juice form helps in reducing blood glucose levels across the body due to its insulin-like property. It is known to be a go-to weight loss food source, being low in calories and fats but rich in vitamins, antioxidants and minerals. For instance, 100 grams of *kalmi saag* carries only nineteen calories. This green is also known to help prevent osteoporosis and anemia caused by iron-deficiency.

CULINARY BENEFITS

One of the comfort foods in Bengal, it is stir-fried with garlic, green chillies and bengal gram. But the sweet, sour and spicy *anne soppu* chutney made with kalmi shak, lahsun, onion, tomato and green chillies, in Karnataka, is a great immune booster.

COSMETIC CURES

In terms of cosmetic use, kalmi shak juice is beneficial for hair growth and prevents hair loss besides improving the quality and texture of your hair. It is also used as a cosmetic ingredient for hair conditioning. A great source of vitamins A and C, regular consumption of the plant helps rejuvenate the skin and has an anti-aging effect.

Kalmi shak is said to have helped sustain and save several lives during the Great Bengal Famine of 1943–44 and also during World War II in Japanese-occupied Singapore.

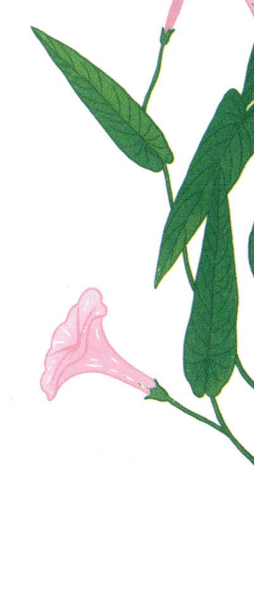

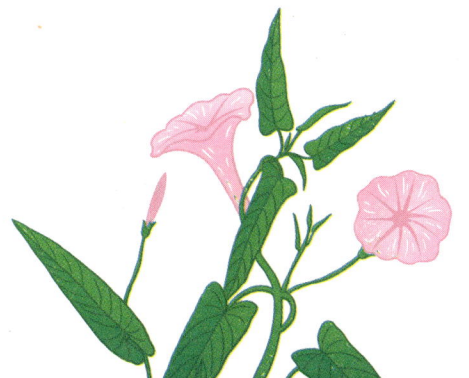
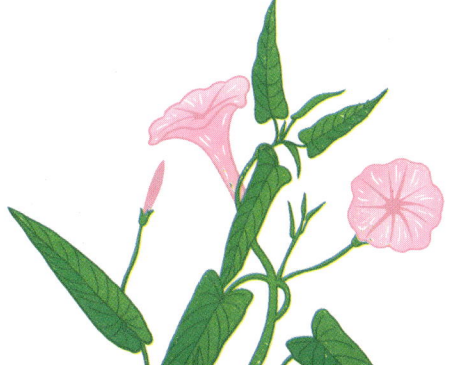

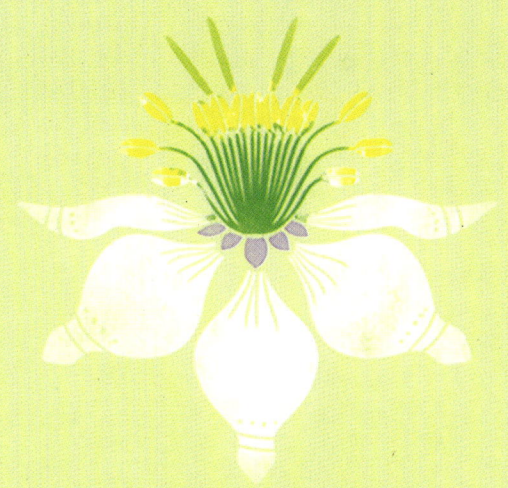

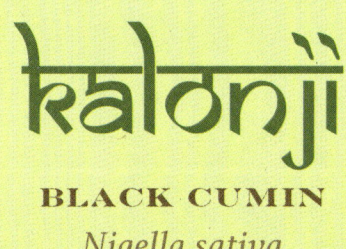

kalonji

BLACK CUMIN

Nigella sativa

KALONJI *Hindi, Punjabi* . **KAUNG SEERAGAM** *Tamil* .
KALE JEERE *Marathi* . **NALLA JEELAKARA** *Malayalam*

MEDICINAL PROPERTIES

Kalonji contains effective therapeutic agents that help in combating infectious and non-infectious skin conditions including different types of allergy, skin inflammations and vitiligo. Kalonji acts as a remedy for chronic headaches and migraines, and has also been extensively used because of its therapeutic potential as a bronchodilator, and its gastro-protective, hepatoprotective and renal protective properties. Kalonji also contains anti-inflammatory properties that help in preventing chronic inflammations, and help maintain a healthy heart as it manages cholesterol and blood pressure. Chew on a few kalonji seeds daily for stronger teeth and gums. Alternatively, one could mix half a teaspoon of kalonji oil in yogurt and apply it on the gums and teeth twice a day.

CULINARY BENEFITS

Kalonji is widely grown for its flavourful seeds and leaves, and is used as a culinary spice in many different ways in the Indian subcontinent. Sometimes used as a topping in Indian breads like naan, it is also a regular component of the typically Bangla combination of five spices called *paanch phoron*.

COSMETIC CURES

Kalonji serves as a relief for afflictions such as pimples, abscess, alopecia, eczema, freckles and leucoderma. A mixture of kalonji oil and olive oil, is applied on the skin for 10-15 minutes, and then washed away. Repeat this twice a week to improve skin texture and prevent acne. It is also great for hair growth in combination with methi in hair oils.

Kalonji seeds have traditionally been used in the Southeast Asian and Middle East countries for the treatment of diseases such as asthma, bronchitis, rheumatism and other inflammatory diseases.

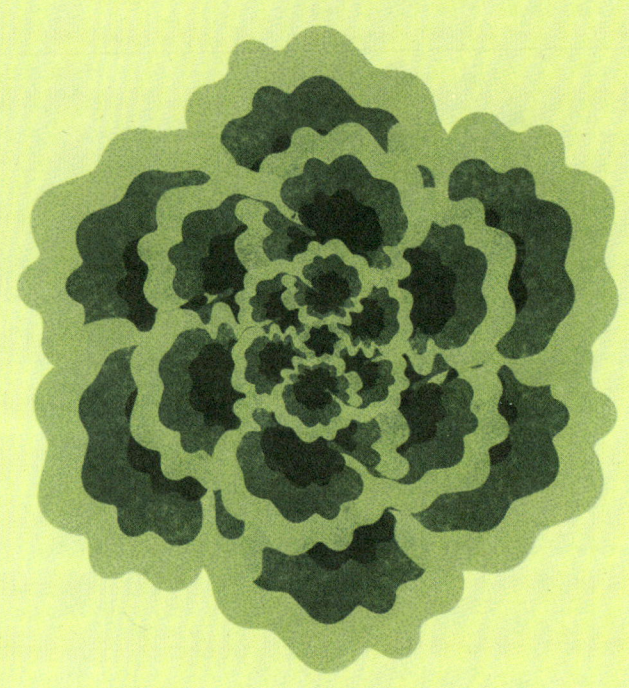

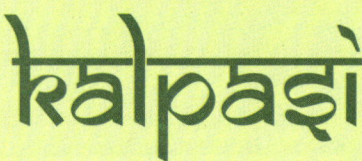

kalpasi

BLACK STONE FLOWER

Parmotrema perlatum

KALPASI *Tamil* . DAGAD PHOOL *Marathi* .
CHARILA/CHADILA *Hindi* . DAGAD DA PHOOL *Punjabi* .
SHAILAJ *Bangla* . KALLU HUVU *Kannada* .
SHAILEYA/SHAILAPUSHPA *Sanskrit*

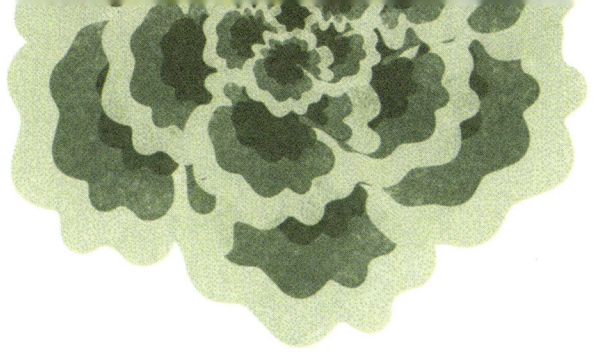
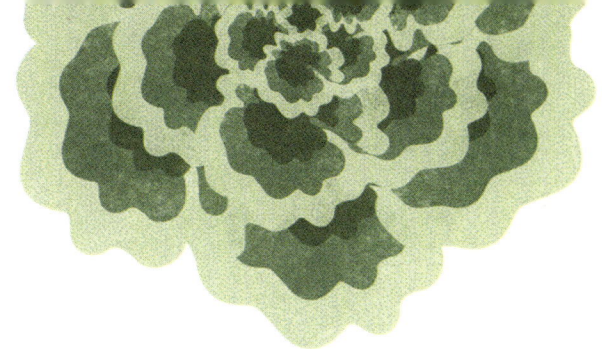

Kalpasi is an edible lichen, a symbiotic association of algae and fungi that sprouts amid tree trunks, mountains and rocks in the hilly areas.

MEDICINAL PROPERTIES

Kalpasi is widely applied in traditional Ayurvedic formulations as an effective remedy for urolithiasis (formation of stones in the bladder or urinary tract) as well as to treat urinary tract infections and for pacifying cases of dysuria (painful urination). The plant carries several wound-healing properties, when applied topically – thanks to its strong antimicrobial and anti-inflammatory traits. The lichen also carries superb capabilities in balancing the exacerbated kapha and pitta doshas, besides relieving asthma symptoms and curing respiratory illnesses, owing to its decongestant qualities. The dried powder of kalpasi combined with honey and water helps in keeping the airways open at all times.

CULINARY BENEFITS

While Kalpasi dominates traditional Chettinad products, this edible lichen is also widely used in Hyderabad and Maharashtrian cuisines. These black-purple flowers do not have their own flavour, yet they add a mysterious tang to whatever food they are added to, hence they are equally used in cooking dals (lentils) and meat. The plant, generally, lends a signature black colour to whatever it is mixed with.

Kalpasi's core medicinal quality is believed to be its ability to deal with kidney stones, hence its name in Hindi and other languages, 'patthar ke phool', refer to that quality.

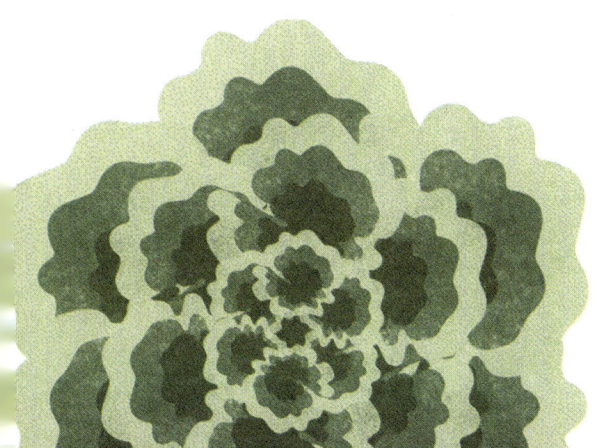
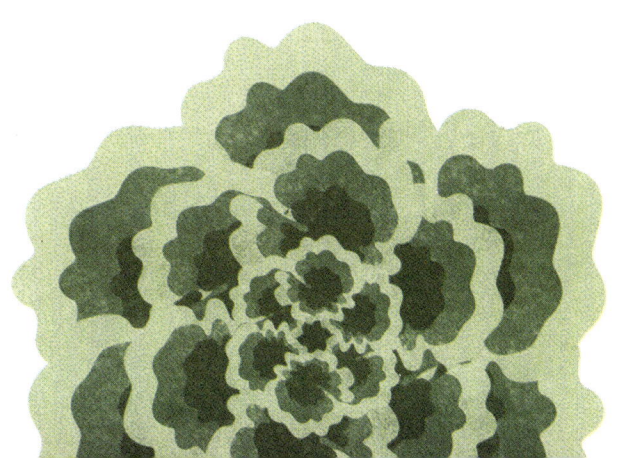

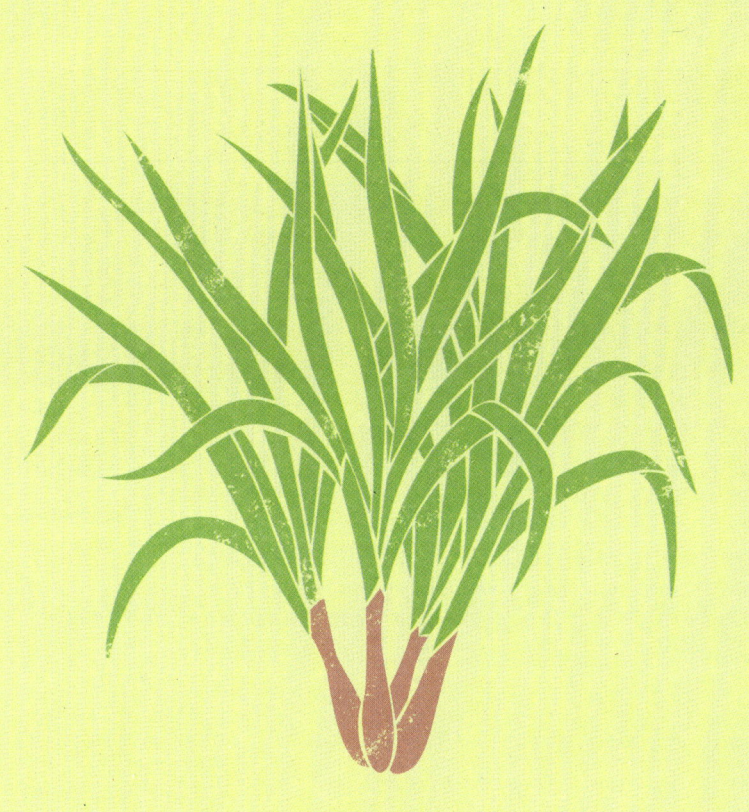

karppurappul

LEMONGRASS

Cymbopogon citratus

KARPPURAPPUL Tamil . **INCHI PULLU/VASANA PULLU/SUGANDHA
BHOOTHRANA/THAKRA THUNI** Malayalam . **NIMMA GADDI/VASANA
GADDI** Telugu . **MAJJIGE HULLU/PURVALI HULLU** Kannada .
CHAIPATT Hindi . **GANDHA BENA** Bangla . **LILLY-CHAYA** Gujarati .
CHAHAVECHE THAN Konkani . **SUGANDHICHAHA/BHUSTRIMA** Marathi

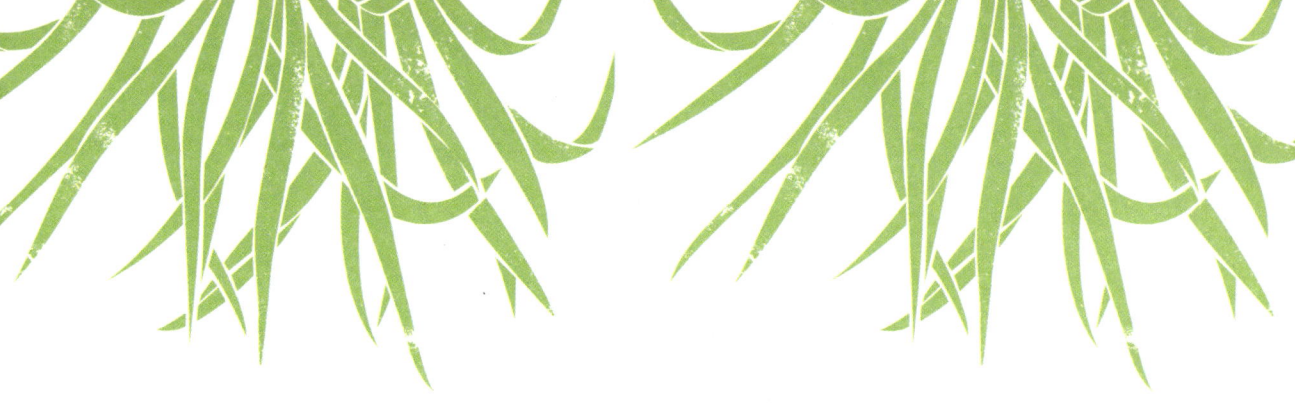

MEDICINAL PROPERTIES

Folk healers make a paste of karppurappul's leaves, mixed with buttermilk, and apply it on ringworm. The oil mixed with twice its bulk of coconut oil is a stimulating embrocation for rheumatism, lumbago, neuralgia, sprains and other painful affections. This healing aspect of the oil has become most accessible now, with it being available and applied directly onto the body.

CULINARY BENEFITS

Karppurappul is increasingly being used in teas, especially in urban households in the past couple of decades. A part of the culinary traditions followed in many parts of the country, its availability in metros now makes it possible to follow those recipes. Being a part of many southeast Asian cuisines, their popularity in India today also brings it closer to Indian tables.

COSMETIC CURES

Karppurappul is good for the hair and skin. The essential oil in its leaves is its most precious and valuable constituent. It is advised, however, that the same be used in combination with either almond or coconut oil. Washing the face, in lukewarm water, with a karppurappul-based cleanser helps clean pores of dirt and germs, and get rid of acne-causing bacteria.

A decoction of the leaves of the grass is used in several different ways: in the form of an infusion, locally over rheumatic joints, lumbago and sprains; with aromatics it is given as a diaphoretic; with black pepper the infusion is used in congestive and neuralgic forms of dysmenorrhoea, vomiting and diarrhoea.

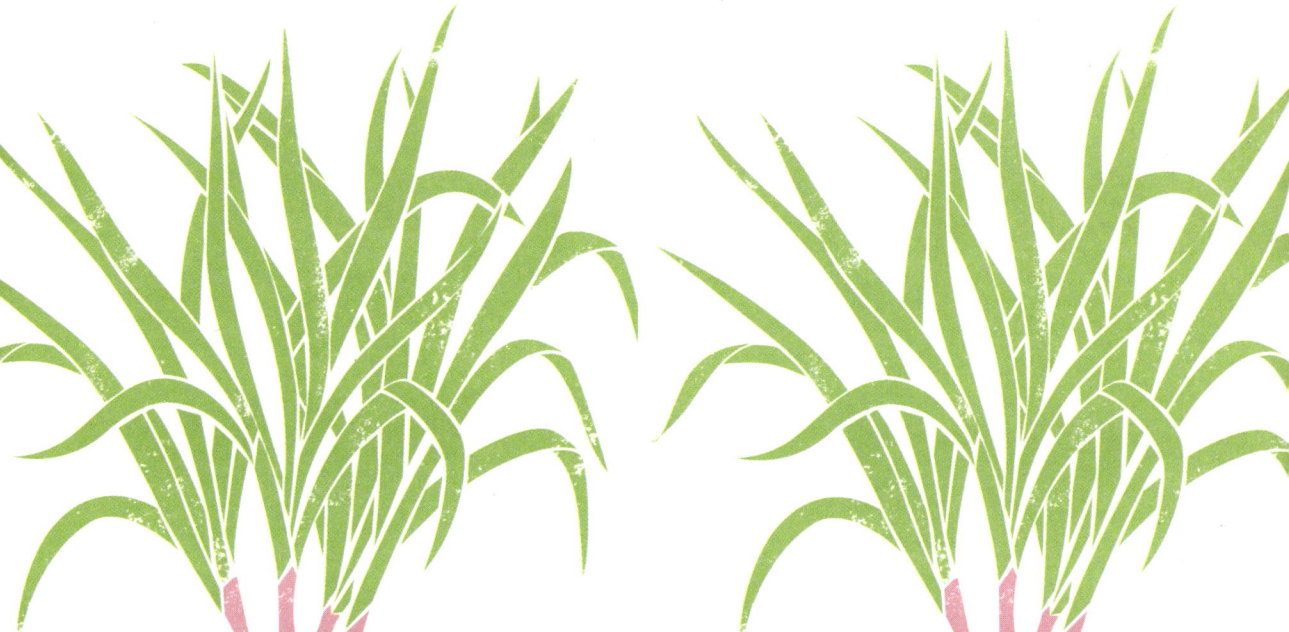

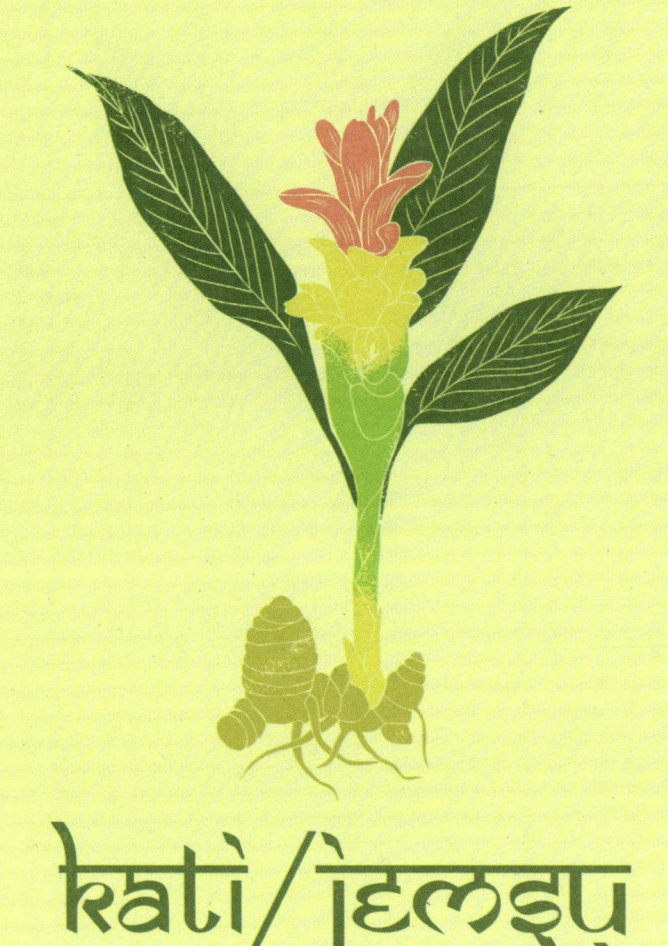

kati/jemsu naro tepetila

ZEDOARY

Curcuma zedoaria Roscoe

KATI/JEMSU NARO TEPETILA *Zeilang*

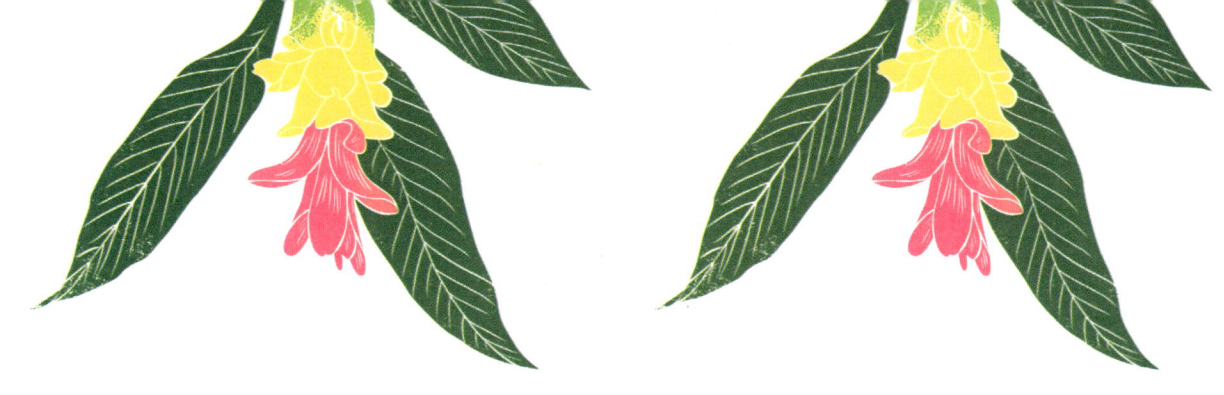

MEDICINAL PROPERTIES

Kati's effect on digestive organs is similar to ginger yet milder. The plant is used to treat flatulence and disorders of urinary system, spleen and liver. Along with other therapeutic applications, the Ayurvedic Pharmacopoeia of India demonstrated the use of its roots in the treatment of goitre. The plant is utilized customarily to treat inflammation pain, and a variety of skin ailments including wounds and ulcers as well as menstrual irregularities.

CULINARY BENEFITS

The edible root of the plant has a white inside and an aroma reminiscent of mango, though its flavour is more like ginger with an exceptionally harsh trailing sensation. At times, it is also used as a vegetable, and the powder is used to make curry pastes. It is also used in pickling and salads, and in flavouring dals and chutneys.

COSMETIC CURES

Kati's dried roots produce an essential oil which is used in perfumery and soap fabrication.

The roots of this plant are also a source of Shoti starch, primarily used as food for babies and convalescents recovering from chronic stomatitis.

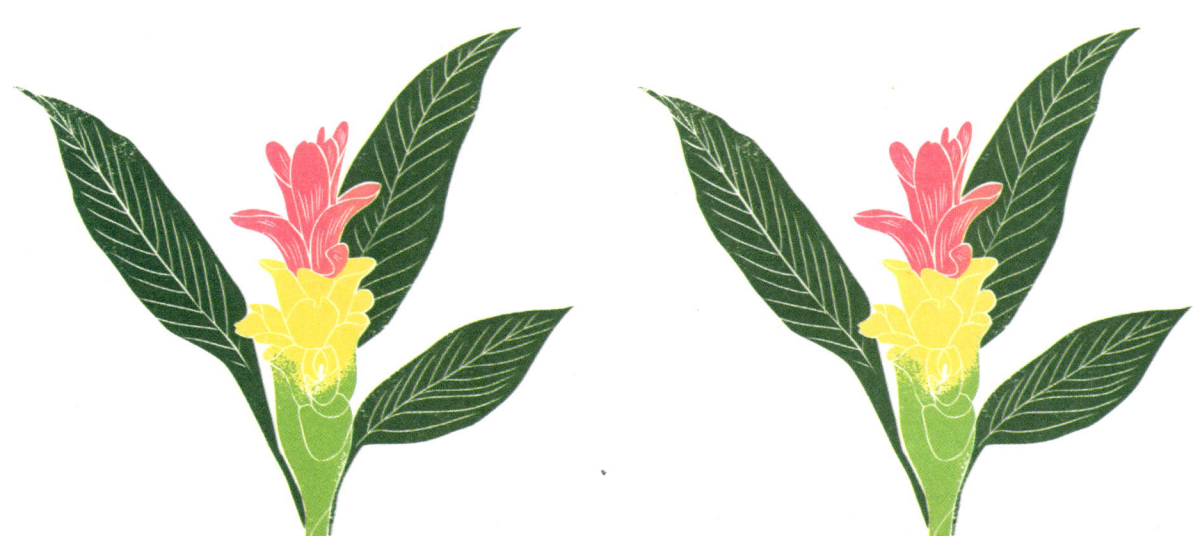

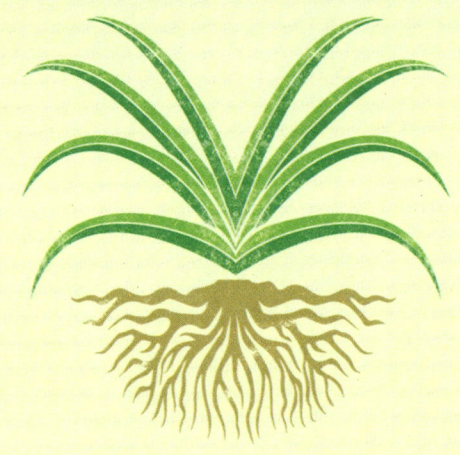

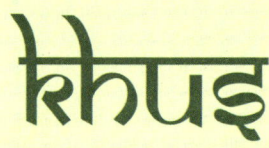

VETIVER

Vetiveria zizanioides

KHUS *Hindi* . MUDIVALA/LAAMANCHA *Kannada* . RAMACHHAM
Malayalam . AVVURU-GADIVERU/KURUVAERU *Telugu* . PANNI *Punjabi* .
BHITIBHARA *Bangla* . VALA VALA *Marathi* . KHAS-VALO *Gujarati*

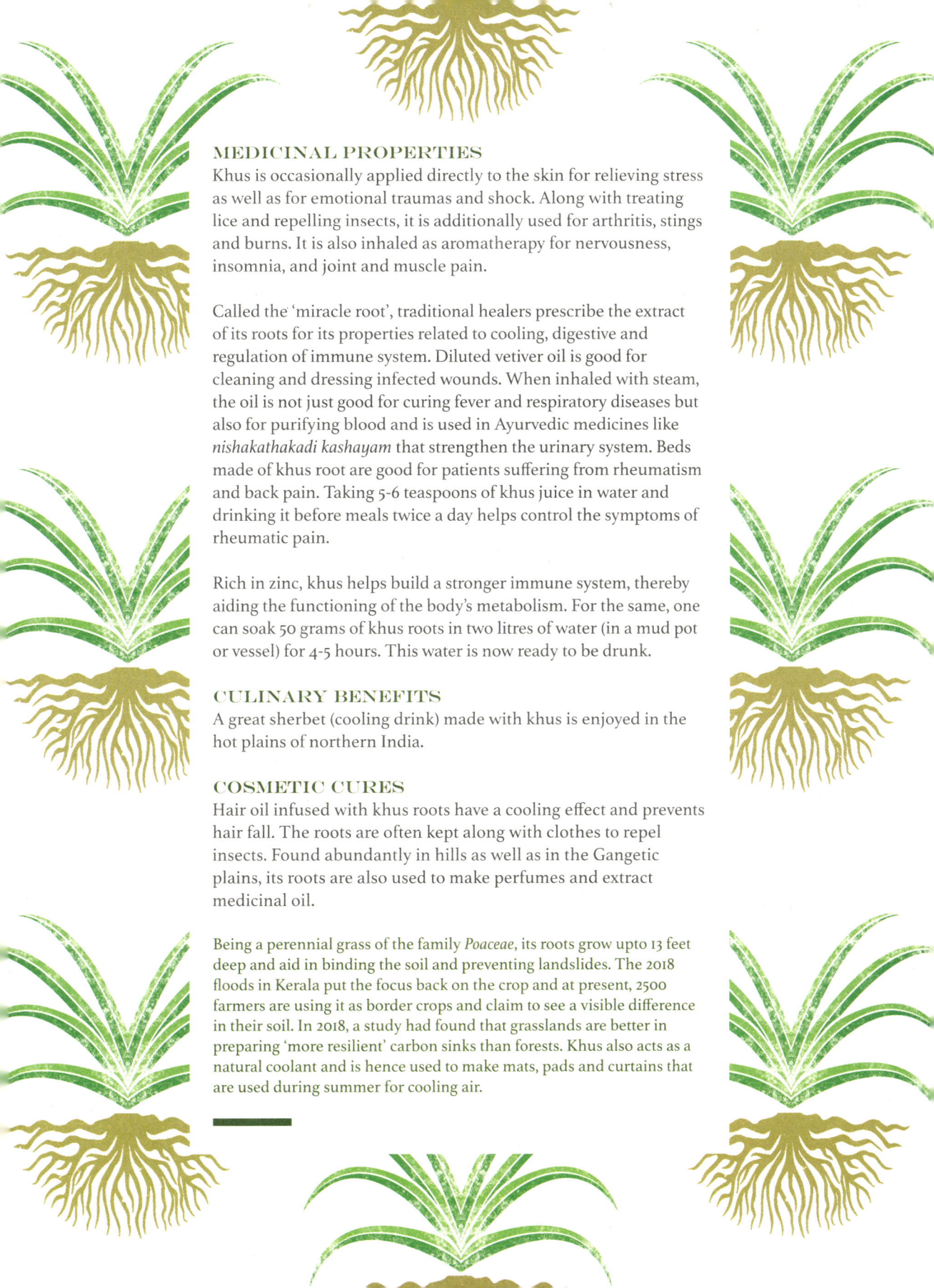

MEDICINAL PROPERTIES

Khus is occasionally applied directly to the skin for relieving stress as well as for emotional traumas and shock. Along with treating lice and repelling insects, it is additionally used for arthritis, stings and burns. It is also inhaled as aromatherapy for nervousness, insomnia, and joint and muscle pain.

Called the 'miracle root', traditional healers prescribe the extract of its roots for its properties related to cooling, digestive and regulation of immune system. Diluted vetiver oil is good for cleaning and dressing infected wounds. When inhaled with steam, the oil is not just good for curing fever and respiratory diseases but also for purifying blood and is used in Ayurvedic medicines like *nishakathakadi kashayam* that strengthen the urinary system. Beds made of khus root are good for patients suffering from rheumatism and back pain. Taking 5-6 teaspoons of khus juice in water and drinking it before meals twice a day helps control the symptoms of rheumatic pain.

Rich in zinc, khus helps build a stronger immune system, thereby aiding the functioning of the body's metabolism. For the same, one can soak 50 grams of khus roots in two litres of water (in a mud pot or vessel) for 4-5 hours. This water is now ready to be drunk.

CULINARY BENEFITS

A great sherbet (cooling drink) made with khus is enjoyed in the hot plains of northern India.

COSMETIC CURES

Hair oil infused with khus roots have a cooling effect and prevents hair fall. The roots are often kept along with clothes to repel insects. Found abundantly in hills as well as in the Gangetic plains, its roots are also used to make perfumes and extract medicinal oil.

Being a perennial grass of the family *Poaceae*, its roots grow upto 13 feet deep and aid in binding the soil and preventing landslides. The 2018 floods in Kerala put the focus back on the crop and at present, 2500 farmers are using it as border crops and claim to see a visible difference in their soil. In 2018, a study had found that grasslands are better in preparing 'more resilient' carbon sinks than forests. Khus also acts as a natural coolant and is hence used to make mats, pads and curtains that are used during summer for cooling air.

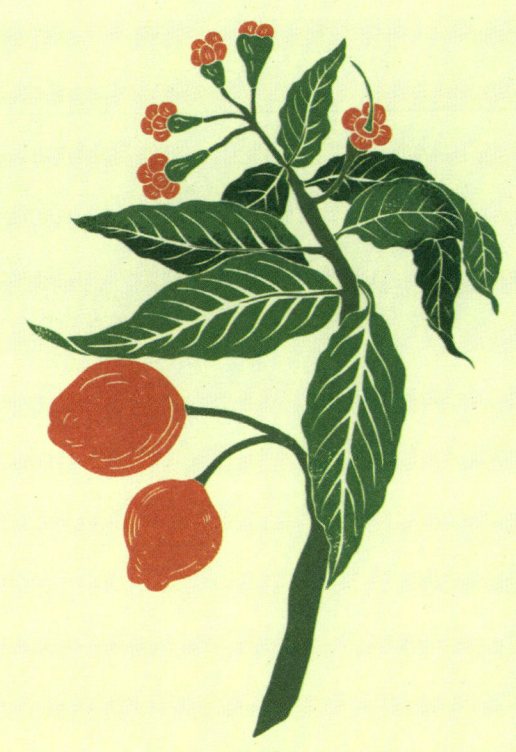

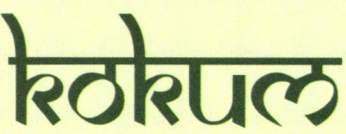

BUTTER TREE

Garcinia indica

KOKUM *Konkani* . **MURUGALU** *Kannada* . **BHERANDA** *Marathi* .
VRIKSHAMALA *Sanskrit* . **PUNARPULI** *Tulu* . **MURGAL-MASALA** *Tamil*

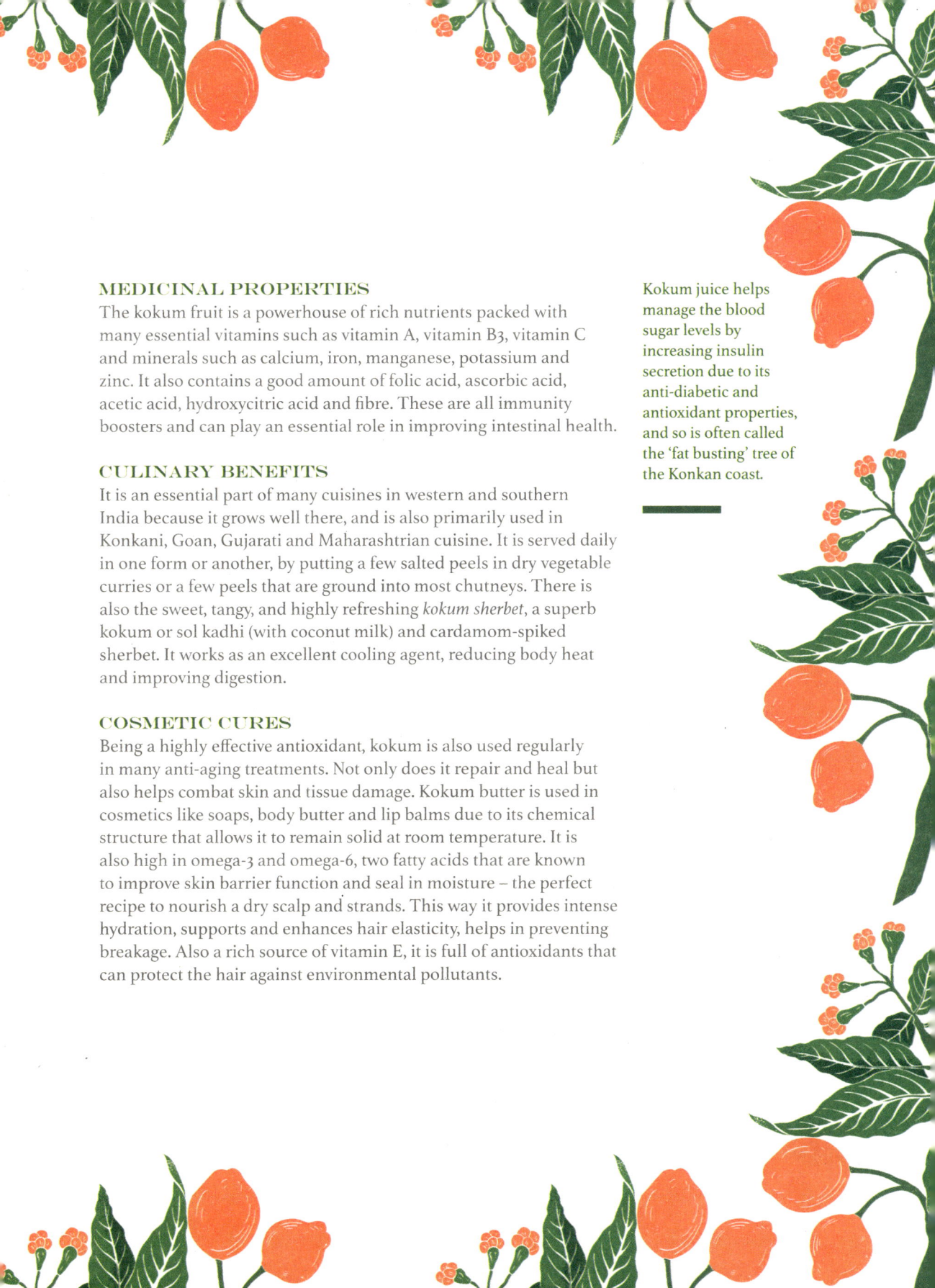

MEDICINAL PROPERTIES

The kokum fruit is a powerhouse of rich nutrients packed with many essential vitamins such as vitamin A, vitamin B3, vitamin C and minerals such as calcium, iron, manganese, potassium and zinc. It also contains a good amount of folic acid, ascorbic acid, acetic acid, hydroxycitric acid and fibre. These are all immunity boosters and can play an essential role in improving intestinal health.

CULINARY BENEFITS

It is an essential part of many cuisines in western and southern India because it grows well there, and is also primarily used in Konkani, Goan, Gujarati and Maharashtrian cuisine. It is served daily in one form or another, by putting a few salted peels in dry vegetable curries or a few peels that are ground into most chutneys. There is also the sweet, tangy, and highly refreshing *kokum sherbet*, a superb kokum or sol kadhi (with coconut milk) and cardamom-spiked sherbet. It works as an excellent cooling agent, reducing body heat and improving digestion.

COSMETIC CURES

Being a highly effective antioxidant, kokum is also used regularly in many anti-aging treatments. Not only does it repair and heal but also helps combat skin and tissue damage. Kokum butter is used in cosmetics like soaps, body butter and lip balms due to its chemical structure that allows it to remain solid at room temperature. It is also high in omega-3 and omega-6, two fatty acids that are known to improve skin barrier function and seal in moisture – the perfect recipe to nourish a dry scalp and strands. This way it provides intense hydration, supports and enhances hair elasticity, helps in preventing breakage. Also a rich source of vitamin E, it is full of antioxidants that can protect the hair against environmental pollutants.

Kokum juice helps manage the blood sugar levels by increasing insulin secretion due to its anti-diabetic and antioxidant properties, and so is often called the 'fat busting' tree of the Konkan coast.

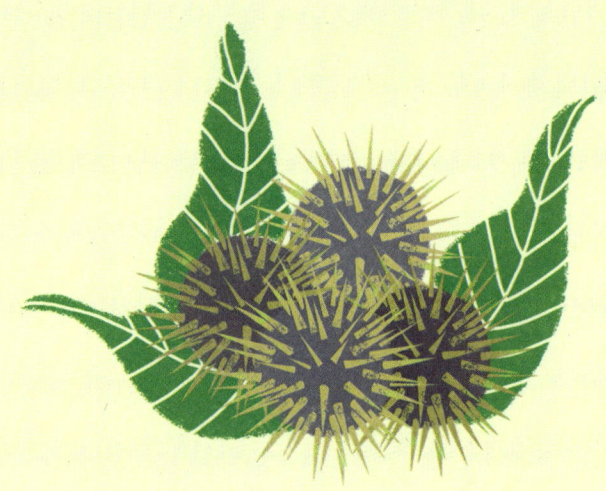

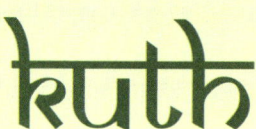

INDIAN COSTUS ROOT

Saussurea costus

KUTH *Punjabi* . KUTHA *Hindi* . KOOD *Bangla* . CHANGLUVA/KOSHTU/
KUSHTAM *Telugu* . KOTTAM/SEYUDDI *Malayalam* . KUDU/UPALET
Gujarati . KOSHTA *Kannada* . KUTH *Kashmiri* .
QUST *Urdu* . KUST-E-TALKH *Persian*

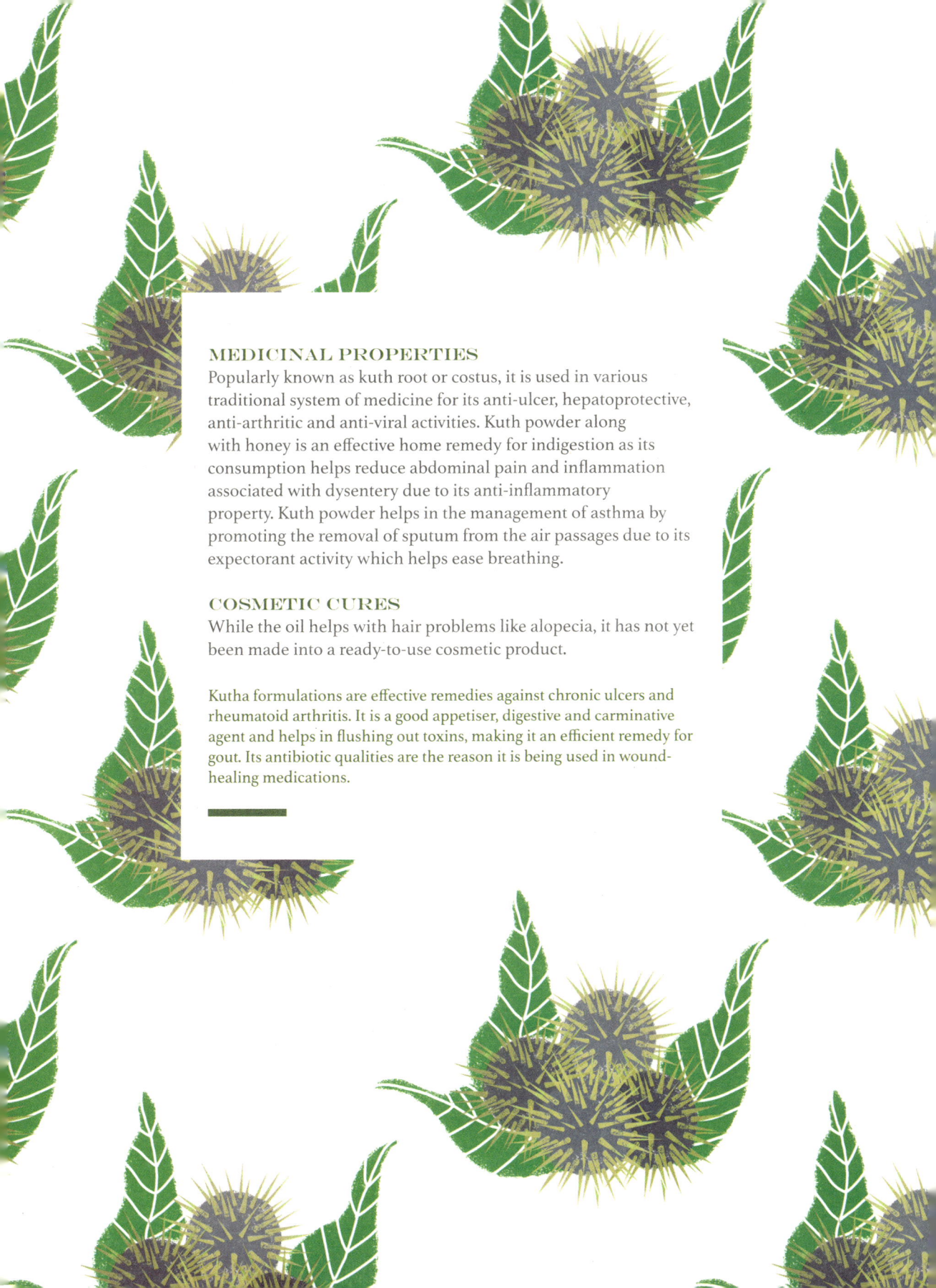

MEDICINAL PROPERTIES

Popularly known as kuth root or costus, it is used in various traditional system of medicine for its anti-ulcer, hepatoprotective, anti-arthritic and anti-viral activities. Kuth powder along with honey is an effective home remedy for indigestion as its consumption helps reduce abdominal pain and inflammation associated with dysentery due to its anti-inflammatory property. Kuth powder helps in the management of asthma by promoting the removal of sputum from the air passages due to its expectorant activity which helps ease breathing.

COSMETIC CURES

While the oil helps with hair problems like alopecia, it has not yet been made into a ready-to-use cosmetic product.

Kutha formulations are effective remedies against chronic ulcers and rheumatoid arthritis. It is a good appetiser, digestive and carminative agent and helps in flushing out toxins, making it an efficient remedy for gout. Its antibiotic qualities are the reason it is being used in wound-healing medications.

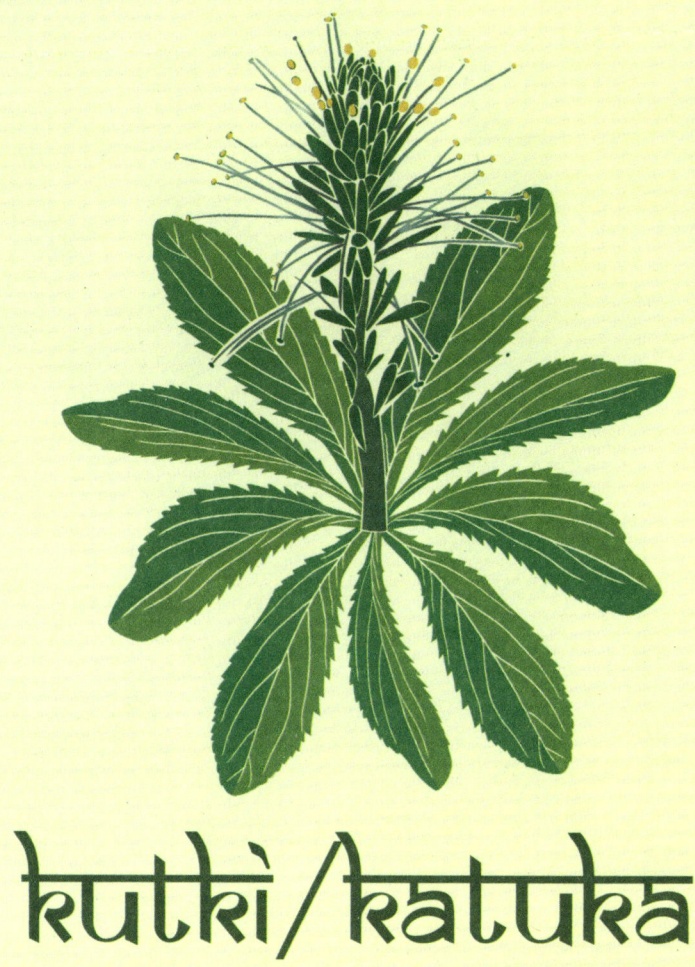

kutki/katuka

YELLOW GENTIAN

Picorrhiza kurroa

KUTKI/KATUKA *Hindi* . **KADU/ KUDU/UPALET** *Gujarati* . **KATUKI** *Bangla* . **KATUKAROHINI** *Telugu* . **LOSHT/KADUGUROHINI** *Tamil* . **KOTTAM/ SEYUDDI** *Malayalam* . *Gujarati* . **KATUKA ROHINI** *Kannada* . **KUTH** *Kashmiri* . **KATUKI** *Urdu* . **KALI KATUKI** *Marathi*

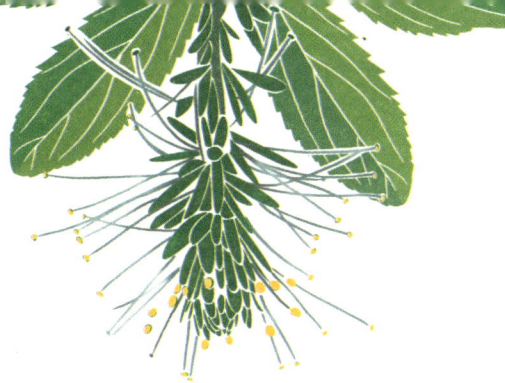
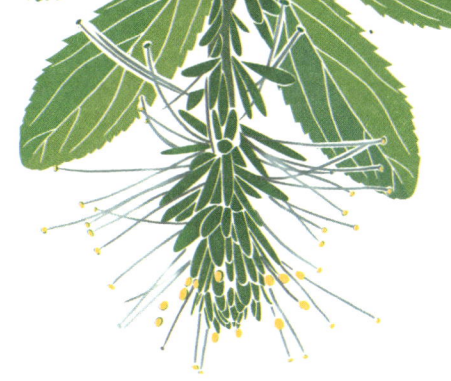

MEDICINAL PROPERTIES

Traditionally used for liver disorders, the plant has also been included in the treatment of upper respiratory tract, fevers, dyspepsia and chronic diarrhoea. It is used to treat fevers that are caused due to vitiated pitta and kapha dosha in the human body. Combining 10 grams of kutki with a few grams of honey helps break the fever. Sanctified with antioxidant, antimicrobial and anti-inflammatory properties, it helps in removing toxins from the blood and hence help manage skin diseases.

COSMETIC CURES

Kutki not only helps in shielding the skin from oxidative radical damage due to the harmful UVA and UVB rays – thereby reducing the risk of the various signs of aging like wrinkles, blemishes, spots, fine lines, and dark circles – but also treats conditions like acne, pimples, zits, psoriasis and scabies. The paste of the leaf is used to relieve burning sensations, so these qualities can combine to make them effective for cosmetic use as well.

The plant is among the several globally significant medicinal plants in the Himalayas, which are highly sensitive to climate change and are under threat, due to their narrow distribution range and small population size. A study aimed to identify the most critical environmental variables affecting *P. kurroa* distribution, and to find suitable habitats for it, found the Rudraprayag, Tehri and Uttarkashi districts of the state of Uttarakhand most suitable.

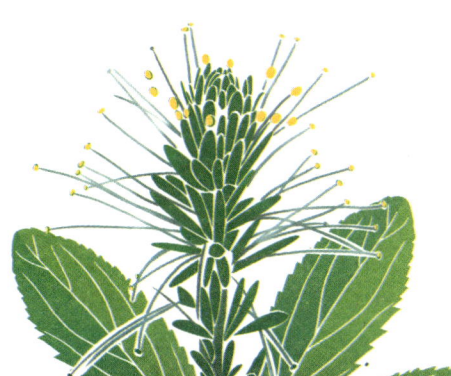
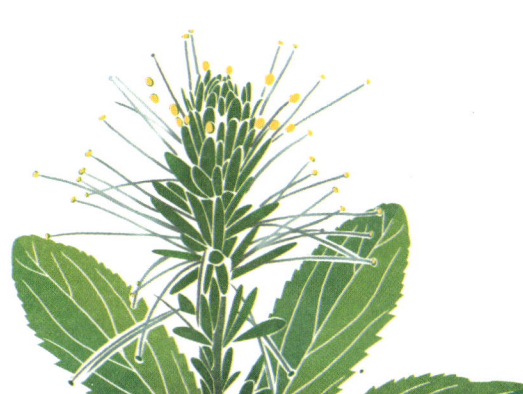

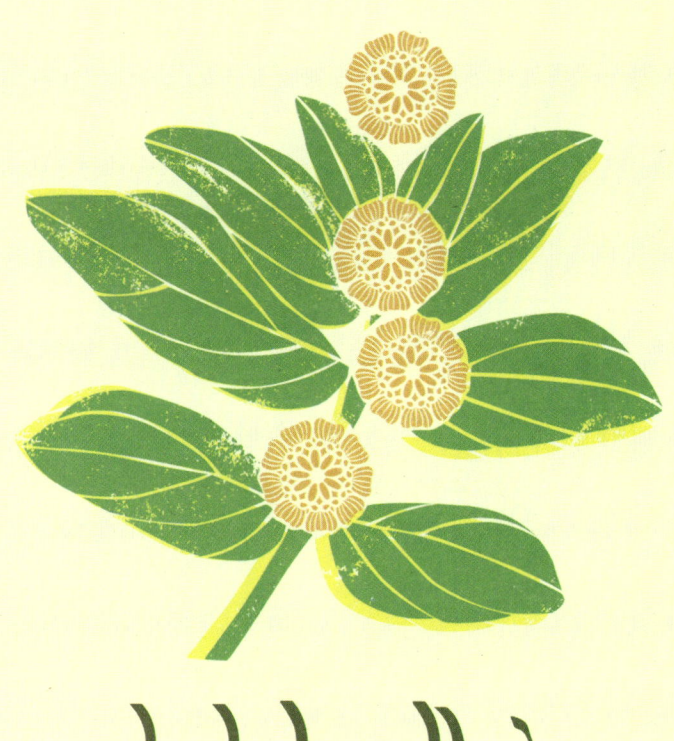

laldodhi

COMMON SPURGE/SNAKE WEED

Euphorbia hirta L.

LALDODHI *Nyishi* . **GAKHIROTI BON** *Assamese* . **BAROKARNI** *Bangla* .
NASHRAI KHORO *Bodo* . **DUDHI** *Hindi* . **PACHAIKUDHUCHEDI** *Irula* .
AKKIGIDA/ACHCHEDIDA/KEMPUNENEYAKK *Kannada* . **DUDURLI** *Konkani*
. **KUZHINAGAPPALA/NILAPPAALA** *Malayalam* . **PAKHAMBA MATON** *Meitei* .
KSIRA/DUGDHIKA/NAGARI/NAGARJUN *Sanskrit* .
AMMAN PACHARISI *Tamil* . **NANAPALA** *Telugu*

MEDICINAL PROPERTIES

The plant is an effective remedy for bronchial diseases and asthma and hence also called the 'asthma plant'. The resin or sap of this plant is mixed with any type of drink and used for this purpose. A milky latex is released when the plant is broken at any point – useful as a galactagogue for lactating mothers who make a decoction with the root. At the same time, it is considered useful to treat intestinal worms and other disorders – for which a paste made with the leaves and seeds are used.

CULINARY BENEFITS

While the young shoots and leaves are used as a vegetable, the fruits are eaten raw by the Bodos, the largest minority group in Assam. One of the most interesting examples of culinary usage of this herb is that it is used, along with a hundred others, to make a very special dish at the harvest festival of Assam, the Bohag Bihu, in April. The first day of the Bohag Bihu is called Goru (cow) Bihu and in that particular day, these are collected and 'Akhoh ata sak', a special dish believed to have medicinal values, is prepared.

COSMETIC CURES

The plant contains a high amount of phenol and flavonoid content which are known as an antioxidant in plants, the extract of which is used in the formulation of anti-aging cream.

When combined with a couple of other herbs, made into a fine paste, and added to a glass of milk with sugar, it becomes an effective home remedy for jaundice. The paste of the leaves combined with tulasi leaves is a fine remedy for pimples.

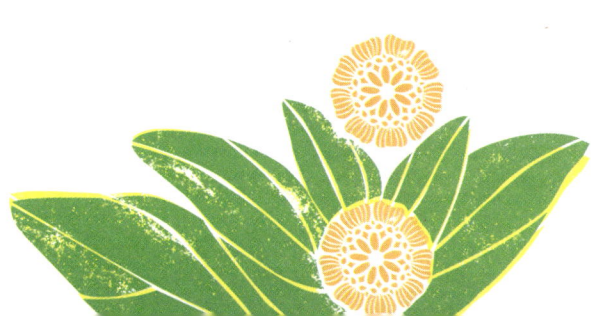
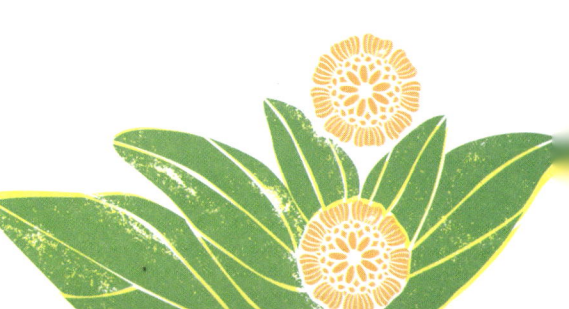

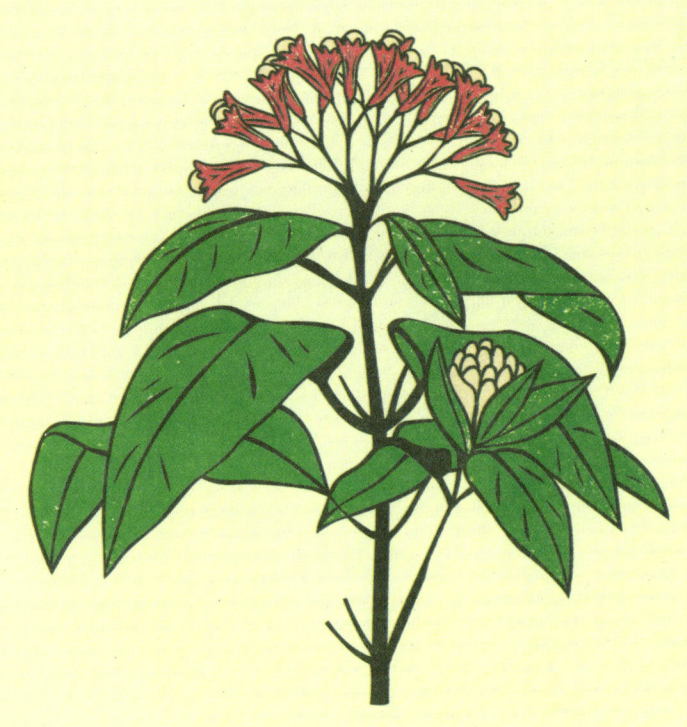

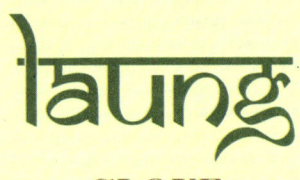

laung

CLOVE

Syzygium aromaticum

LAUNG *Hindi, Assamese, Punjabi* . **LAUBONGO** *Bangla* . **LAVANG** *Gujarati, Marathi* . **RUNG** *Kashmiri* . **KARAMPU/KARAYAMPOOVU/GRAMPU* *Malayalam* . **KIRAMBU** *Tamil* . **DEVAPUSHPA** *Sanskrit*

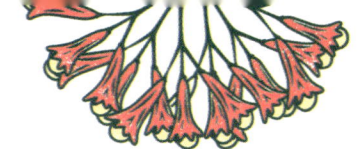

MEDICINAL PROPERTIES

Laung is carminative in nature, which means it prevents the formation of gas in the gastrointestinal tract, thus aiding digestion. Laung is also naturally a topical anaesthetic and carry antimicrobial, anti-inflammatory and antioxidant properties. Hence, it is widely used routinely for a number of everyday maladies. Using laung for clearing up a cold and congestion with a healing brew of laung, cinnamon and some whole cardamoms infused in tea has been an ancient natural remedy. Inhaling the vapours of laung oil also helps with clearing up the nasal tract. In aromatherapy, it is used as an antiseptic and pain reliever, especially for toothaches and stomach pain.

Laung oil is also often mixed with other oils to treat various disorders. For instance, those who have trouble sleeping, can apply some warm laung oil along with sesame oil on the forehead to feel calm and relaxed.

CULINARY BENEFITS

Laung is an important component of that ubiquitous combination of spices and herbs in Indian cuisine, 'garam masala'. Whether it is the Bengal/Odisha freshly wet ground combination of cardamom, cinnamon and laung or the dry ground combination of these three along with peppercorns and cumin, it is a must. It is common practice to add laung while cooking foods like kidney beans or black gram that tend to cause flatulence. At the same time, their pungent and strong flavour make them equally attractive in most food, as a complement or addition to other flavours. Hence it is extensively used in Indian culinary traditions. There is a sweet made in Bengal, Lobongo Lotika, in which it is – quite literally – the centre-piece!

RITUAL USE

Like with many medicinal plants and herbs, laung is an essential ingredient in the mix used for 'homa' – a Hindu ritual practice of lighting and making offerings to fire within the house – done with the intent to purify the surrounding physically as well as spiritually.

Laung is is also a great freshener. Tie some laung in a small muslin bag and, hang it up in a corner of your wardrobe. Additionally, a paste with cloves, some honey and a drop of lime, makes for a great face pack for glowing skin.

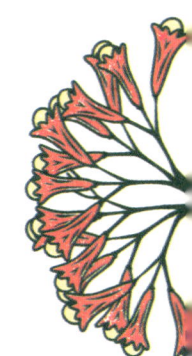
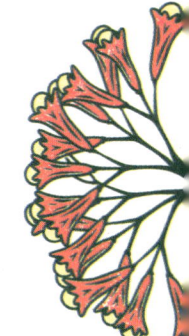
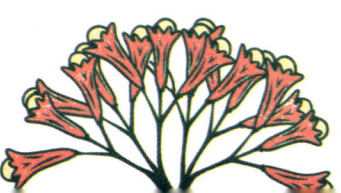
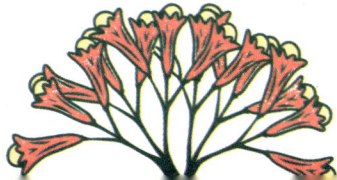

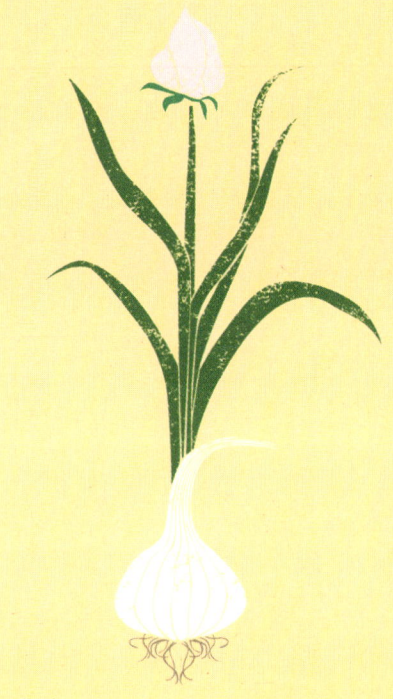

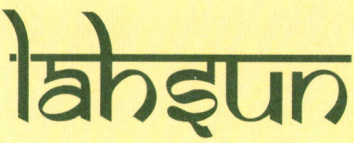

lahsun

GARLIC

Allium sativum

LAHSUN *Hindi* . CHUMERIE *Angami* . NAHARU *Assamese* .
ROSHUN *Bangla* . BELLULI *Kannada* . RUHUN *Kashmiri* . VELLULI
Malayalam . CHANAM *Meitei* . PURUNVAR *Mizo* . ACHANAM/POONDU
Tamil . VELLULI *Telugu* . HANAM *Tungkhul*

MEDICINAL PROPERTIES

Lahsun is a wonderful medicinal plant, owing to its preventive characteristics in cardiovascular diseases, regulating blood pressure, lowering blood sugar and cholesterol levels, effective against bacterial, viral, fungal and parasitic infections, enhancing the immune system and having antioxidant features. Lahsun exerts these effects thanks to more than 200 chemicals – broad-spectrum therapeutic effect with minimal toxicity. It is also used as an antiseptic lotion for washing wounds and ulcers.

CULINARY BENEFITS

Lahsun paste is extensively used in Indian cuisine along with onions and ginger, as a base of many gravies, especially in north India. But it is used peeled and crushed as a flavouring in many other parts of the country as well. It is very commonly pickled, made into dry and wet chutneys – standard accompaniments to Indian food, lending itself to a number of different spice combinations. Highly nutritious, lahsun has very few calories and is a good source of manganese and vitamins B6 and C. Easy to include in any kind of diet, lahsun compliments most savoury dishes, especially soups and chutneys.

In Ayurveda, the assessment of lahsun's effect on the human body is that of producing heat – *tamsic*. That is why there are many norms about its usage. Not only those that vary according to weather and climate, but also on certain days of the year when fasting is observed for religious and spiritual reasons. Some communities even forbid it entirely on the grounds of it being incompatible with their overall religious and spiritual outlook.

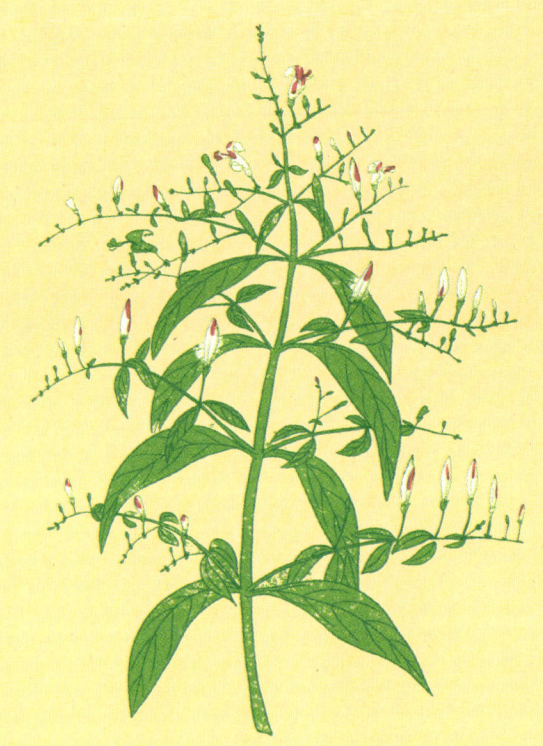

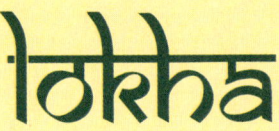

GREEN CHIRETTA/KING OF BITTERS
Andrographis paniculata

LOKHA *Vaiphei*

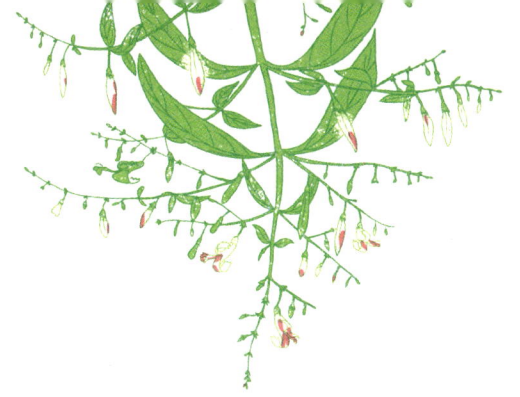
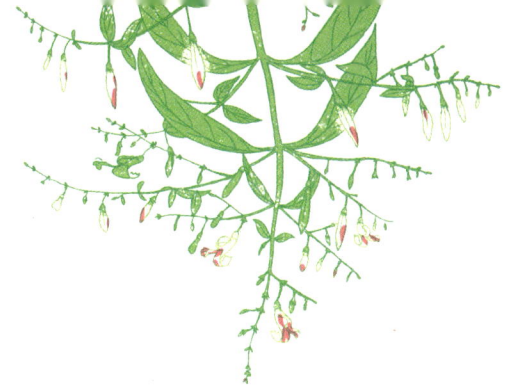

MEDICINAL PROPERTIES

The juice of the lokha leaf is a good remedy against fever and stomach trouble. The juice of the stem taken on an empty stomach, once a day, for 7-10 days helps eliminate worms. Due to the herb's pungent and cooling qualities, it is useful in treating burning sensation in urinary tract infections. Its antipyretic, antiperiodic, anti-inflammatory and expectorant qualities make it good for treating chronic fever, malaria, intermittent fever, inflammation, cough and bronchitis.

Lokha powder can be combined with coconut oil and applied on the skin to oversee eczema, boils and skin infections. A paste of the leaves and haldi can be applied externally to treat infected wounds.

COSMETIC CURES

Lokha is used as astringent and a conditioning agent in skincare products.

Besides working as an immune enhancer, the dried herb also helps in various sicknesses related to digestion and hepatoprotection. It carries vermicide, anti-typhoid and antibiotic activities.

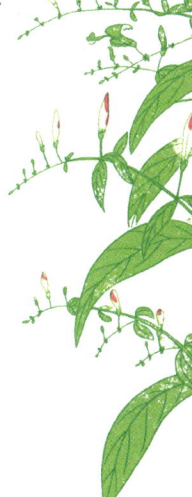

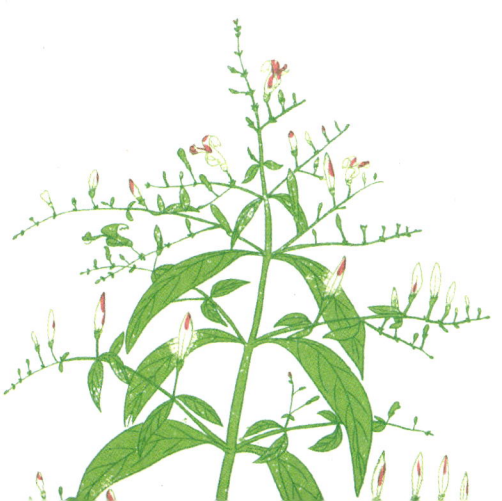
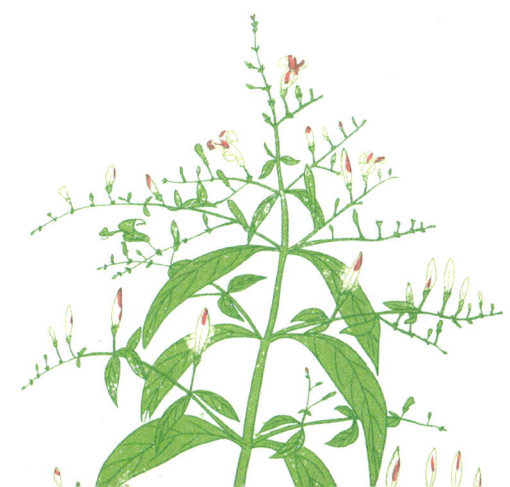

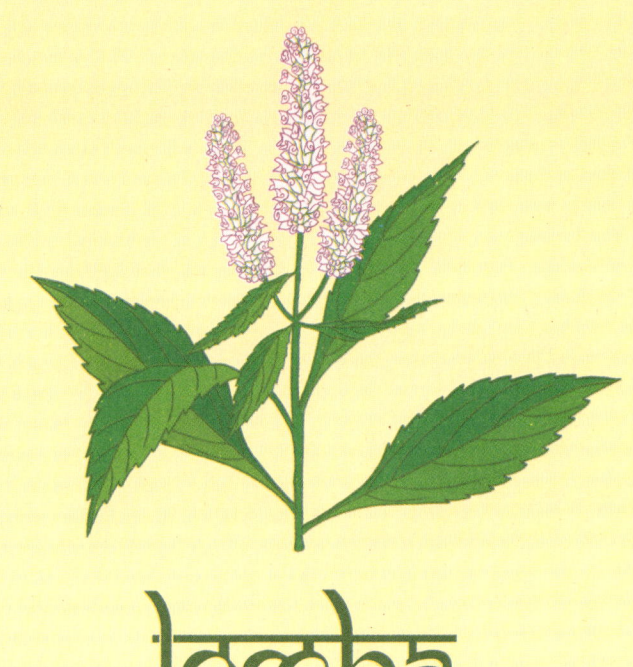

lomba

PLEASANT HIMALAYAN MINT
Elsholtzia blanda Benth

LOMBA *Meitei*

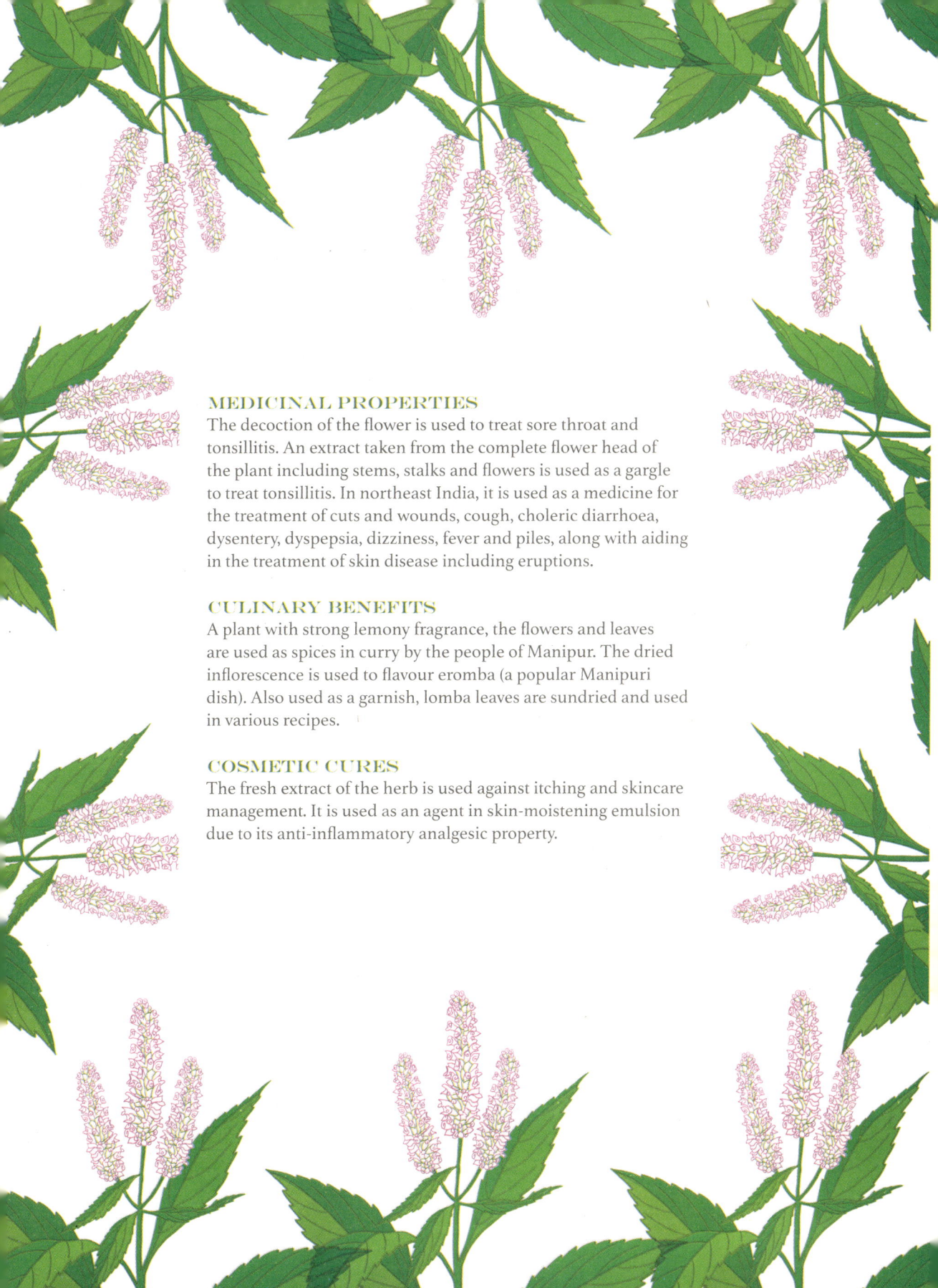

MEDICINAL PROPERTIES

The decoction of the flower is used to treat sore throat and tonsillitis. An extract taken from the complete flower head of the plant including stems, stalks and flowers is used as a gargle to treat tonsillitis. In northeast India, it is used as a medicine for the treatment of cuts and wounds, cough, choleric diarrhoea, dysentery, dyspepsia, dizziness, fever and piles, along with aiding in the treatment of skin disease including eruptions.

CULINARY BENEFITS

A plant with strong lemony fragrance, the flowers and leaves are used as spices in curry by the people of Manipur. The dried inflorescence is used to flavour eromba (a popular Manipuri dish). Also used as a garnish, lomba leaves are sundried and used in various recipes.

COSMETIC CURES

The fresh extract of the herb is used against itching and skincare management. It is used as an agent in skin-moistening emulsion due to its anti-inflammatory analgesic property.

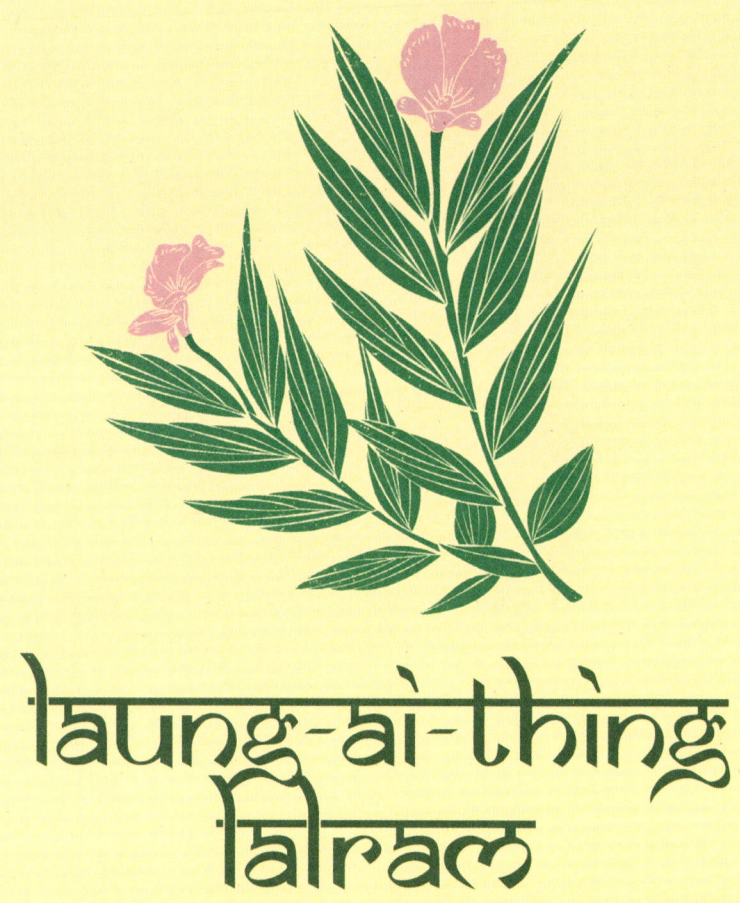

laung-ai-thing lalram

Caulokaempferia linearis

LAUNG-AI-THING LALRAM *Mizo*

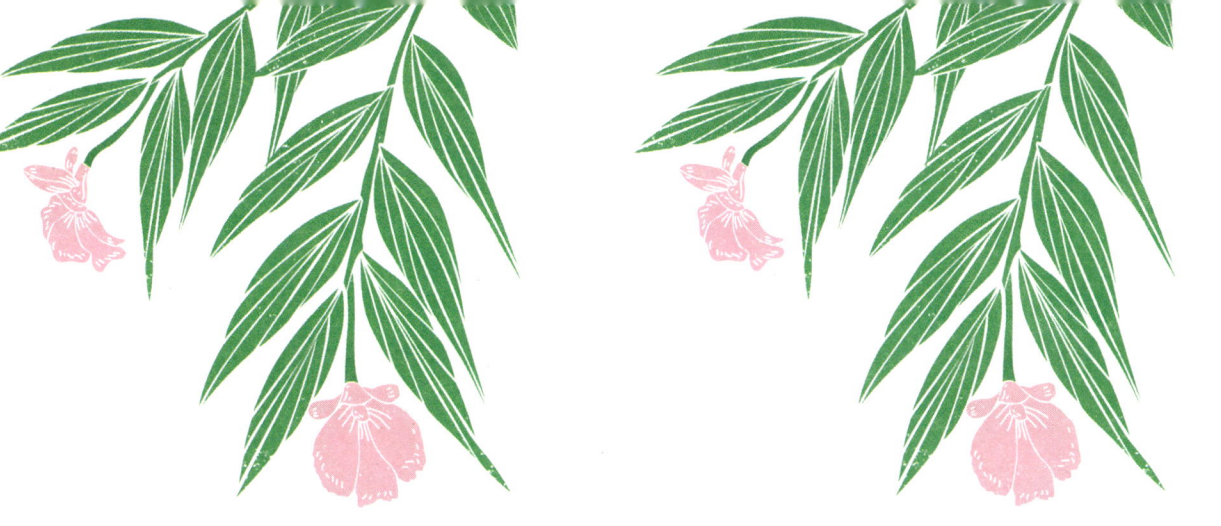

Laung-ai-thing lalram is an uncommon herb that grows in mossy wet rock crevices or boulders in the bank of streams in dark places.

Found in Meghalaya and Mizoram, this plant with its tender roots and leafy stems is a tuberous geophyte and grows primarily in the wet tropical biome – typically in the undergrowth of montane forests, often near mountain streams or on rocky outcrops.

Very little is documented by way of the uses of this plant. It is known however, that the Chakmas, and another local tribe of Mizoram, use crushed leaves on the head to treat vertigo.

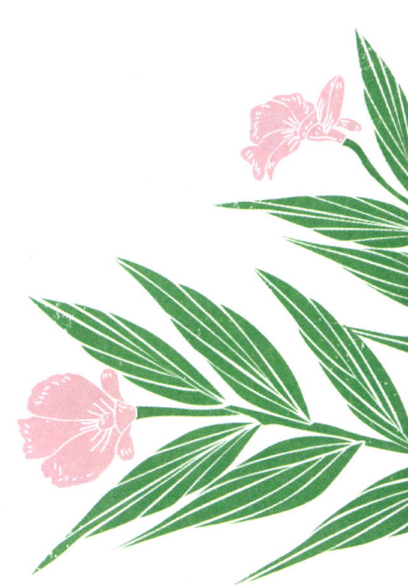

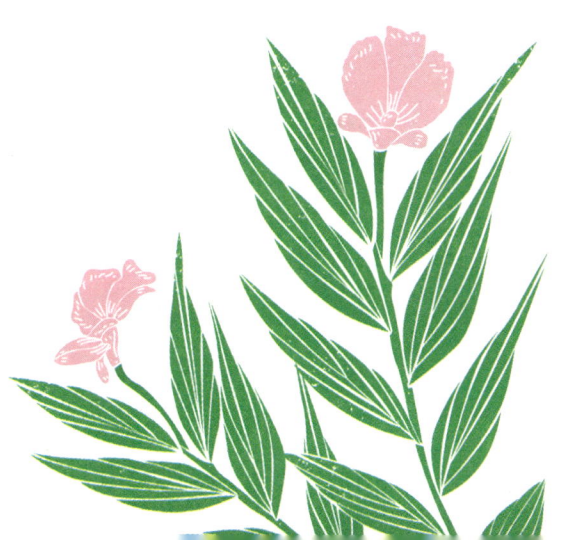

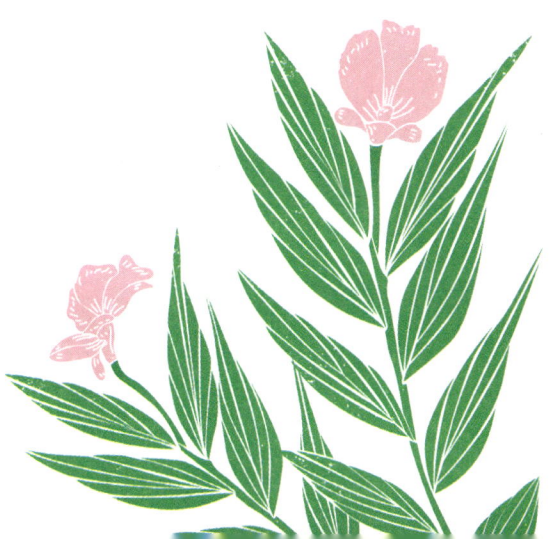

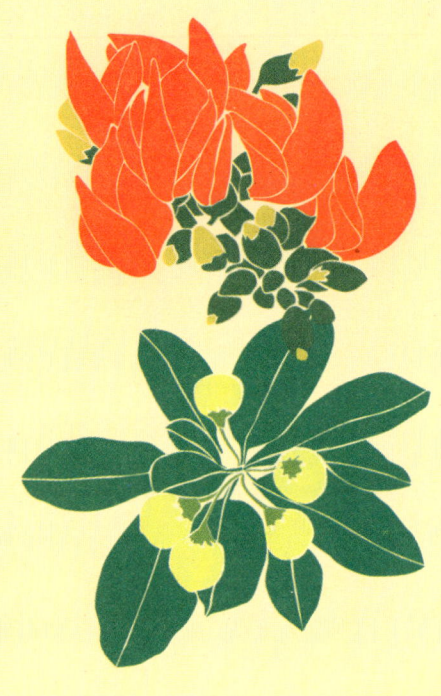

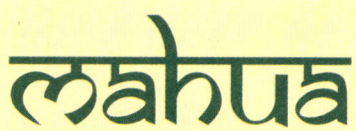

BUTTER TREE
Madhuca Longifolia

MAHUA *Hindi* . MOHULA *Oriya* . DOLMA *Marvari* .
ILUPPAI *Tamil* . VIPPA *Telugu*

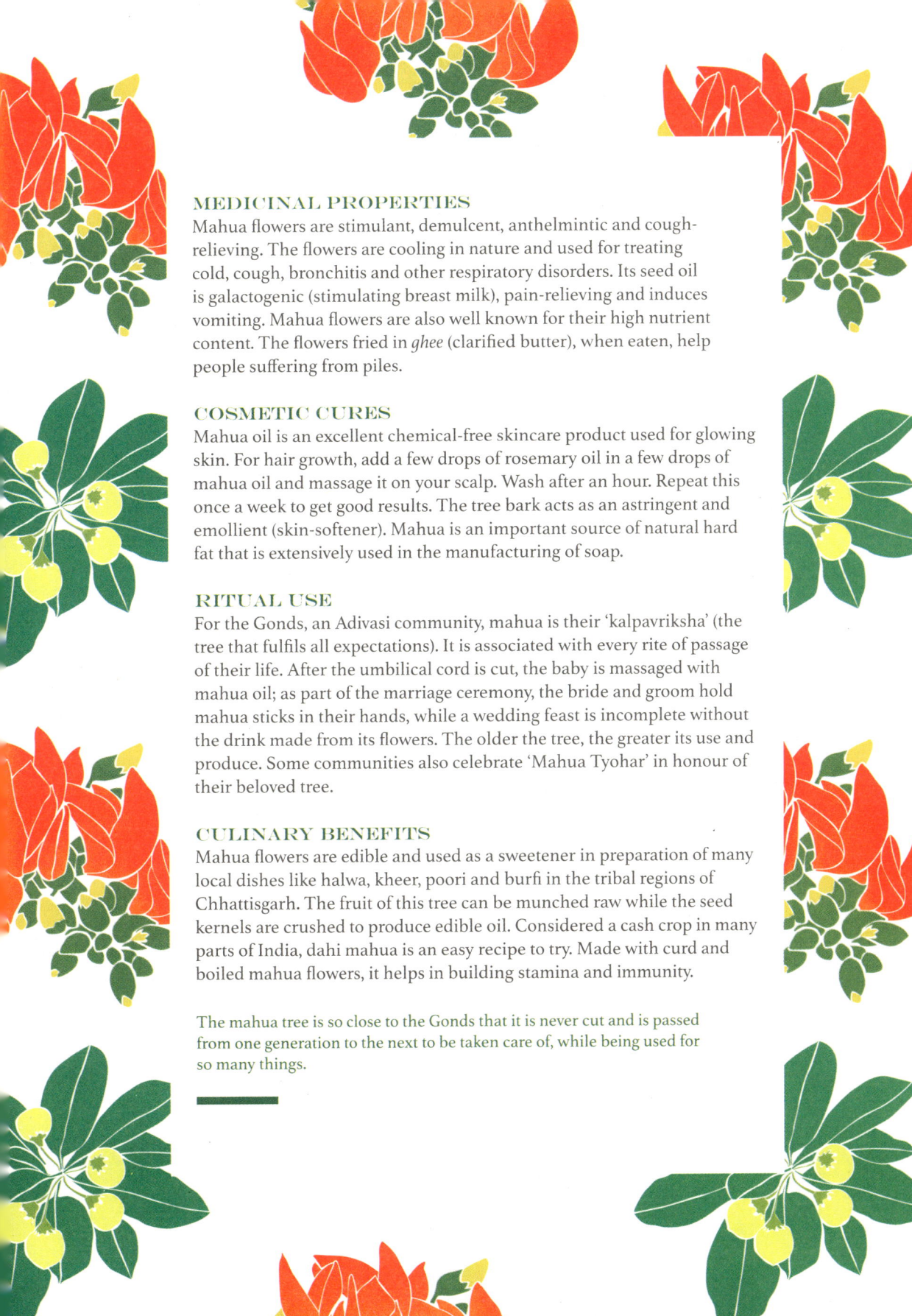

MEDICINAL PROPERTIES

Mahua flowers are stimulant, demulcent, anthelmintic and cough-relieving. The flowers are cooling in nature and used for treating cold, cough, bronchitis and other respiratory disorders. Its seed oil is galactogenic (stimulating breast milk), pain-relieving and induces vomiting. Mahua flowers are also well known for their high nutrient content. The flowers fried in *ghee* (clarified butter), when eaten, help people suffering from piles.

COSMETIC CURES

Mahua oil is an excellent chemical-free skincare product used for glowing skin. For hair growth, add a few drops of rosemary oil in a few drops of mahua oil and massage it on your scalp. Wash after an hour. Repeat this once a week to get good results. The tree bark acts as an astringent and emollient (skin-softener). Mahua is an important source of natural hard fat that is extensively used in the manufacturing of soap.

RITUAL USE

For the Gonds, an Adivasi community, mahua is their 'kalpavriksha' (the tree that fulfils all expectations). It is associated with every rite of passage of their life. After the umbilical cord is cut, the baby is massaged with mahua oil; as part of the marriage ceremony, the bride and groom hold mahua sticks in their hands, while a wedding feast is incomplete without the drink made from its flowers. The older the tree, the greater its use and produce. Some communities also celebrate 'Mahua Tyohar' in honour of their beloved tree.

CULINARY BENEFITS

Mahua flowers are edible and used as a sweetener in preparation of many local dishes like halwa, kheer, poori and burfi in the tribal regions of Chhattisgarh. The fruit of this tree can be munched raw while the seed kernels are crushed to produce edible oil. Considered a cash crop in many parts of India, dahi mahua is an easy recipe to try. Made with curd and boiled mahua flowers, it helps in building stamina and immunity.

The mahua tree is so close to the Gonds that it is never cut and is passed from one generation to the next to be taken care of, while being used for so many things.

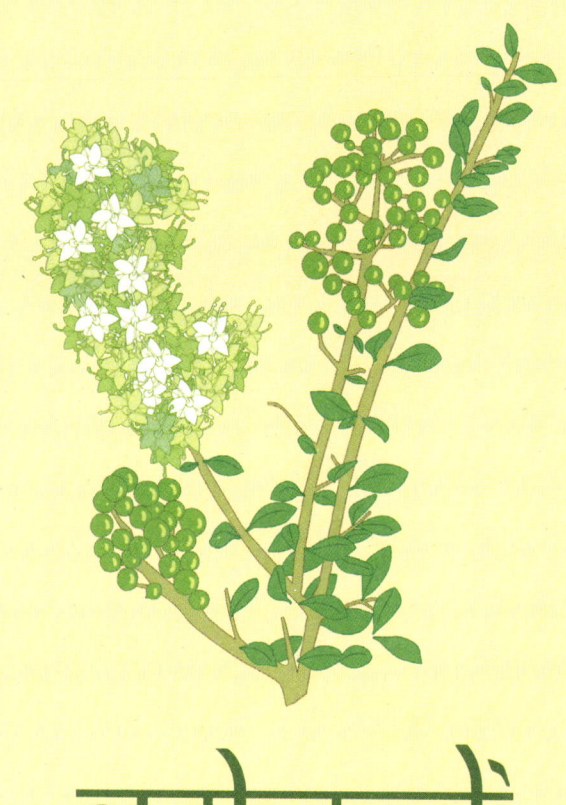

मehendi

HENNA

Lawsonia inermis

MEHENDI *Hindi* . BENJATI *Oriya* . MENDIKA/RAKIGARBHA/
MADYANTI/MEDHINI *Sanskrit* . MAILANCHI *Malayalam* .
MURUTHANI/MARITHONDI/MARUDUM *Tamil* .
MAYILANCHI *Kannada* . MEHEDI *Bangla* . GORANTA *Telugu*

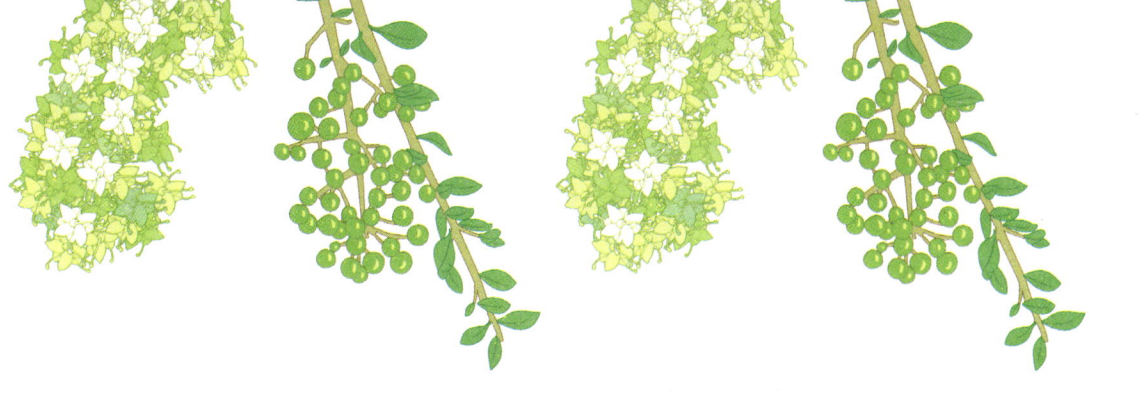

MEDICINAL PROPERTIES

Mehendi is an analgesic, reduces oedema, and is also astringent, anti-inflammatory and anti-dermatosis in nature.

External application of the leaf paste provides relief from headache, joint pains, inflammation, ulcer and skin diseases. A decoction of the leaves is used for gargling in stomatitis and pharyngitis. The juice or decoction of the leaves is used in diseases of the blood and also jaundice. Since the leaf juice is a diuretic, it is combined with sugar and used to treat dysuria and pyuria. It reduces burning in the urine and soothes the urinary tract. Mehendi flowers are used as a refrigerant and in treating insomnia – by putting some dried chamomile flowers in a pillow.

With such a vast list of benefits of mehendi, one can take it on a regular basis by grinding the mehendi seeds and making them into a powder. Take half a teaspoon of the powder mixed with honey after lunch and dinner to get rid of digestive problems. Alternatively, one could juice the leaves and mix the juice with water and honey. This should be taken before meals once or twice a day.

COSMETIC CURES

An essential part of wedding ceremonies in Southeast Asia, mehendi oil is a natural moisturizer and has been used for generations in treating dandruff, split ends and hair fall. Antibacterial and antimicrobial, mehendi-based hair colours are non-toxic and have lately been regaining popularity as chemical-free natural colour for hair.

Mehendi has also been used for dyeing fabrics like silk, wool, and leather.

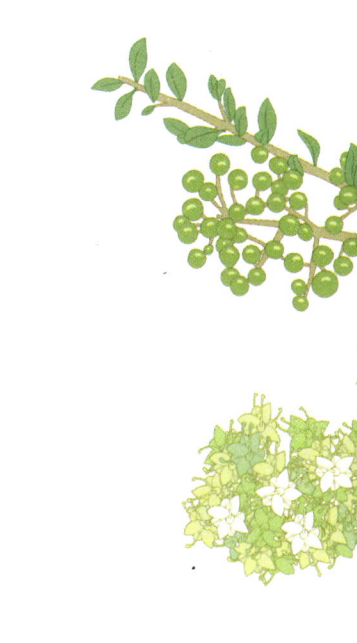

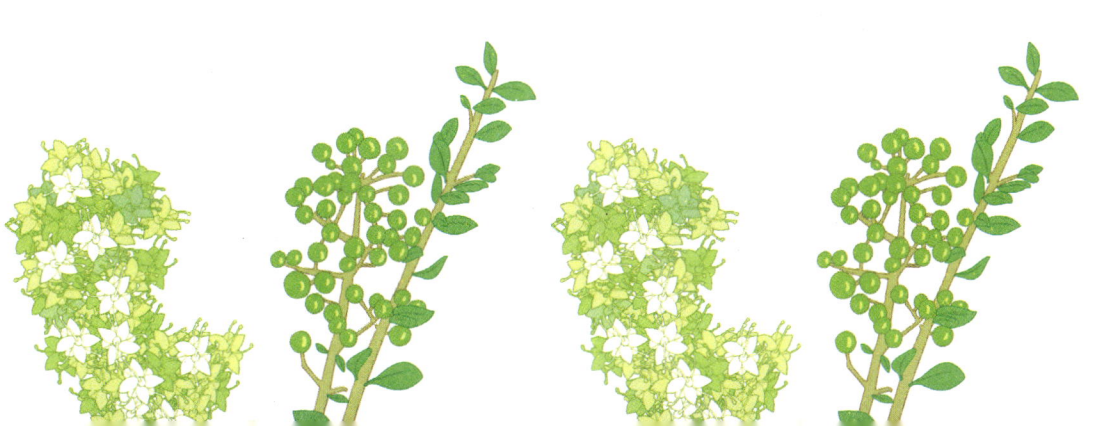

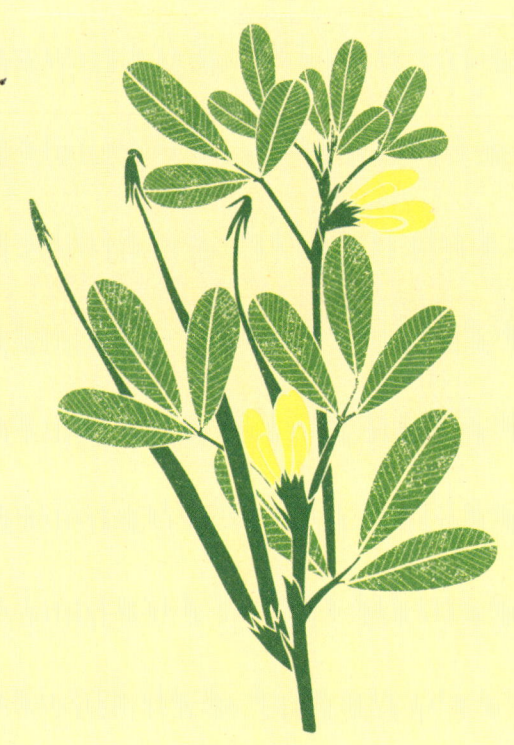

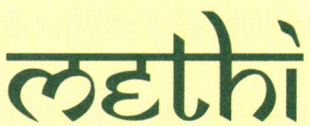

FENUGREEK

Trigonella foenum-graecum

METHI *Hindi, Bangla, Gujarati, Oriya, Punjabi and Urdu* .
MENTHYA *Kannada* . **VENTAYAM/ULUVA** *Malayalam* .
VENDHAYAM *Tamil* . **MENTULU** *Telugu*

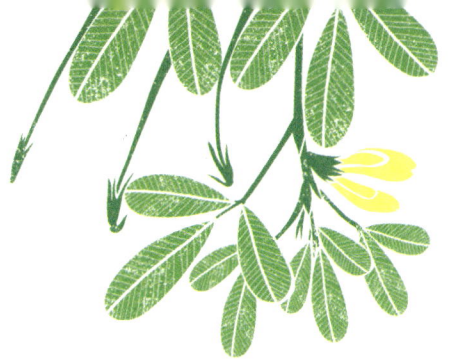
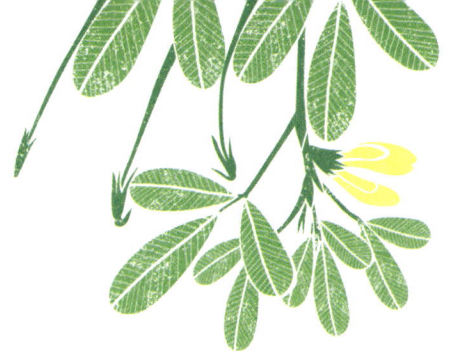

MEDICAL USE

Methi is known to slow sugar absorption in the stomach and stimulate insulin, resulting in the lowering of blood sugar. It also has important anti-arthritic properties – with the seeds soaked in water overnight and that water being drunk in the morning – and the seeds combined with honey to be eaten independently. Methi leaves can also help treat mouth ulcers. Boil a cup of leaves in two cups of water, strain and use the water to gargle.

CULINARY BENEFITS

Leaves and seeds of the methi plant have properties that are known to have a positive impact on the gastro-intestinal tract. Their inclusion in traditional diet and the culinary traditions across the country bears testimony to this common knowledge. The seeds form part of the tempering in different combinations across the country – especially as a component of the Eastern Indian spice 'panch phoran'. Perhaps the most interesting are their usage in pickling during the summer – its property to act as a coolant balances the heat of the other spices used. The seeds are also pickled separately in several Himalayan communities. One can also add methi leaves to parathas and theplas, and enjoy them with a bowl of yogurt for breakfast.

COSMETIC CURES

The paste of methi seeds, soaked overnight in water, has rich anti-oxidant and inflammatory properties that make them an attractive and important component of many a hair mask. They are known to help with cooling the scalp, in fighting dandruff and reducing hairfall. Soak the seeds in water overnight, drain the water and mash the seeds into a paste. Apply the paste on the scalp. Rinse it off after an hour with shampoo. Another standard practice is to put a few seeds into a glass jar of coconut oil and keep it in the sun regularly for ten days. This helps the oil absorb the properties of the seeds, making it that much more nourishing for the hair.

The plant typically matures from early winter in north India and hence becomes a regular part of winter meals. Methi leaves and tender stems are typically cooked in combination with a number of other vegetables.

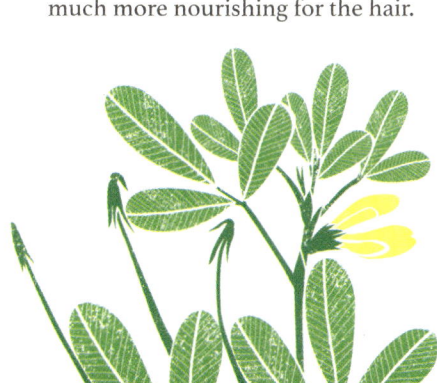
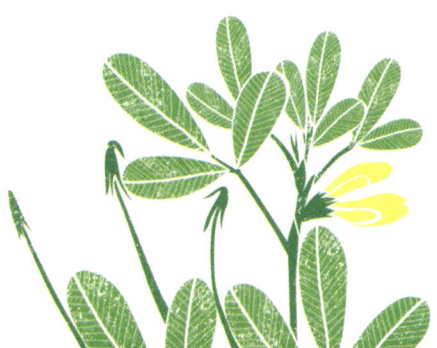

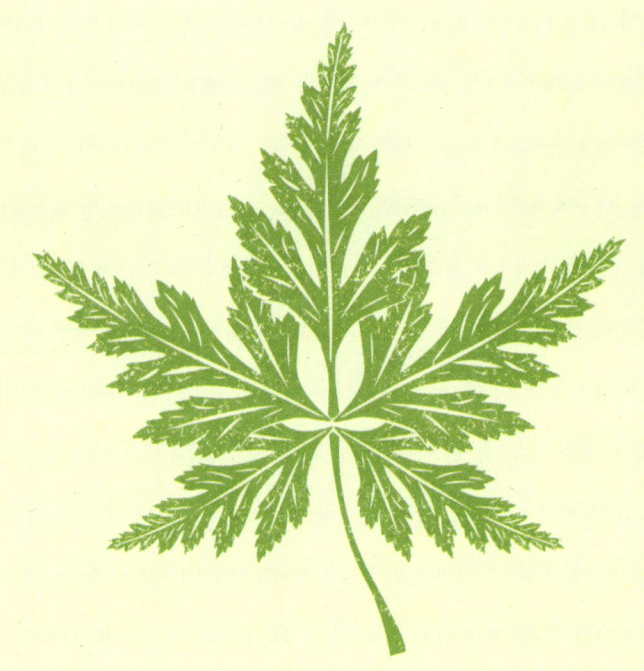

mishmi teeta

GOLDEN THREAD

Coptis teeta Wall (Ranunculaceae)

MISHMI TEETA *Assamese* . **MAMIRA** *Hindi* . **PITMULA HALDIYA**
BACHNAG *Marathi* . **CHIRETA** *Punjabi* . **VISHATEETEE** *Kannada* .
SUPITA *Sanskrit* . **PITAROHINI** *Tamil*

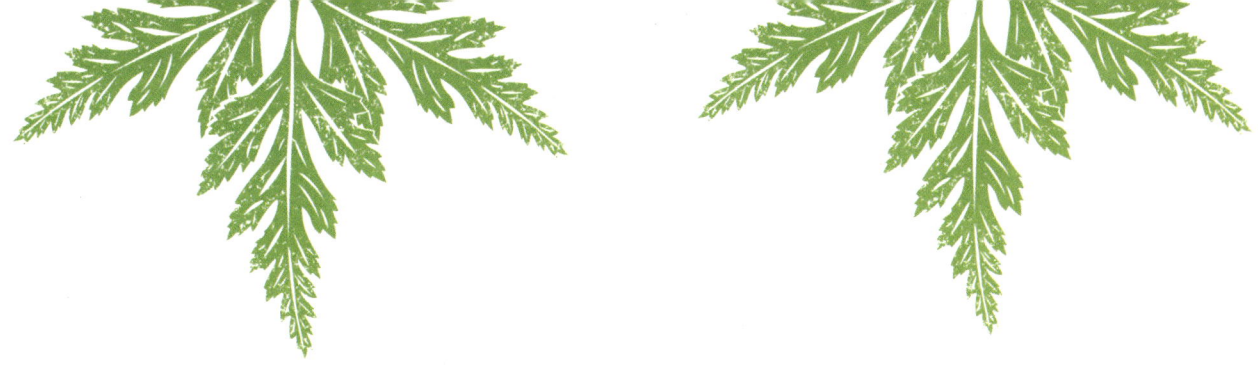

MEDICINAL PROPERTIES

This plant was used by the Mishmis and other tribes of Arunachal Pradesh to treat malaria, stomach ache and dysentery. Since it is bitter in taste and was known from the Mishmis, in all likelihood gave it the name 'Mishmi teeta'. The part of the plant that is used are its rhizomes (root stalks). Well-dried rhizomes can be used for upto twenty years. It is a cooling and potent bacteriostatic herb.

The dried rhizomes of this plant contains significant dynamic compounds that are utilized for the treatment of various conditions. Crushed, ground together with black peppercorn, and formed into pea-sized pellets, it helps in the treatment of bronchitis. A thick paste formed from ground roots, when applied around the eyes, helps cure soreness and other eye problems. A mixture of the roots, crushed together with a bit of sap from gawarpatha leaves or sap from mayoe (*Calotropis procera*) is applied topically to snakebites. It is also used as an all-round general tonic.

COSMETIC CURES

Mishmi teeta used in combination with other herbs is known to have anti-aging properties and also helps treat discolouration of the skin.

Mishmi teeta is prized in Ayurveda, Unani and Siddha – and hence has been increasingly collected from the wild for commercial purposes. However, due to its slow growth rate, this has resulted in it becoming endangered. Efforts at cultivation have been unsuccessful in any other soil type and climatic conditions than temperate climates, making it difficult to be produced in other parts of the country.

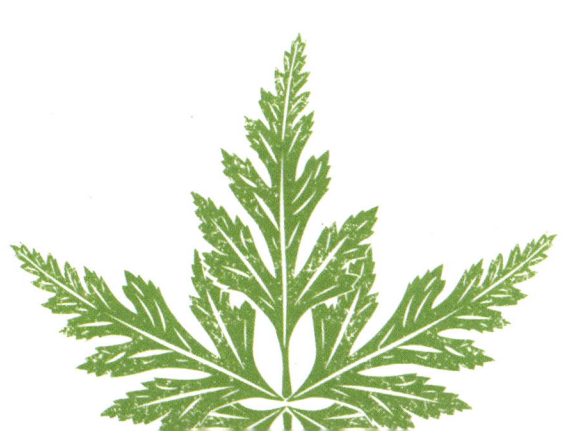

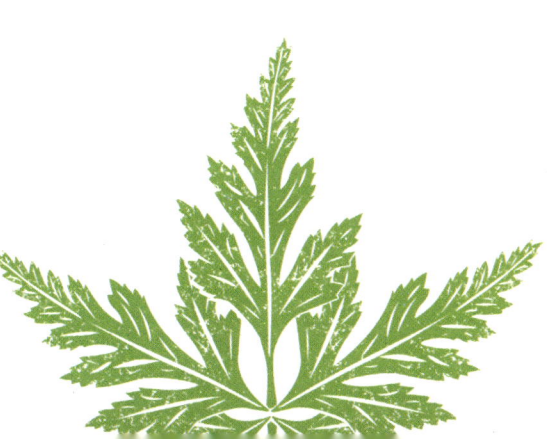

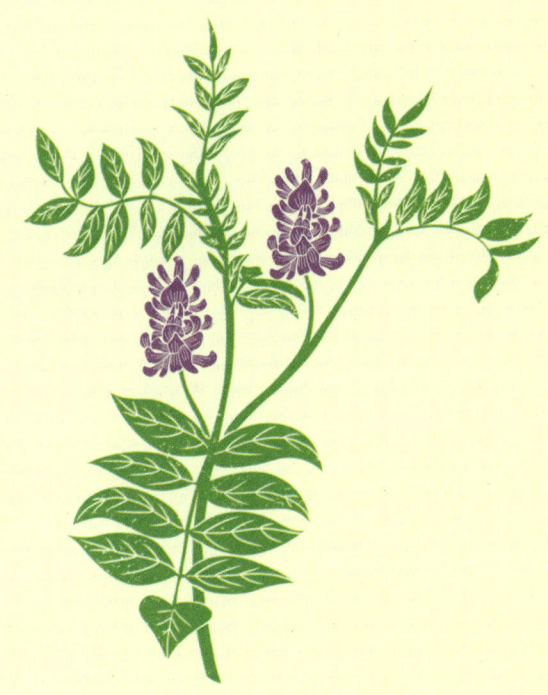

mulethi

LIQUORICE

Glycyrrhiza glabra

MULETHI *Hindi, Urdu* . **JOSHTIMODHU** *Bangla* .
IRATTIMADHURAM *Malayalam* . **JESHTIMADH** *Marathi* .
YASHTIMADHU *Sanskrit* . **ATIMADHURAM** *Tamil*

MEDICINAL PROPERTIES

Traditionally, this was a go-to herb for whenever there was a throat infection of some kind. Either a bit of the stem was chewed independently or it was powdered and used in combination with some other herb like ginger or tulasi, as its roots have anti-microbial qualities. In case of respiratory troubles, a kadha prepared by boiling a few mulethi sticks in water and taken several times a day helps treat cough and cold. The root extract also has the power to control influenza and even helps in the treatment of sores.

CULINARY BENEFITS

Tea made by the root or stem of the mulethi plant is very common at the first hint of a sore throat. It is also used as a sweetener in many desserts, and is a great substitute for sugar.

COSMETIC CURES

Mulethi powder is very versatile for a good complexion, even for very different skin types. While for dry skin, it is recommended to be combined with kumkumadi taila (saffron oil), for oily skin, it is great on its own or combined with red sandalwood powder and some water. It has elements that help fight the effect of UV rays on the skin and hence also helps in brightening the skin. Its regular use also helps protect the skin from various harmful environmental elements such as pollution.

Mulethi's capacity to increase the production of lymphocytes and macrophage helps in minimizing autoimmune complications. Its supportive effect on the adrenal gland indirectly stimulates the brain, decreasing the effects of amnesia, improves learning and also renders a shielding effect on the brain cells. It fights ulcers, protects the liver and is a great digestive aid.

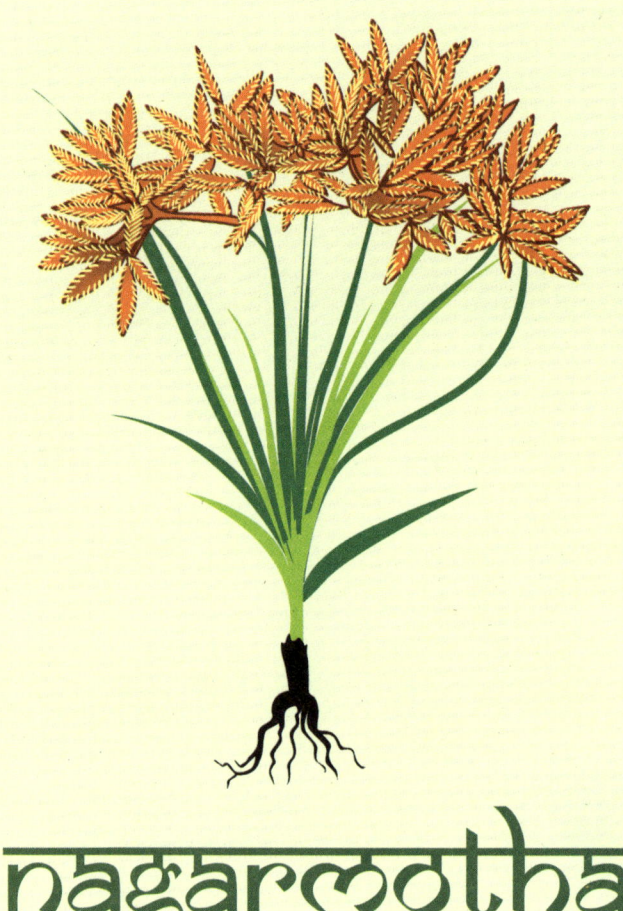

nagarmotha

NUTGRASS/JAVA GRASS

Cyperus scariosus

NAGARMOTHA *Hindi* . **NAGARMOTHAYA** *Gujarati* . **TUNGE
GADDE** *Kannada* . **TUNGA MUSTALU** *Telugu* . **MUTHAKACH** *Tamil* .
KRODESHTA/HIMA/VARIDA *Sanskrit*

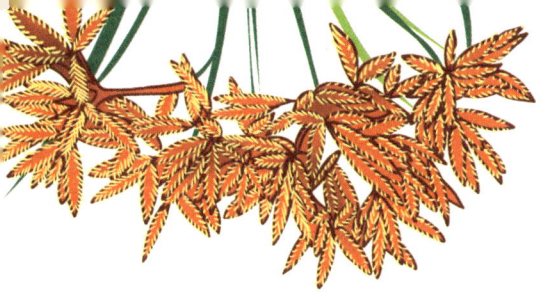
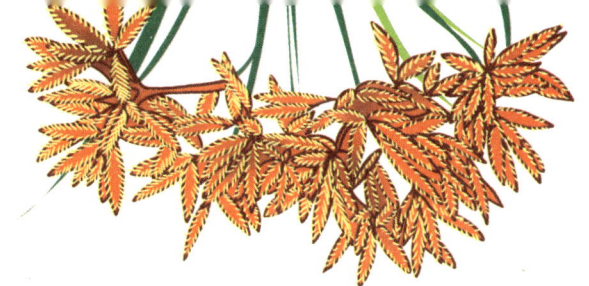

Nagarmotha, also known to be in modern literature as 'the world's worst weed', grows rapidly, filling the soil with its tangle of roots and rhizomes.

MEDICINAL PROPERTIES

Nagarmotha is an important ingredient for several prescriptions used in indigenous system of medicine to treat various diseases and a number of practices are known to utilize this. The rhizomes are used as an antidote to snake bite. A paste made from nagarmotha is used in treating skin-related ailments like scabies and eczema. The extract from the roots is instilled into eyes in conjunctivitis to reduce the pain, redness and ocular discharges. When taken in powdered form, it improves digestive system and removes worms from the gastro-intestinal tract. Where it grows, it is considered to be the best herb for treating any type of fever.

COSMETIC CURES

The roots of this plant yield an essential oil that is used extensively in perfumery. The oil extracts from the rhizomes is used by perfumers as a fixative. It forms a good substitute for patchouli oil in making soap and other perfumes. The rhizomes are used to wash hair and the oil is also used as hair tonic. A paste made with two tablespoon nagarmotha powder and one tablespoon coconut oil can be applied over the face and left for two hours. Wash off with cool water and repeat on alternate days to improve skin quality and complexion.

It is often used as an insect repellent for perfumed clothing.

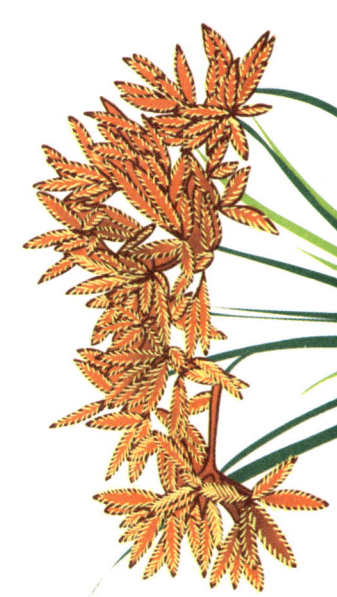

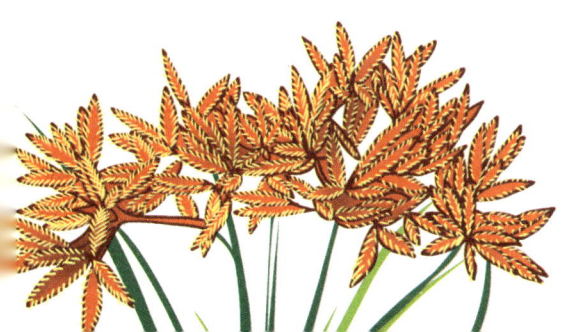
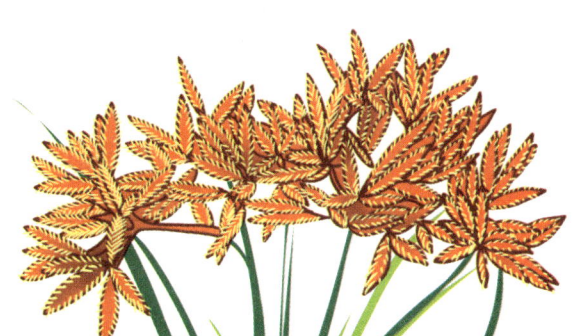

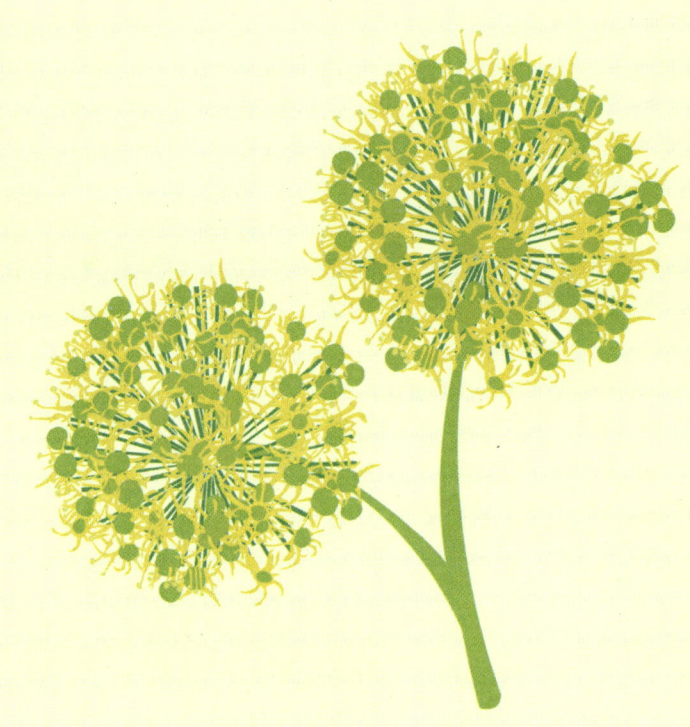

napakpi

HOOKER CHIVES

Allium hookeri Thaw

NAPAKPI *Meitei*

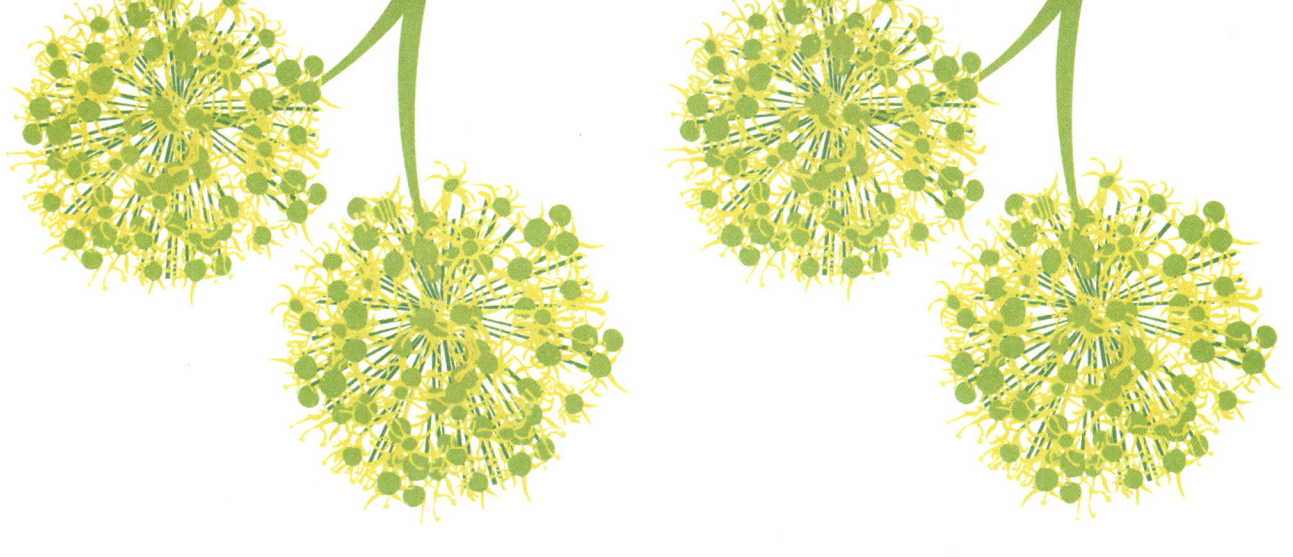

MEDICINAL PROPERTIES

Napakpi is used as a folk medicine for cough, cold, painful swellings and skin eruptions. The herb contains a good amount of nutritious compounds like ascorbic acid, proteins, sugar, fibre, phytosterols, and phenols. It also tones up the digestive system and regulates the circulatory system. In Manipur, people use the fresh green leaves for reducing temperatures and blood cholesterol and improving appetite. The juice of its leaves, when taken with salt, can also help treat ulcers and stomach ailments.

CULINARY BENEFITS

The fibrous root of this plant is used almost every day in all the preparation of a special dish of Manipur called eromba, paknam (baked delicacy), vegetable stew (kangsoi) and chicken curry. In Meghalaya, the leaves and roots of this plant are often consumed fresh. While the leaves add punch to broth and vegetables, the roots go well with potatoes and other vegetables, enhancing their taste and flavour.

Local healers in the state of Manipur preserve napakpi by sun-drying it. They also often send this preserved form to their out-of-state relatives so that their dear ones can continue to savour the herb's benefits.

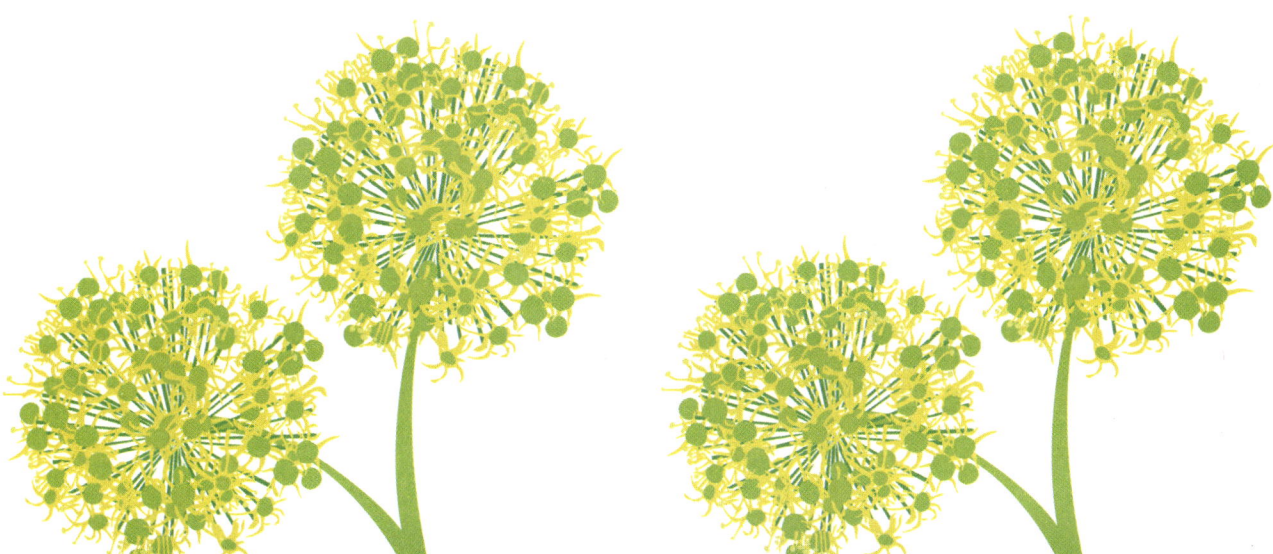

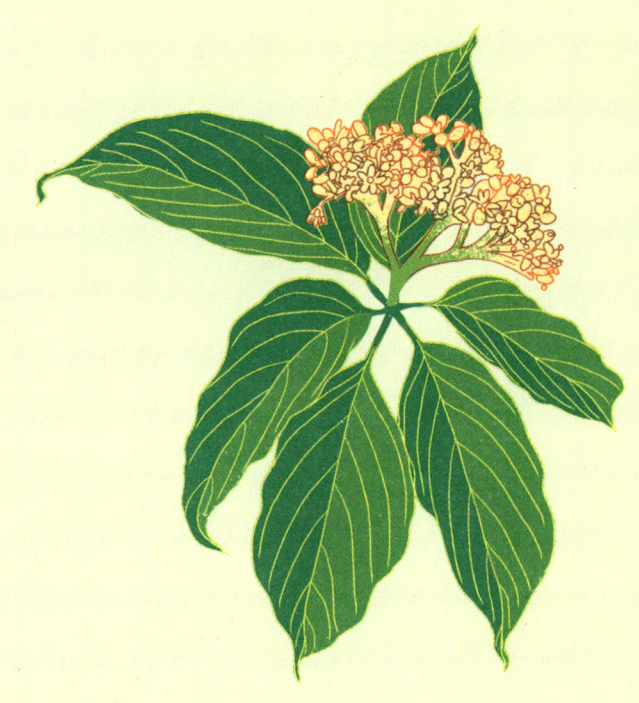

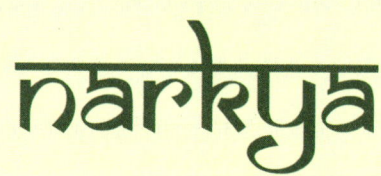

narkya

STINKING TREE

Nothapodytes nimmoniana

NARKYA *Marathi* . DURNAATHADA MARA *Kannada* .
GHANERA *Konkani* . PEENARI *Malayalam* .
AMRITA/KALAGURA *Marathi* . ARALI/PILLIPICCU *Tamil*

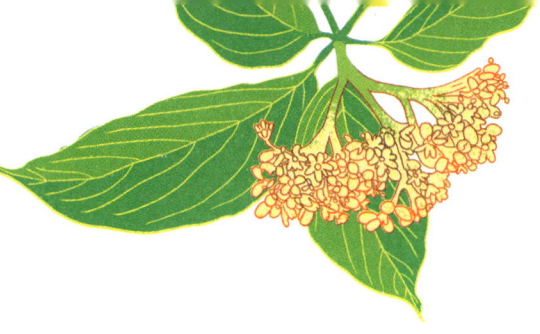
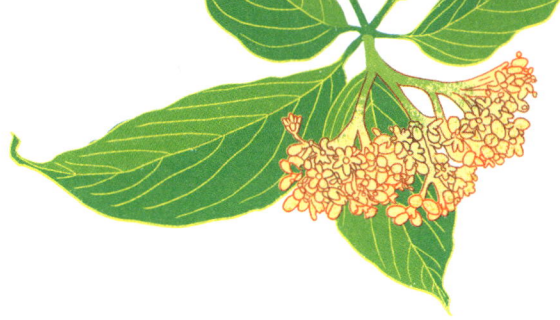

MEDICINAL PROPERTIES

Narkya is an imperative medicinal plant, the foremost source of a potent alkaloid, namely camptothecin, of a wide spectrum of pharmacological activities like anti-malarial, antibacterial, anti-oxidant, anti-inflammatory, anti-fungal, and is also applied in the treatment of anemia.

The plant contains camptothecin (CPT) which is a well-known anti-cancer drug, possibly the maximum proportion among all plants that have it. Hence, this plant has been explored for its phytochemical, biotechnological and pharmacological aspects. Given the huge global demand for CPT, overexploitation of *N. nimmoniana*, unplanned deforestation along with reduction of seed germination and high market cost has us optimistic in investigating this plant in a systematic manner.

This valuable and medicinally important tree is being over exploited due its commercial importance. The only alternative is to cultivate the tree and avoid wild collections. However, large-scale plantations depend upon the availability of planting stocks. Natural regeneration is through seeds and is curtailed by several factors leading to low percentage of germination. Vegetative propagation through rooting the cuttings is also not successful, posing a problem for planting stocks.

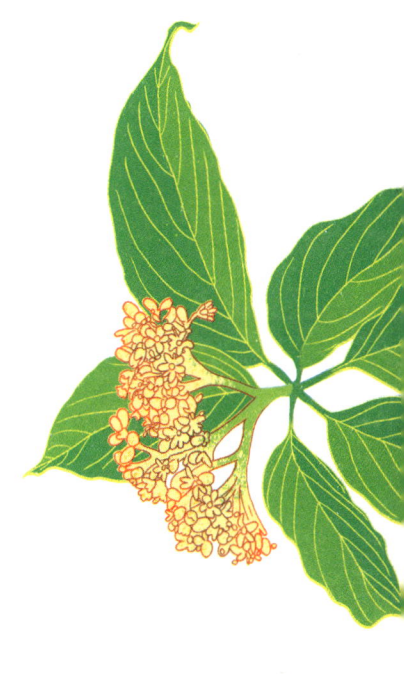

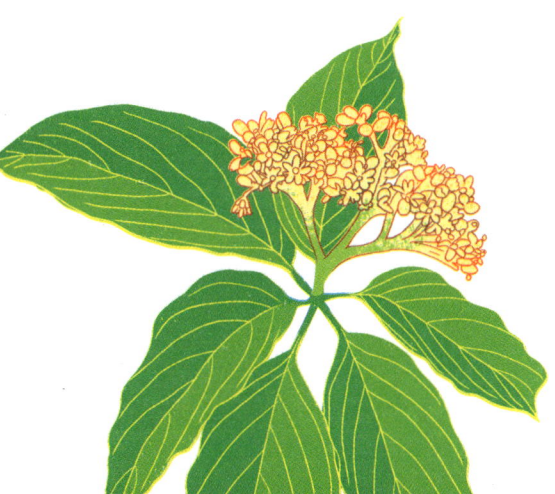
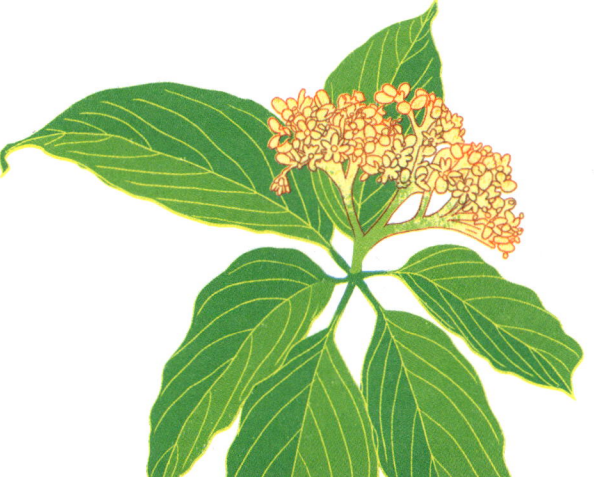

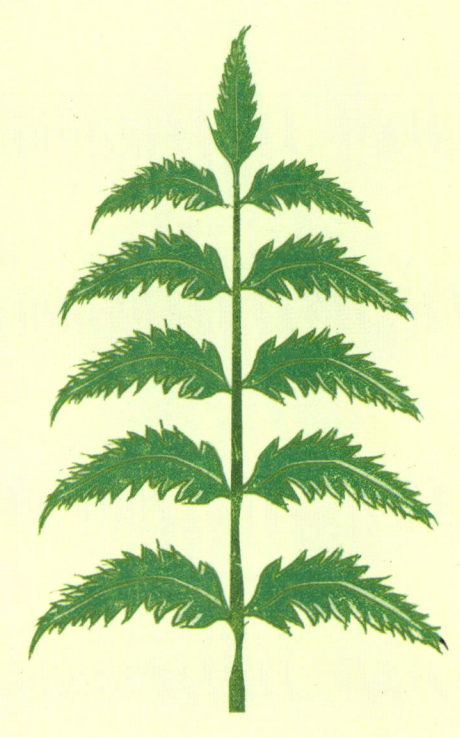

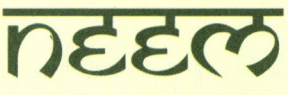

INDIAN LILAC
Azadirachta indica

NEEM *Assamese, Hindi, Bangla, Oriya* . **VEMPU** *Tamil* . **KADULIMBA**
Marathi . **BEVU** *Kannada* . **VEPA** *Telugu* . **LIMADO** *Gujarati*

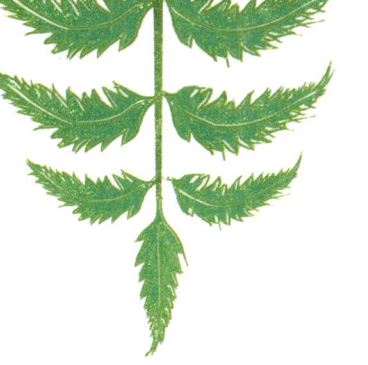
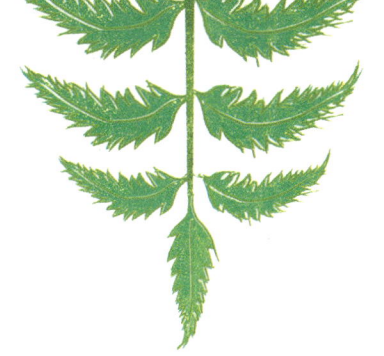
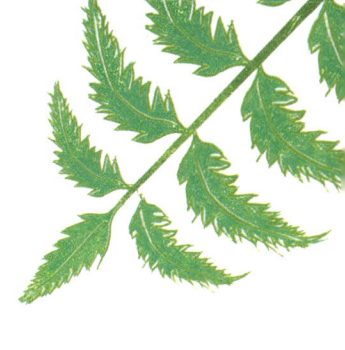

MEDICINAL PROPERTIES

Known as a wonder herb, neem's main quality is its cleansing property, hence it is very useful in a range of conditions – clearing up skin diseases, improving liver function, detoxifying the blood, pest and disease control, fever reduction, dental treatments, cough, asthma, ulcers, piles, intestinal worms, urinary diseases etc. Neem leaf paste is applied to the skin to treat acne, and in a similar vein is used by those suffering from measles and chicken pox. Chewing neem leaves daily is believed to help balance one's insulin level. Practitioners of traditional Indian medicine recommend that patients suffering from chicken pox should sleep on neem leaves and also be administered a decoction prepared from neem leaves to relieve fever. Bathing with water that has had neem leaves soaked in it, is both very refreshing and protective of the skin.

COSMETIC CURES

Neem oil is used in soaps, shampoos, balms and creams as well as toothpaste. While tender branches of the tree are used as a toothbrush, neem oil is also directly useful for skincare such as acne treatment, and maintaining the skin's elasticity. It is also a great insect repellent – a few drops of oil in a diffuser helps keep mosquitoes and flies at bay. Applying neem oil on the belly button is considered to be beneficial for skin health.

CULINARY BENEFITS

There are several variations of neem chutney made in different regions of India. The leaves are rich in minerals and vitamins. Traditionally, in Bengal, tender leaves and flowers are fried in ghee or mustard oil, and relished with steamed rice. In the state of Tamil Nadu, the new year is celebrated with neem flowers and raw mangoes to symbolize prosperity. A special rasam made on this occasion, with dried neem flowers, tamarind and pigeon peas is paired with rice.

In many parts of the country, when the first neem leaves appear, at the very beginning of summer, it is a practice to fry them lightly and eat at the beginning of every meal for about a fortnight, as a measure of cooling the body and building immunity for the harsh summer months.

It is one of the five trees recommended to be planted next to water bodies meant to serve human settlements, since it would keep the air and the water clean. Ancient religious texts and beliefs underline its significance, urging that planting a neem tree is a sure path to liberation.

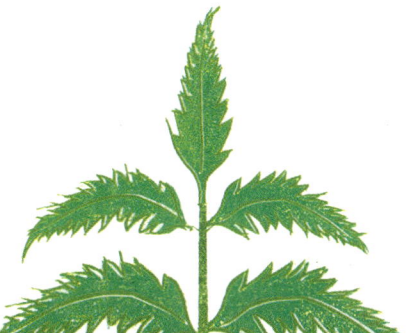
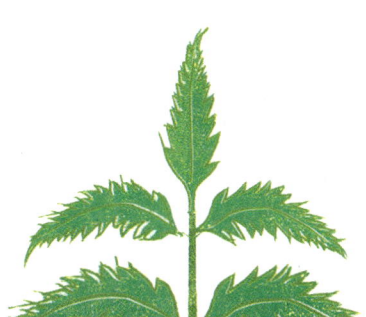
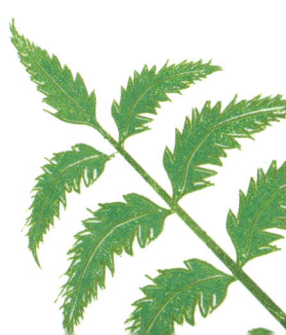

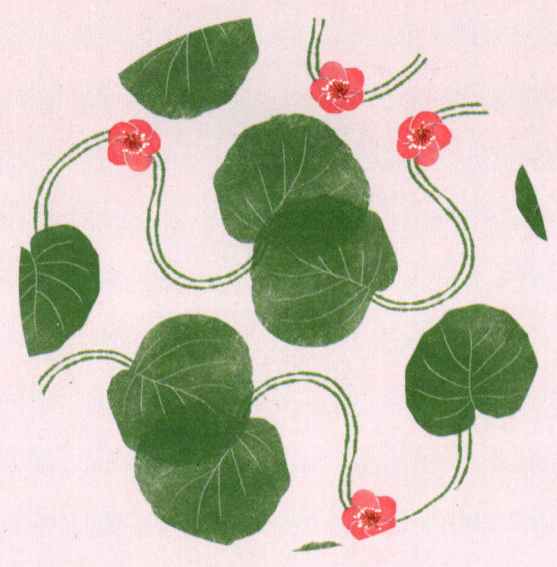

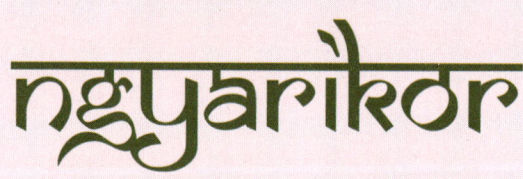

ngyarikor

ASIATIC PENNYWORT

Centella asiatica L.

NGYARIKOR *Apatani*

MEDICINAL PROPERTIES

Ngyarikor has been considered a significant therapeutic plant and also been utilized generally in Ayurvedic medication for diseases of the central nervous system including memory loss, insomnia, stress as well as epilepsy, leprosy, wounds, malignant growth, fever, inflammations, asthma, tuberculosis. Ngyarikor is used to treat stomach and urinary tract infections due to its antibacterial characteristics – by boiling ngyarikor water, adding honey to it and drinking it on an empty stomach. It is also good for healing wounds. A paste of the same helps in healing wounds.

CULINARY BENEFITS

The leaves and shoots are used as vegetables. It is advised to be eaten in the morning directly once properly washed. In Manipur, it is believed that taking seven leaves of ngyarikor in the morning just after waking up improves brain function and makes it sharper. It is also taken as a salad along with other vegetables, and is often eaten raw as it is believed to be good for digestion. One of the most appetizing dishes made with ngyarikor is a pakoda-like snack called sankuni patal bora, made with mashed ngyarikor, onions, lentils and green chillies.

COSMETIC CURES

The use of ngyarikor or its components are known to be valuable in the treatment of psoriasis and scleroderma. *Centella asiatica* is a typical element of cosmetics applied on aging skin as well as a treatment for cellulite and stretch marks. The whole plant boiled with rice water is also used as a hair moisturizer or cleanser.

Ngyarikor can also be used as one of the many ingredients of eromba – a famous Manipuri dish where vegetables, spices and herbs are boiled with or without *ngari* (small fermented fish), then made into a mash.

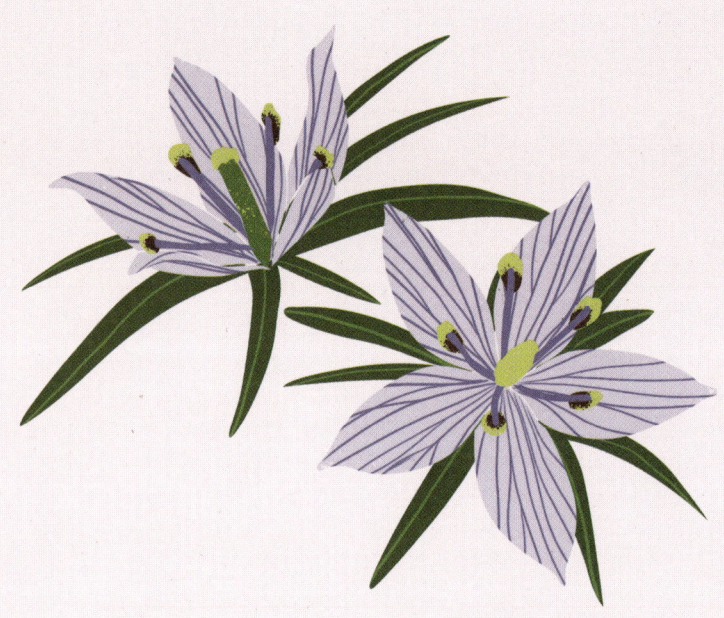

nilavembu

INDIAN ECHINACEA

Andrographis paniculata

NILAVEMBU *Tamil* . KALMEGH *Assamese, Bangla* .
KALA CHIRAYATA *Dogri* . HARA CHIRAYATA *Hindi* . KARIYATU
Gujarati . NILO KIRIYATO *Kachchhi* . VUBATI *Meitei* . HNAKAPUI *Mizo*
. BHADRATIKTA/BHUI NIMBA/HAIMA/SHANKINI/STHALAPUSHPI
Oriya . KIRATHAKADDI *Tulu*

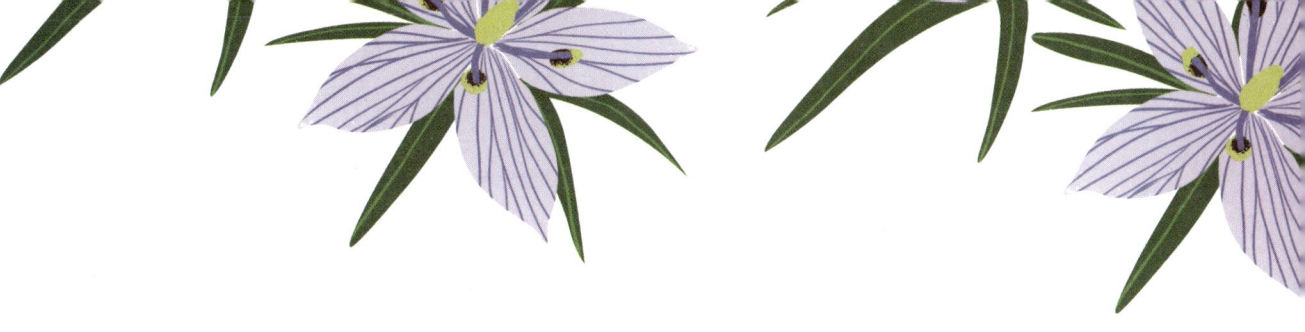

MEDICINAL PROPERTIES

Nilavembu leaf paste is used to treat poison bites, and is specially considered to be an antidote to snake venom. Before antibiotics were introduced, it was used to fight infections, especially those of the gastro-intestinal tract and also of the throat. It is also an important medicine for liver health, because it has been shown to help fight free radicals around the liver that cause damage to it. It is also considered good to help reduce fatty liver as well as lower the risk of gallstone formation.

Essentially, this herb has a cleansing and purifying action, especially of the blood and treats a variety of fevers including malaria and filaria. Filarial fever has the effect of obstructing the lymph nodes, preventing lymphatic circulation and hence leading to gross swelling in different parts of the body, commonly called elephantiasis. Nilavembu helps restore lymphatic circulation and so is highly recommended for this condition. Due to its laxative properties, a decoction is taken in small amounts daily to help regulate bowel movements and overall immunity. In Ayurvedic practice, the use of a small quantity of nilavembu churna to manage arthritis is prescribed.

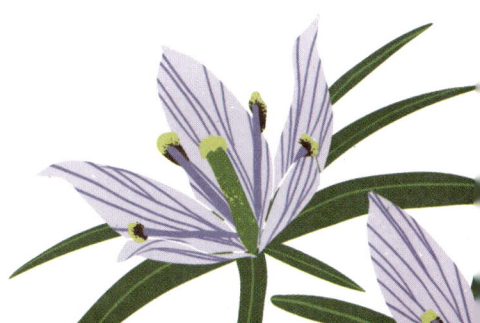

CULINARY BENEFITS

In West Bengal and possibly other parts of eastern India, small pills or 'badis' are made with the paste of nilavembu leaves that are sun-dried. It is considered beneficial to eat one of these at the beginning of the meal, especially during summer due to its cooling and cleansing properties.

COSMETIC CURES

Nilavembu powder along with coconut oil can be applied on the skin to manage eczema, boils and skin infections due to its antioxidant, antimicrobial and anti-inflammatory properties.

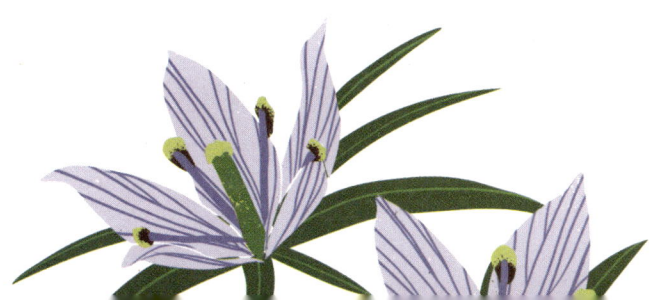

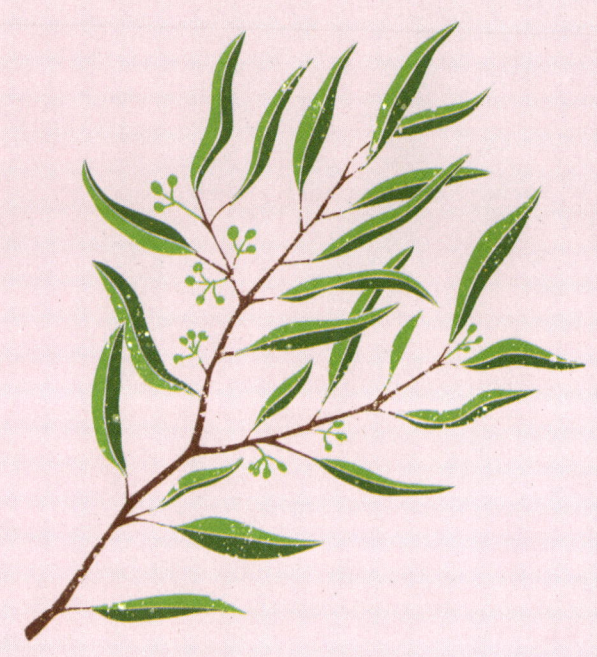

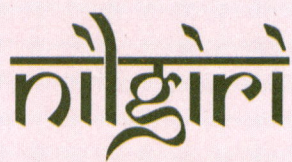

BLUE-GUM EUCALYPTUS
Eucalyptus globulus

NILGIRI *Hindi* . **NASIK** *Meitei* .
TAILAPATRA/TAILAPARNA/SUGANDHPATRA *Sanskrit* .
JAMAOIL/NEELAGIRI *Telugu, Konkani, Marathi and Kannada*

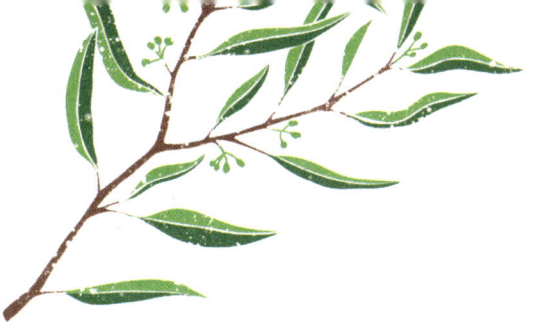
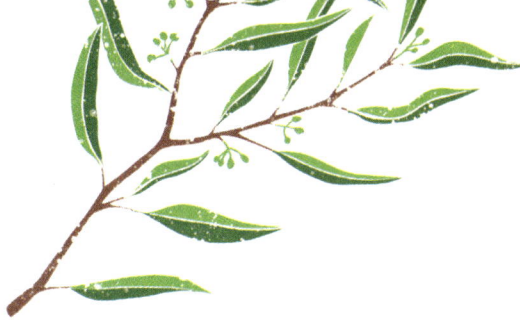

MEDICINAL PROPERTIES

Nilgiri leaves are used in a number of different ways. The oil that is made from them is used as a decongestant and stimulant. It is ideal for clearing the nasal and breathing pathways. Even more simply, gargling with water in which the leaves have been boiled is known to relieve throat infections.

The strong antiseptic qualities in this plant make it ideal for supporting the healing of cuts and wounds. Due to its analgesic and anti-inflammatory properties, nilgiri oil is also an excellent choice for pain relief when diluted with a carrier oil and massaged onto sore muscles and joints. It is a common remedy for colds and congestion. Soak a clean cloth in the infusion, then apply it directly on your chest or back to help ease that hacking cough. Sinus congestion can be cleared up by inhaling the steam of fresh nilgiri leaves in boiled water. The leaves also help freshen one's breath as they are used to fight germs that cause mouth odour.

CULINARY BENEFITS

Nilgiri leaves can be used to make a syrup, and is a great flavouring for cocktails or desserts. The leaves can also be used to make an infusion, in olive oil or vinegar that can be drizzled over salads or other dishes to add flavour.

COSMETIC CURES

The benefits of nilgiri oil are best accessed when it is added to carrier oils. Its anti-bacterial properties help the skin to attain a soft and healthy glow. A few drops of nilgiri oil added to coconut or olive oil gives dry hair a nice pick-me-up, while warding off dandruff and an itchy scalp. Nilgiri is also an effective natural alternative to synthetic chemical treatments for head lice. Apart from its essential oil being added to a diffuser, one can also add nilgiri leaves to one's bath for a relaxing and refreshing experience.

Dried nilgiri leaves bring a fresh fragrance to potpourri or a fresh stem with leaves too in a vase. Nilgiri oil combined with lemon and peppermint oils and water in a spray bottle is a great household cleanser, an effective green alternative to harsh spray-on disinfectants.

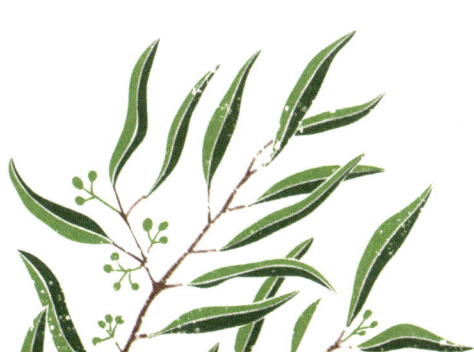
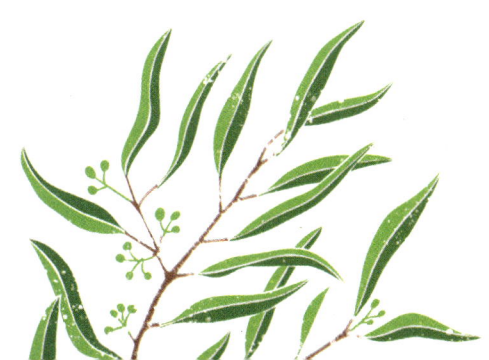

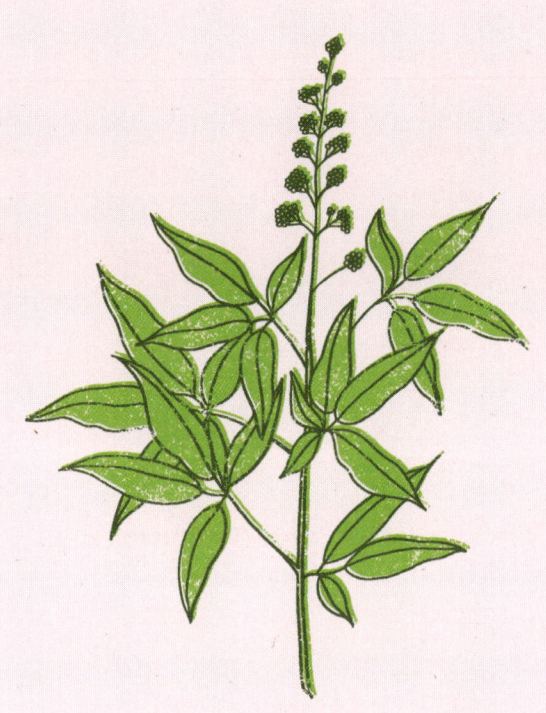

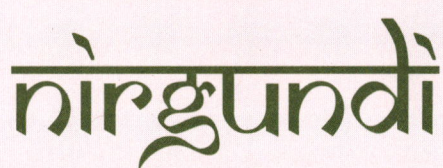

FIVE-LEAVED CHASTE TREE

Vitex negundo

NIRGUNDI *Bangla* . **POCHOTIA** *Assamese* . **SAMBHALU/NISINDA/
MEWRI** *Hindi* . **BILE-NEKKI/LAAKKI SOPPU/LAKKI GIDA** *Kannada* .
BANNA/MARWAN/SWANJAN TORBANNA *Punjabi* . **SHEPHALIKA/
SUVAHA/NILAMANJARI/HUTAKESHI** *Sanskrit* . **CHINDUVARAM** *Tamil* .
INDHUVARA/VAVILI/LEKKALI *Telugu*

158

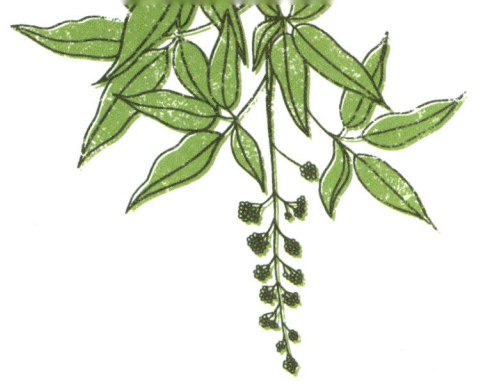
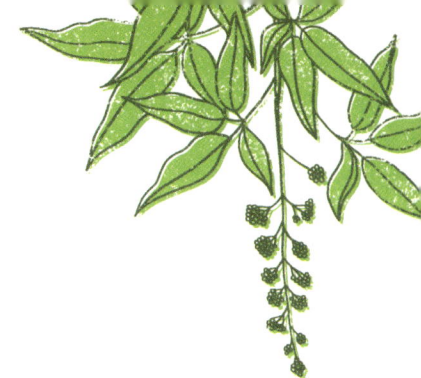

MEDICINAL PROPERTIES

Nirgundi is a part of the treatment of various types of ailments and diseases like leprosy, tuberculosis, piles, intestinal worms, constipation, leucorrhoea and fever. It is a primary constituent in treating typhoid and malarial fever. Its analgesic properties can be accessed by boiling the leaves in water and tied as a poultice over the affected part. For osteoarthritic conditions and lumbago, the root of the plant is powdered, and used to great effect.

It has immense value in improving the circulation of blood – especially in improving menstrual flow for those suffering from irregular menstrual cycles. The powder of the leaves also helps in conditions like endometriosis – a condition that many women suffer from. The leaves are ground along with garlic, rice and jaggery, and eaten to treat worms.

The leaves, when soaked overnight in cold water, can be used to gargle with for treating toothache, gingivitis, bleeding gums, halitosis and excessive salivation as well as for general cleansing.

COSMETIC CURES

The oil of this herb is used in making soaps. Its anti-inflammatory properties are useful in external applications. The oil is also known to be a hair tonic, when mixed with sesame oil and massaged on the scalp, as well as applied from roots to ends.

Sleeping on a pillow stuffed with dried nirgundi leaves helps to reduce headache.

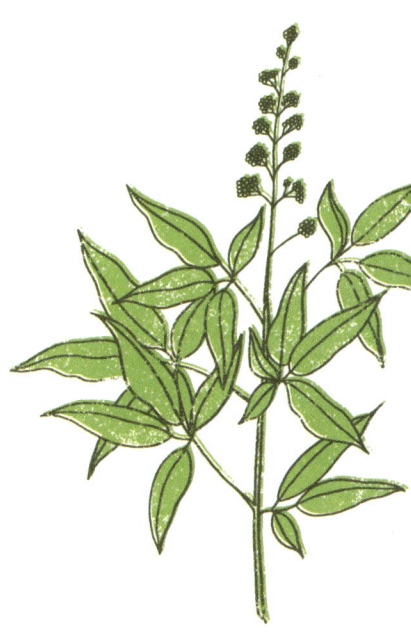
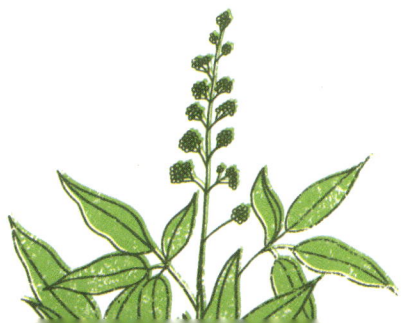
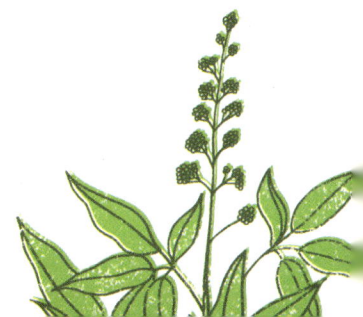

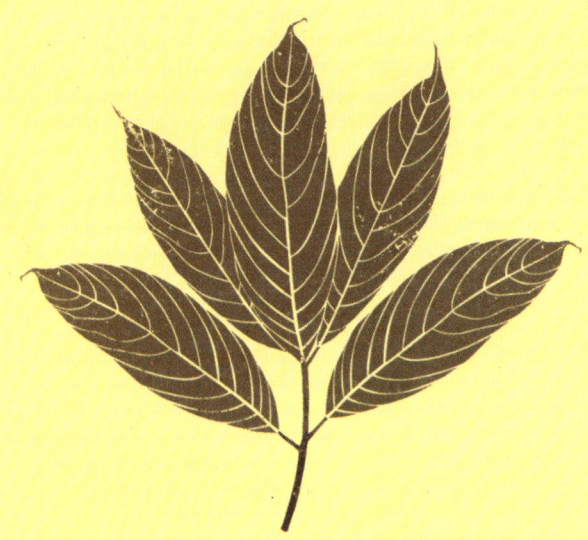

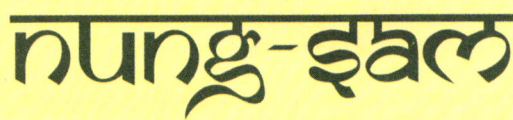

NUNG SAM

Lemanea australis Atkins [Lemaneaceae]

NUNG-SAM *Meitei*

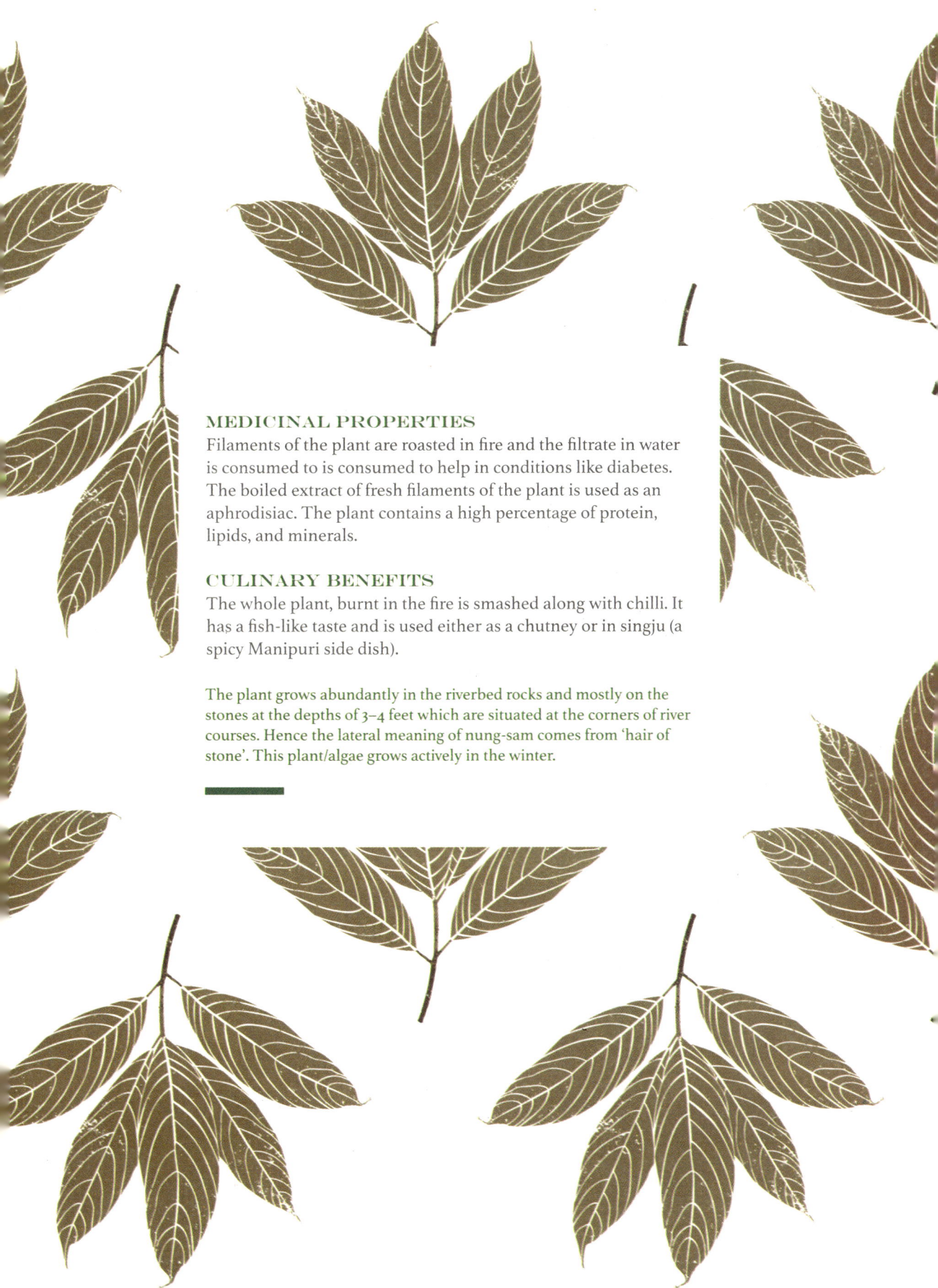

MEDICINAL PROPERTIES

Filaments of the plant are roasted in fire and the filtrate in water is consumed to is consumed to help in conditions like diabetes. The boiled extract of fresh filaments of the plant is used as an aphrodisiac. The plant contains a high percentage of protein, lipids, and minerals.

CULINARY BENEFITS

The whole plant, burnt in the fire is smashed along with chilli. It has a fish-like taste and is used either as a chutney or in singju (a spicy Manipuri side dish).

The plant grows abundantly in the riverbed rocks and mostly on the stones at the depths of 3–4 feet which are situated at the corners of river courses. Hence the lateral meaning of nung-sam comes from 'hair of stone'. This plant/algae grows actively in the winter.

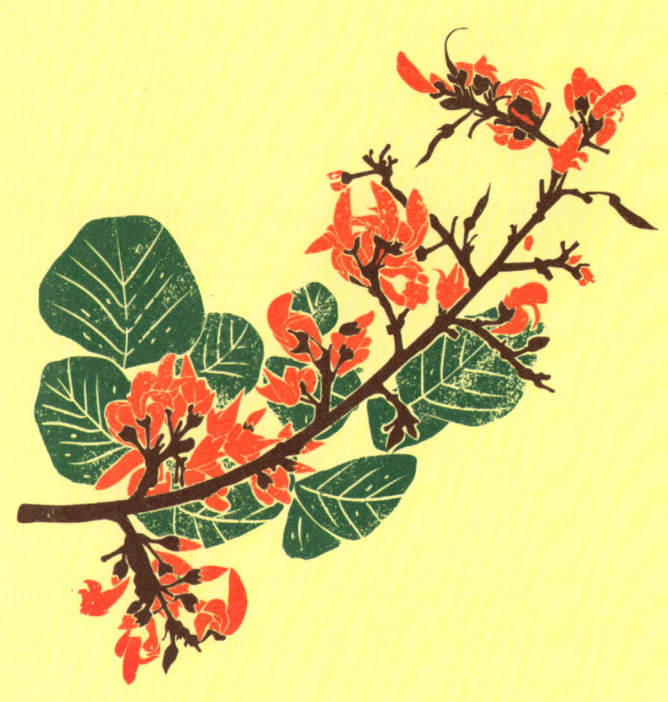

palash

FLAME OF THE FOREST

Butea monosperma

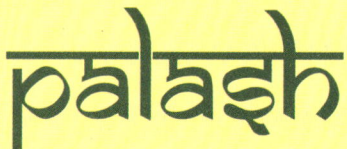

PALASH *Bangla* . BIPORNOK *Assamese* . DHAK *Hindi, Urdu* .
KESUDO *Gujarati* . MUTTUGA *Kannada* . CHMATA/KINSUKAM
Malayalam . PANGONG *Meitei* . BAKRA PUSHPA/BRAHMA BRUKSHA/
RAKTA BARGA *Oriya* . MURUD *Santhali* . KAMPIRAM *Tamil* . RGY
SKYEGS SIN *Tibetan* . MUTTAKA *Tulu*

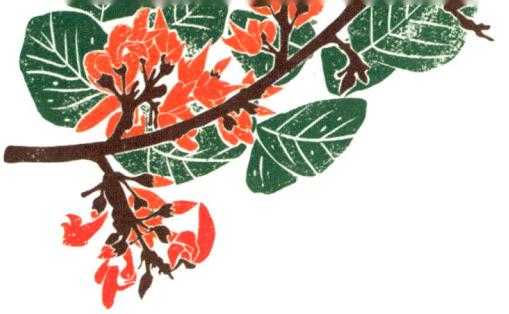
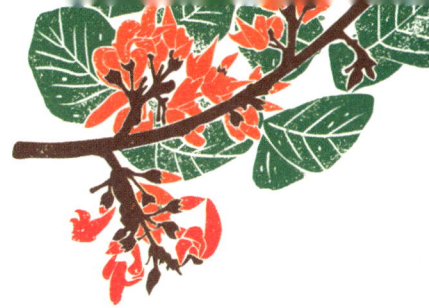

MEDICINAL PROPERTIES

Various parts of the tree like its flowers, bark, leaf and seed gum are used for medicinal purposes. The astringent bark is used to treat piles and menstrual disorders. Gum from the trunk called Butea gum, is also astringent and used in diarrhoea. A powder of the palash seeds is mainly used for deworming due to its anthelmintic activity. It also helps in managing liver disorders due to its antioxidant properties along with managing blood sugar levels by improving the glucose metabolism in the body.

The brilliant colour obtained from an infusion of the flowers may be used into water-paint (during the festival of Holi) or made into a dye. Both the lucid oil obtained from the seeds and the gum from the stems are useful to leather workers. One of the most important uses of the young roots of the tree is that it can make a very strong fibre, which has been used for making rope sandals. Because of their strength, the leaves of the tree are also used for wrapping anything that needs to be carried.

CULINARY BENEFITS

Once considered the best coolant with nutritional and healing properties, the blooming of this flower heralds the spring season. During summer months, a cold infusion of the dried flowers is consumed as sherbet. Tea prepared from the dried flowers can be taken with or without milk.

Sacred utensils are made from Palash wood. It is believed that the tree is a form of Agni, the God of fire and war. In the state of Telangana, these flowers are specially used in the worship of Shiva on the occasion of Shivaratri.

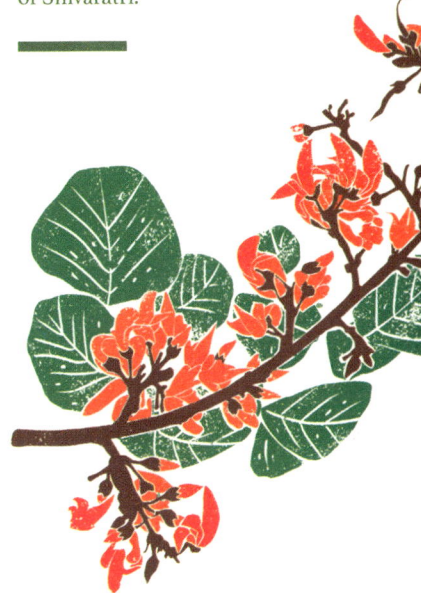
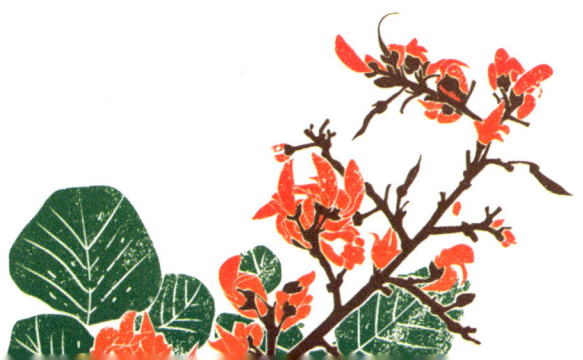
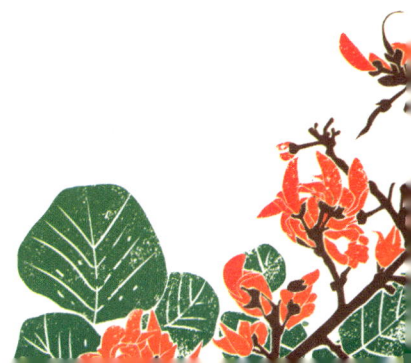

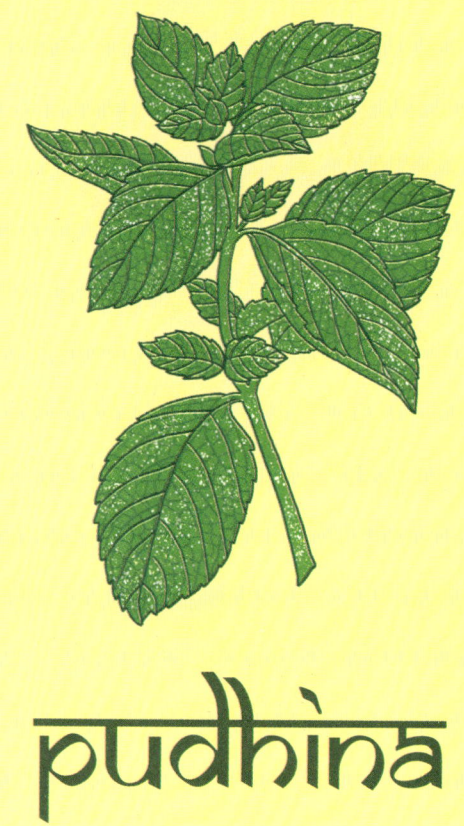

pudhina

MINT

Mentha arvensis

PUDHINA *Hindi, Marathi, Bangla, Punjabi, Gujarati, Tamil, Telugu .*
PUDINIH *Kashmiri .* **PUTHINA** *Malayalam .*

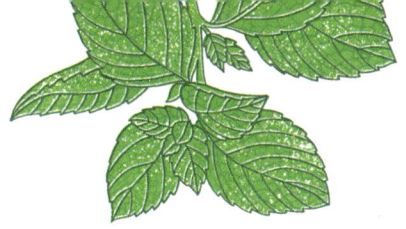
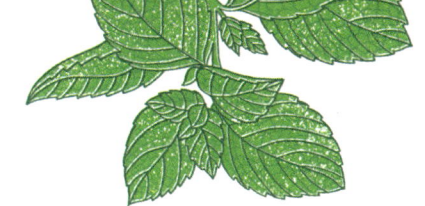

MEDICINAL PROPERTIES

The strong smelling, aromatic leaves of pudhina are mainly used to cure coughs and also been used in Ayurvedic healing of digestive disorders, respiratory problems, menstrual discomfort and skin problems like acne, itching and rashes. Its oil helps with digestion. A paste of the leaves simply covering a wound would help heal it. Chewing the leaves at night helps with reducing cholesterol and strengthens the bones. Having a decoction of the leaves, three to four times a day manages anything that causes irritation or a burning sensation, for example a urinary tract infection.

CULINARY BENEFITS

Due to its highly cooling property, the leaves of this plant are used to make cold beverages and chutneys. For as long as it has been known, pudhina has been used as a powerful ingredient for cooking primarily due to its countless medicinal properties. A cooling drink made with the leaves in the summer helps fight the effects of the 'loo' winds.

COSMETIC CURES

Pudhina has a great deal of menthol with many other minerals and hence is great for oral health. Chewing fresh leaves every day for a month or so helps kill bacterial growth in the mouth. Also, a small quantity of the dried leaves, mixed with a pinch of sea salt can be used to massage the gums for great oral health. It is hence used widely in toothpastes and mouthwashes.

Pudhina is also traditionally used to treat skin problems like acne and rashes, with a cooled decoction made with the leaves simply patted on the face with cotton and left to dry for about fifteen minutes to completely clear skin plagued by pimples or any kind of allergies. Added to a paste of yogurt and oatmeal, it is great for oily skin. It is now known to be a great source of energy for skin cells and so now being used in face cleansers, soaps and body wash. For the hair, mint oil added to a carrier oil regularly raises the Ph level of the scalp, enhancing hair growth and reducing dandruff. Combined with fresh dhaniya and raw mango or lemon juice, the popular green chutney is part of street food and chaats of India.

Keeping a bunch of fresh leaves under one's pillow helps the brain work well to keep fresh and alert, apart from improving one's sleep.

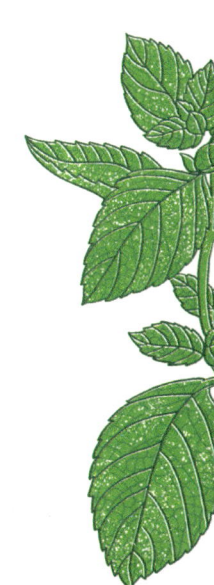
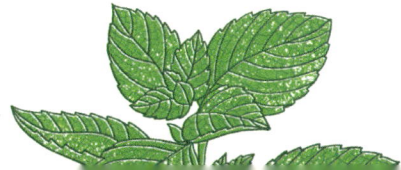
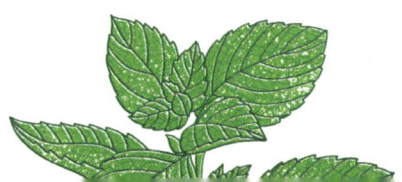

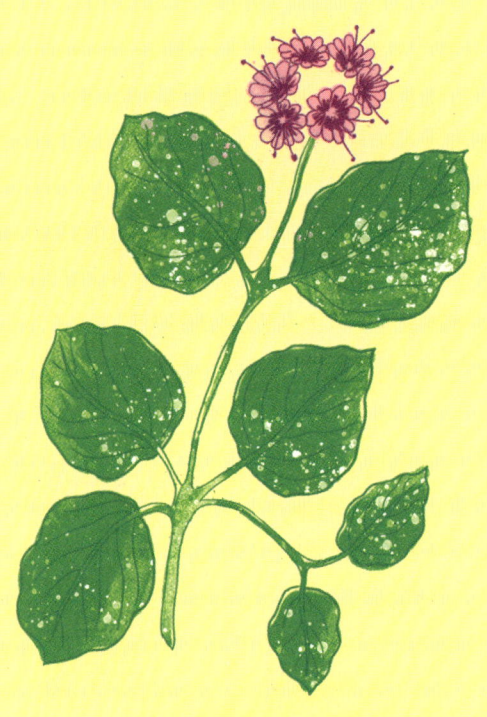

punarnava

MIRACLE LEAF/SPREADING HOGWEED

Boerhavia diffusa

PUNARNAVA *Hindi* . **GHETULI** *Marathi* . **SHOTHAGNI** *Sanskrit* .
ATAVASA/MIDI *Telugu* . **SATODI/BASEDO** *Gujarati* .
PANFUTI/PATHARCHUR *Hindi*

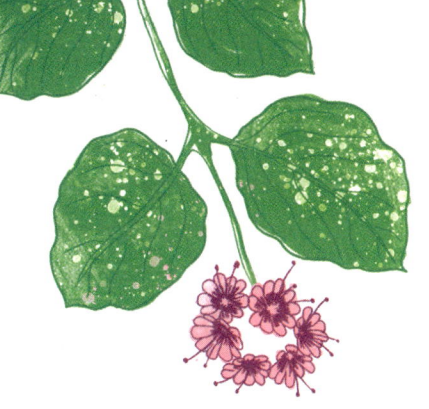
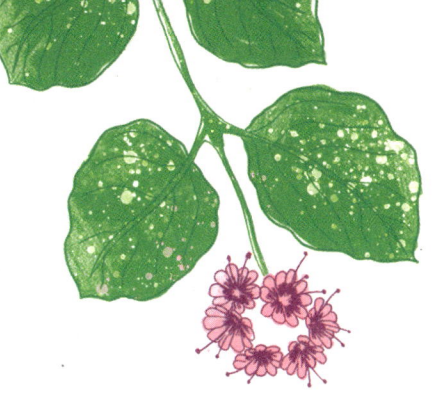

MEDICINAL PROPERTIES

Punarnava means 'new birth', and many feel the plant is rightly named so, as it is believed to bring back vigour and vitality. Many Ayurveda experts call it the miracle herb for its health benefits. This plant is best identified by its flowers. The flowers are seasonal, but are very useful for making a powder for pain relief. Even though it is slightly bitter, the entire plant is edible. Punarnava is ideal for detoxing as it flushes out toxins from the body. It is an excellent diuretic and also tones up the urinary tract and supports the body's natural ability to expel fluids, thus preventing water retention. This reduces urea levels in the body very effectively and makes it useful for treating all disorders of the kidneys. Chewing a bit of the root helps treat mouth ulcers, and a decoction of the roots helps with lack of sleep. The paste of the root also serves as a local application to reduce swelling due to painful joints.

CULINARY BENEFITS

The leaves and stems are routinely cooked and eaten like many greens in Indian cuisine. When combined with either moong dal (split yellow lentil) or kaala chana (Bengal gram), it makes for a great dish. When boiled and mashed, it is mixed with yogurt for typical North Indian raita, or a chutney on its own. Cooked dry with coconut, it is enjoyed as thoran or poriyal in Kerala and Tamil Nadu, respectively.

Traditionally, a syrup used to be made with boiling down this plant in water and mixed with mishri (rock sugar) used to be kept in homes. It was a ready-to-drink kind of remedy for a variety of ailments and administered according to the age and condition of the patient.

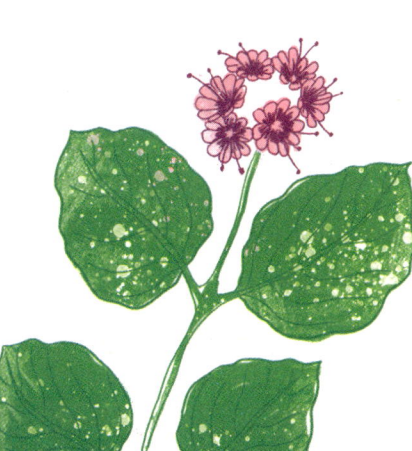
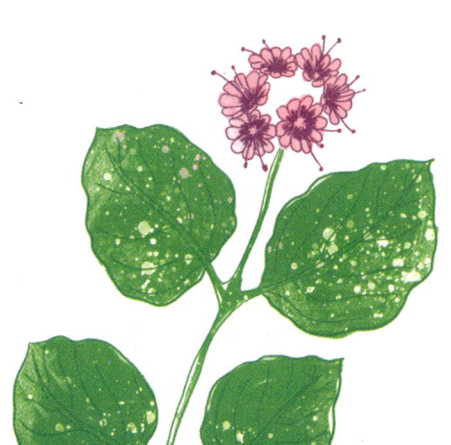

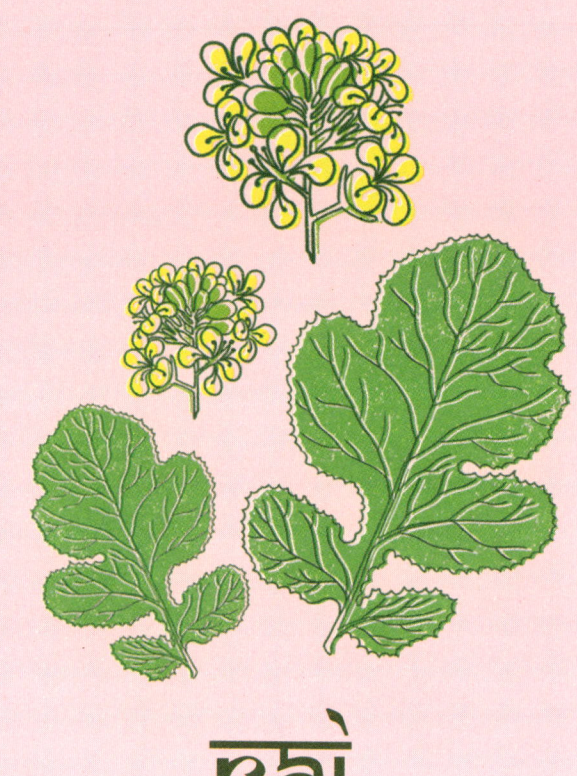

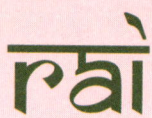

rai

BLACK MUSTARD
Brassica nigra

RAI *Hindi* . KALO SHORSHE *Bangla* . SASIVE *Kannada* . KADUGU
Malayalam . KRISHNAKA *Sanskrit* . AVALU *Telugu* . DASEMI *Tulu*

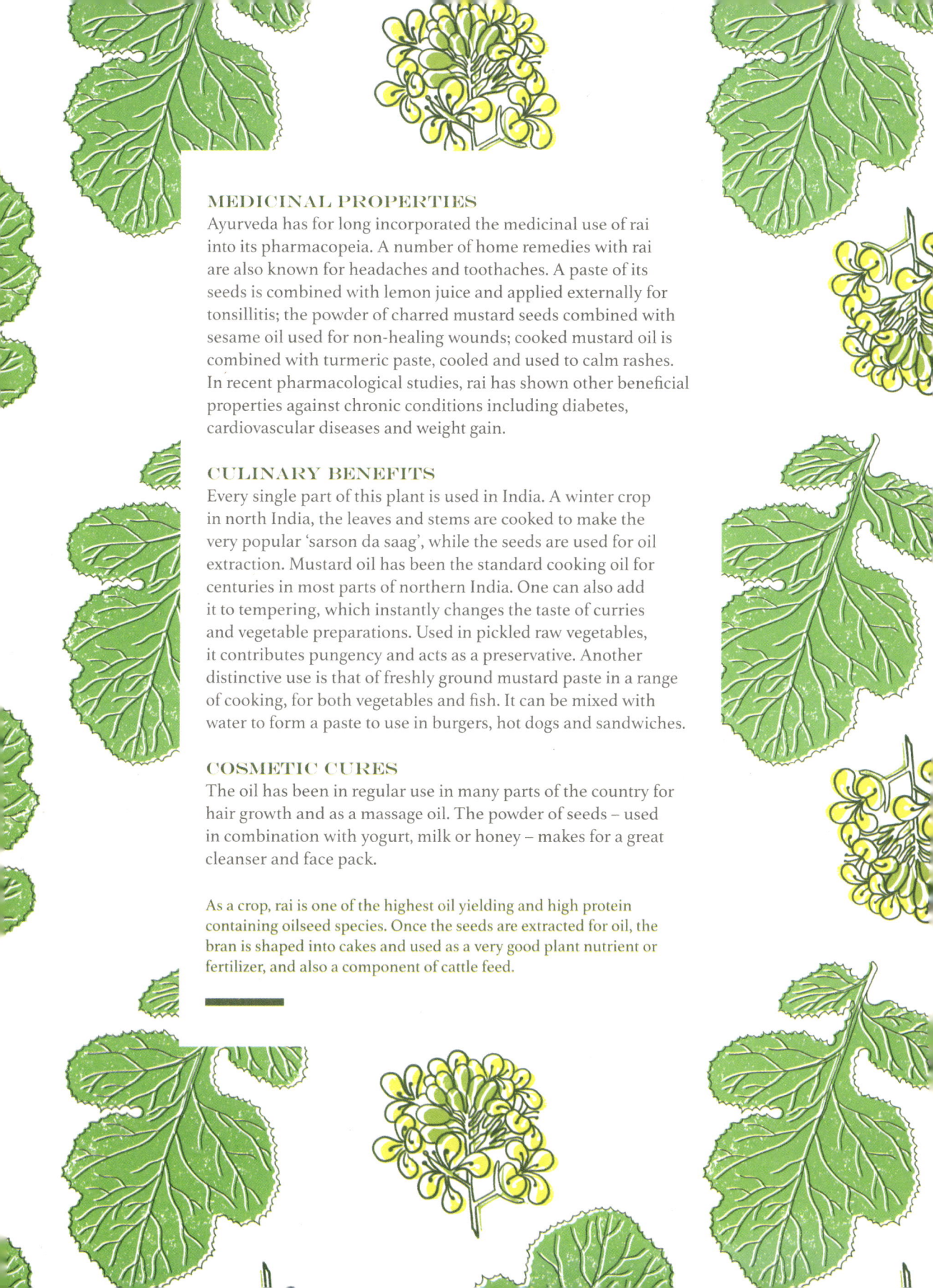

MEDICINAL PROPERTIES

Ayurveda has for long incorporated the medicinal use of rai into its pharmacopeia. A number of home remedies with rai are also known for headaches and toothaches. A paste of its seeds is combined with lemon juice and applied externally for tonsillitis; the powder of charred mustard seeds combined with sesame oil used for non-healing wounds; cooked mustard oil is combined with turmeric paste, cooled and used to calm rashes. In recent pharmacological studies, rai has shown other beneficial properties against chronic conditions including diabetes, cardiovascular diseases and weight gain.

CULINARY BENEFITS

Every single part of this plant is used in India. A winter crop in north India, the leaves and stems are cooked to make the very popular 'sarson da saag', while the seeds are used for oil extraction. Mustard oil has been the standard cooking oil for centuries in most parts of northern India. One can also add it to tempering, which instantly changes the taste of curries and vegetable preparations. Used in pickled raw vegetables, it contributes pungency and acts as a preservative. Another distinctive use is that of freshly ground mustard paste in a range of cooking, for both vegetables and fish. It can be mixed with water to form a paste to use in burgers, hot dogs and sandwiches.

COSMETIC CURES

The oil has been in regular use in many parts of the country for hair growth and as a massage oil. The powder of seeds – used in combination with yogurt, milk or honey – makes for a great cleanser and face pack.

As a crop, rai is one of the highest oil yielding and high protein containing oilseed species. Once the seeds are extracted for oil, the bran is shaped into cakes and used as a very good plant nutrient or fertilizer, and also a component of cattle feed.

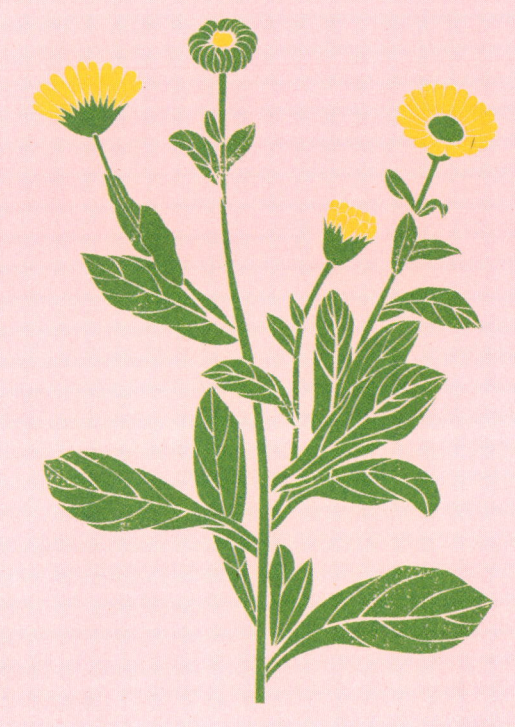

saamanthi

POT MARIGOLD
Calendula officinialis

SAAMANTHI *Tamil* . **GENDA** *Hindi* . **GUL-E-ASHARFI** *Urdu*

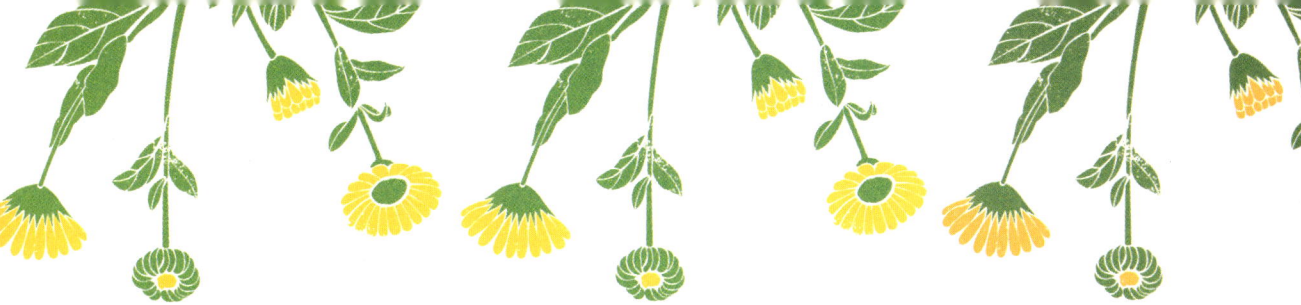

MEDICINAL PROPERTIES

The leaves and flowers of saamanthi are most used for medicinal purposes. The flower of this plant is edible and has analgesic, anti-diabetic, anti-ulcer and anti-inflammatory properties and so has been considered beneficial in reducing inflammation, healing wounds, ulcers, and used as an antiseptic to cure cough and snake-bites.

Given that it is such a common flower, grown all over the country, its medicinal properties for everyday use need to be revived. The decoction of the petals can be used for gargling to relieve a sore throat. A quick crush of the petals is very good to heal fresh wounds and even stubborn skin lesions of any kind.

CULINARY BENEFITS

Saamanthi tea, though not very well known, is excellent for overall gut health, including that of the gall bladder. The tea is delicious and mildly detoxifying. It is also known to help with nausea, stomach ulcers and menstrual discomfort.

COSMETIC CURES

Saamanthi oil, which has many anti-inflammatory properties, is a very good ingredient for cosmetic use. As a component of body butters and face packs, it works wonders for the skin. Generally too, it is excellent for cracked heels or sunburns or calluses.

The word calendula is derived from the Latin word 'Calendae', which means 'little calendar' or 'little clock' because of the promptness of the saamanthi flower appearing on the first day of the lunar month, which is the day of the new moon. The vibrant colour of the flowers is also a very important basis for textile dyes and was traditionally used for colours during the festival of Holi.

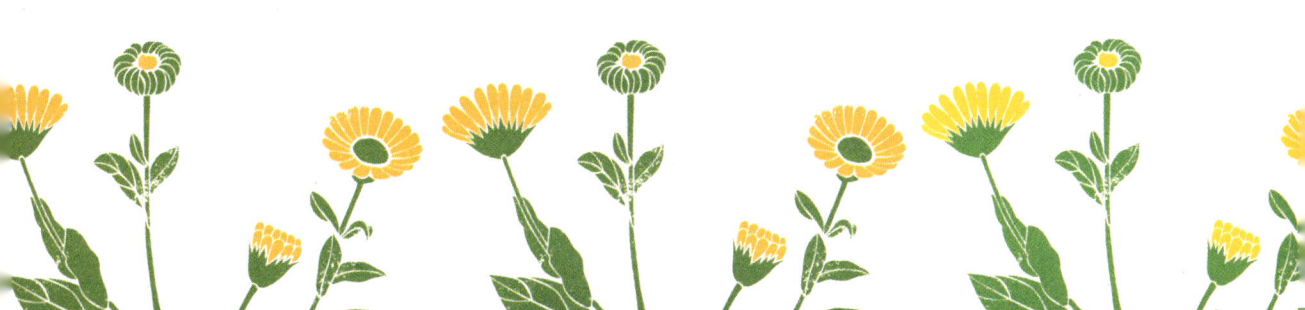

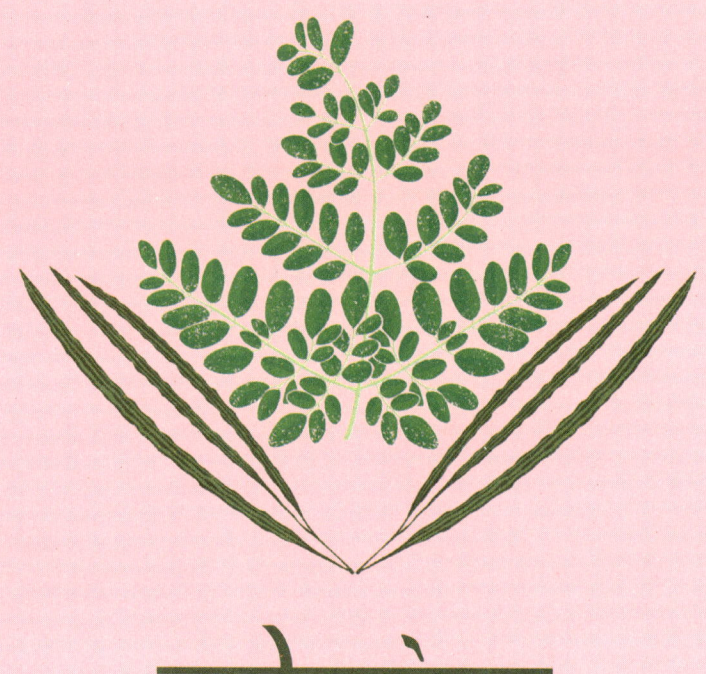

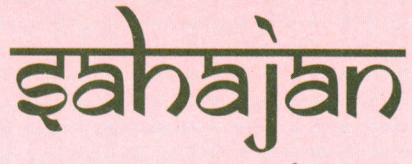

sahajan

DRUMSTICK TREE / MORINGA

Moringa oleifera

SAHAJAN/ BAHU-MUL/DANS-MUL/DRAVIN/MOCHAK/MUNGA/NIL-
KANTH/PRABHANJAN/SANJHNA/SHOBHANJAN *Hindi* . CHAJINA
Assamese . SHOJNE *Bangla* . MITHO SARAGAVO *Gujarati* . NUGGEGIDA/
NUGGE MARA/NUGGE KAI *Kannada* . MASHINGA *Konkani* . MOSING
Malayalam . BADAGA/SHEGAVA/SHENGUL/SHEVAGA *Marathi* . SIGRU/
SHOVANJAN *Nepali* . ACCHIVA *Pali* . SHOBHANJAN/SIGGU *Punjabi* .
AKSIVAH/MUKHAMMODAH/ SHOBHANJAN/SHUBHANJANAKAH/
VANAMPALLAVA *Sanskrit* . MUNAGA *Telugu* . MURUNGAI *Tamil*

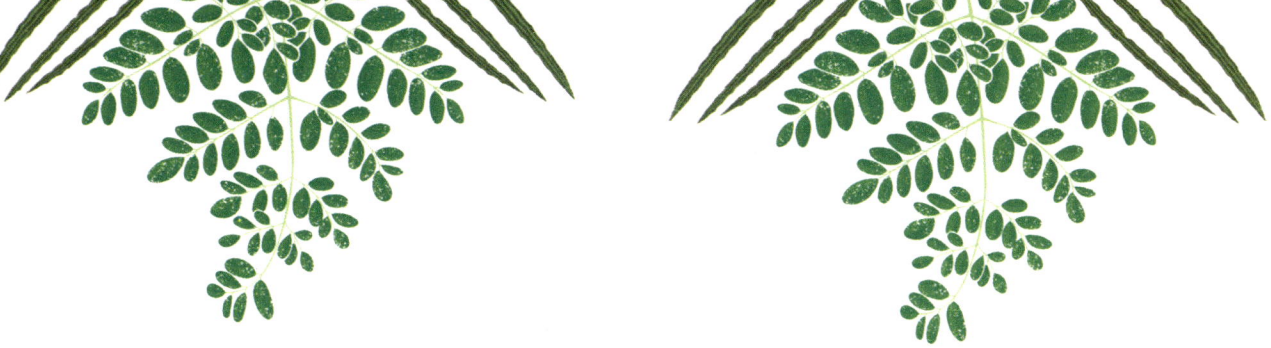

MEDICINAL PROPERTIES

Rich in macro and micronutrients, Sahajan leaves have a high vitamin C content, which are good for immunity building. They are also rich in calcium and phosphorus, crucial for bone health. A decoction of the leaves is advised for those suffering from diabetes because they have a high content of ascorbic acid that increases the secretion of insulin in the body. It is also an important element in controlling diabetes. Its leaves are also beneficial against digestive disorders. Those who suffer from constipation, bloating, gas, gastritis and ulcerative colitis should add fresh leaves to their diet.

CULINARY BENEFITS

The leaves, fruit and drumsticks of this plant all have enormous nutritional value – four times the amount of vitamin A in carrots, four times the amount of calcium in milk and contain all the amino acids, which is very rare for a plant source. So this has been a standard part of the cuisine for deriving nutrition from a plant that grows easily without much care, yields flowers and fruits early. It is great for health and is also used as livestock fodder (it helps the cattle in weight gain and lactation). Sahajan also has seven times more vitamin C than oranges and a dry dish made with its fresh leaves and flowers in considered a delicacy in many regions of India. Its leaves are used in soups, lentils and several other preparations.

COSMETIC CURES

A powder made from the leaves can be used as hand soap due to its anti-bacterial properties. This powder is also a great base for hair masks, made by combining it with coconut milk and some essential oils. The oil made from the seeds is great for hair growth, the amino acids that are all abundantly present helps in this. It also cleanses the scalp without taking away the moisture – which is how it strengthens the hair roots. It needs to be used along with other carrier oils like almond or coconut oil.

The green fertilizer as a spray accelerates growth of young plants. The plants are firmer, more resistant to pests and disease, have a longer lifespan and grow with heavier roots, stems and leaves. Such plants also produce more quantity of fruit as well as larger fruit size, the increase in yield being up to 20–35 per cent.

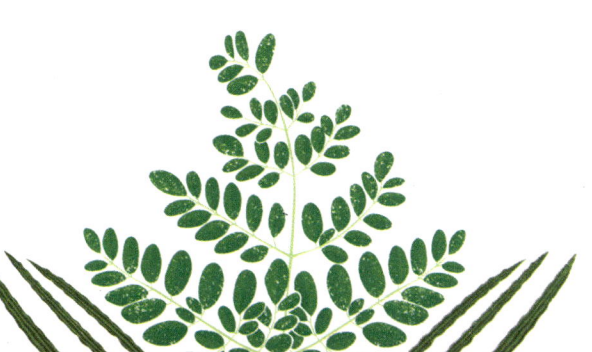

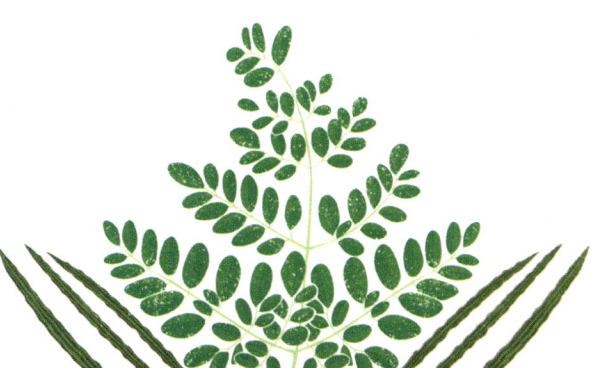

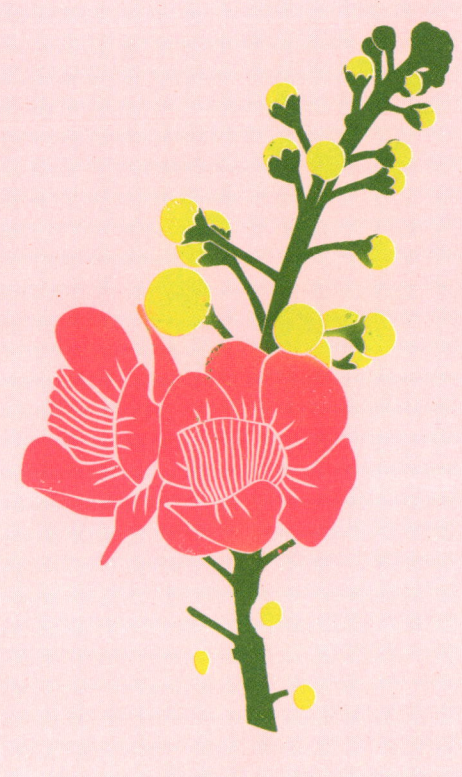

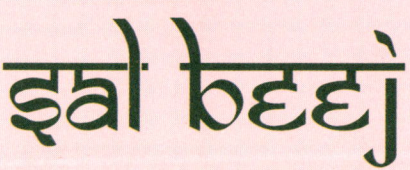

SAL

Shorea robusta

SAL BEEJ *Hindi* . **RAL** *Gujarati* . **SAJARA** *Marathi* .
SAGUA/SARJO *Oriya* . **ATTAM/KUNGILIYAM/SHALAR/TALUR** *Tamil* .
GUGILAMU/SHARJAMU *Telugu*

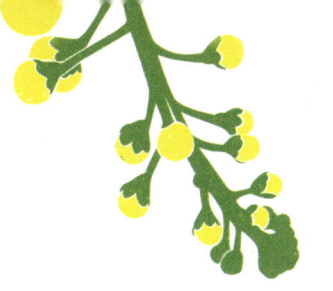
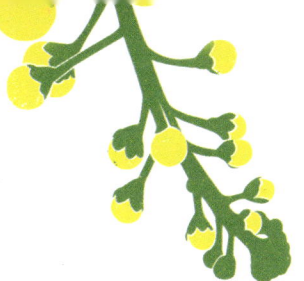

MEDICINAL PROPERTIES

The resin is applied externally to painful and swollen joints and is considered a very effective remedy. Used in Ayurveda with honey or sugar in treatment of dysentery and bleeding piles, it is also used to make complex drugs to treat a variety of diseases including leucorrhoea, gonorrhoea, skin disorders, ulcers, wounds, diarrhoea, burning sensation; it has been used as a treatment regimen for ear disorders too. The leaves and bark are used to treat wounds, ulcers, leprosy, cough and headache. In Unani medicine, the resin is used for treating menorrhagia, enlargement of spleen and for relieving eye irritation. Siddha practitioners recommend this herb to treat ulcers, wounds and menopausal disorders.

COMMERCIAL USE

The sal tree, with its strong, durable wood that is resistant to fire, has for long been used to caulk boats and ships, for building houses, telephone, and electrical poles, railway sleepers, and furniture. While its bark has also been used in tanning, its seeds and fruit are a source of lamp oil and vegetable fat. Its resin is used in paints, varnishes and for sealing joints or seams in boats. For the longest time, its leaves have been widely used for making leaf plates and cups.

RITUAL USE

The resin is burned as incense in Hindu ceremonies, and the oil from the seeds for lamps.

There are various names for this tree in Sanskrit, each name corresponding to one particular feature of the plant. One is Ashwakarna, meaning one whose leaves resemble the ears of a horse; Dhrupavriksha, the tree whose gum resin can be used as an incense. Its various names are evocative of the knowledge that is available about it.

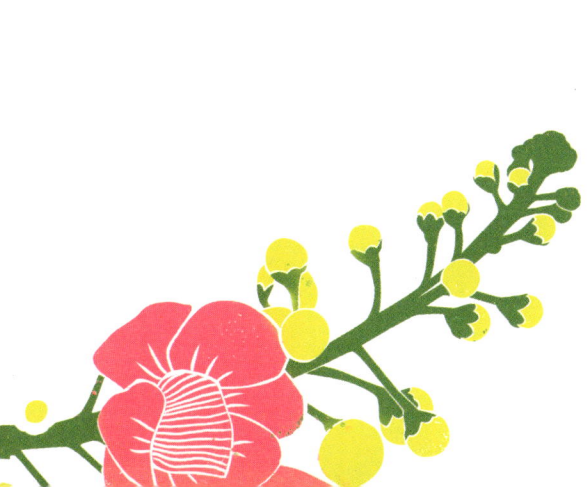
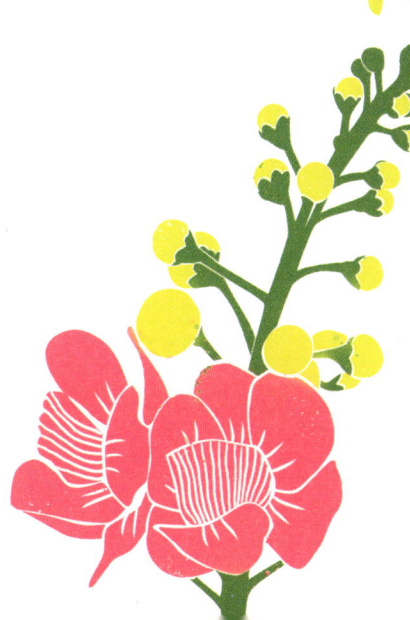

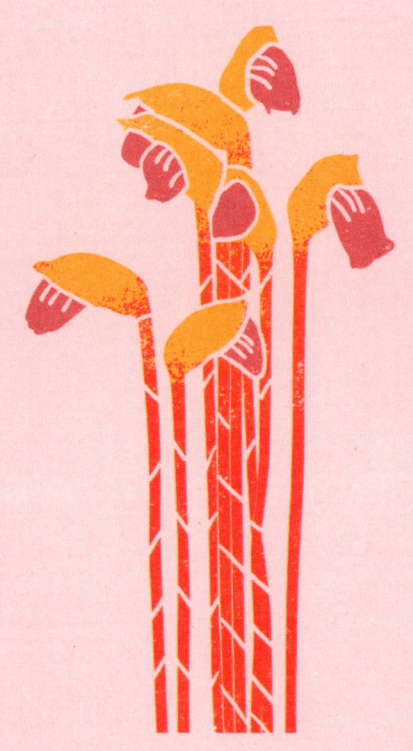

sangharvaibel

FOREST GHOST FLOWER

Aginetica indica L.

SANGHARVAIBEL *Mizo* . **ANKURI BANKURI** *Hindi* .
KEERIPU *Malayalam* . **GULABDANI** *Marathi* . **PUKUSUR** *Nepali*

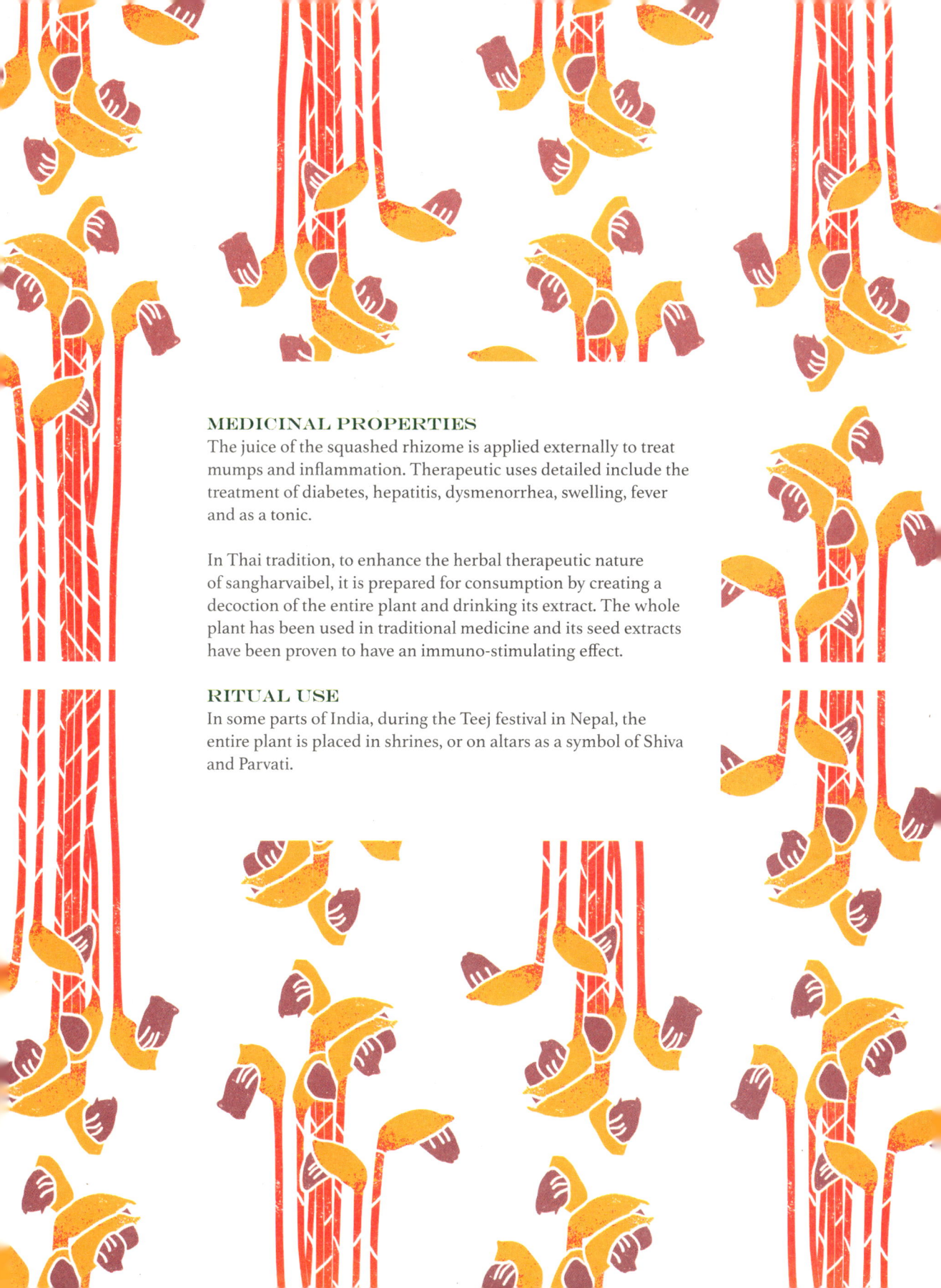

MEDICINAL PROPERTIES

The juice of the squashed rhizome is applied externally to treat mumps and inflammation. Therapeutic uses detailed include the treatment of diabetes, hepatitis, dysmenorrhea, swelling, fever and as a tonic.

In Thai tradition, to enhance the herbal therapeutic nature of sangharvaibel, it is prepared for consumption by creating a decoction of the entire plant and drinking its extract. The whole plant has been used in traditional medicine and its seed extracts have been proven to have an immuno-stimulating effect.

RITUAL USE

In some parts of India, during the Teej festival in Nepal, the entire plant is placed in shrines, or on altars as a symbol of Shiva and Parvati.

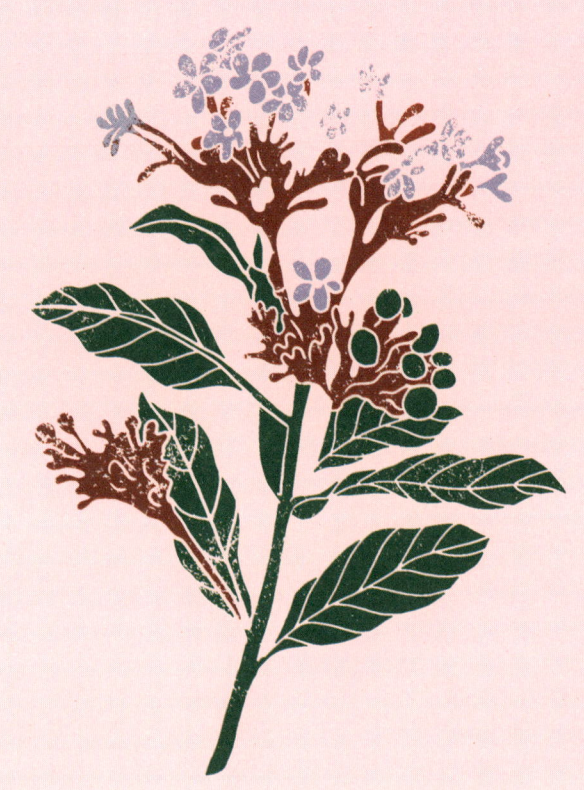

sarpagandha

INDIAN SNAKE ROOT

Rauwolfia serpentina

SARPAGANDHA *Hindi* . **ARACHORITIA** *Assamese* .
SHIVANAABHI/SOOTRANAABHI/HADAKI *Kannada* .
AMALPORI/CHUVANALPORI *Malayalam* . **CHANDRABHAGA** *Meitei* .
HARAKI/NAKULI *Marathi* . **PATAL GARUR** *Oriya* .
CHEVANAMALPODI *Tamil* . **PATALGUNI/PATALGARUDA** *Telugu*

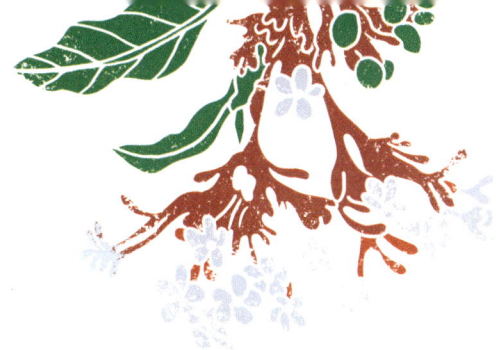
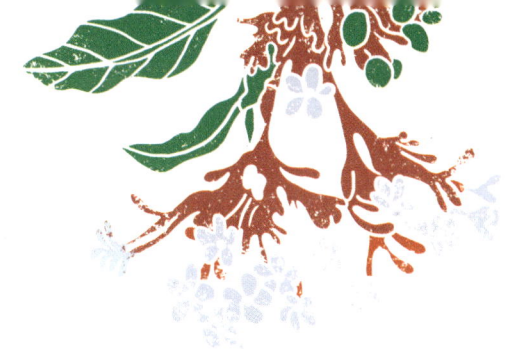

MEDICINAL PROPERTIES

Sarpagandha is known to reduce the tone of the blood vessels and therefore reduces the blood pressure and facilitates the circulation of blood through the heart passages at a normal, healthy pace. It is known to have a stimulatory action on the intestinal musculature. This property may be helpful in the treatment of gut motility disorders. In folk medicine, plant extracts of sarpagandha has been used to treat colic, cholera and fever. The roots of this plant have been used for treating poisonous insect stings and snake bites. Sarpagandha has a depressant action on brain centres and is therefore useful in the treatment of conditions such as anxiety and agitation.

It is also effective in regularizing menstrual cycles, when combined with ginger and black pepper. The juice of the leaves may be applied on the eyes in cases of corneal opacity.

Its various Sanskrit names are evocative of its many uses: chandramara, means one that helps to relieve the tensions of the mind; dhavalavitapa, one that cleanses and purifies mind and body; vishamardhini, one that is antidote to poison. As part of the list of endangered species, the export of this plant from India is restricted by law.

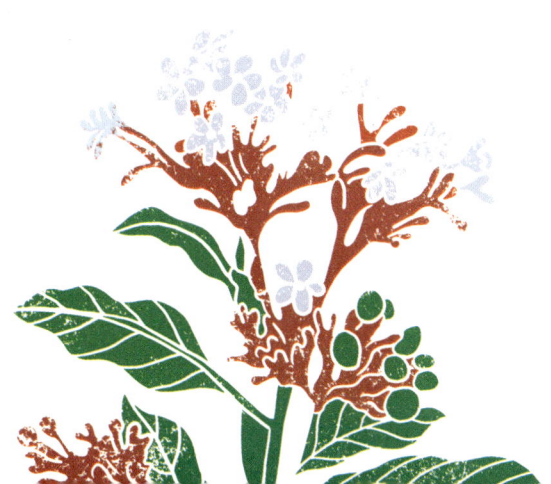
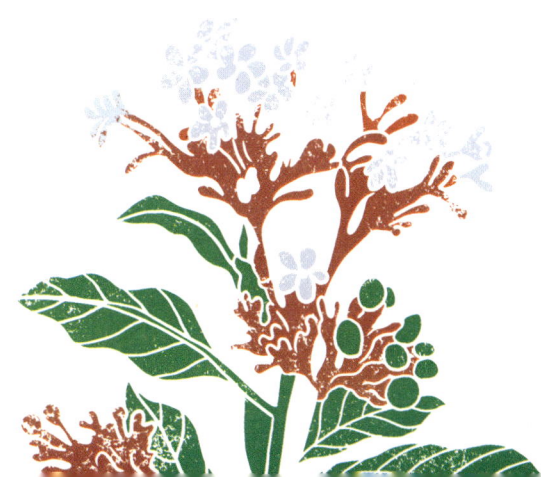

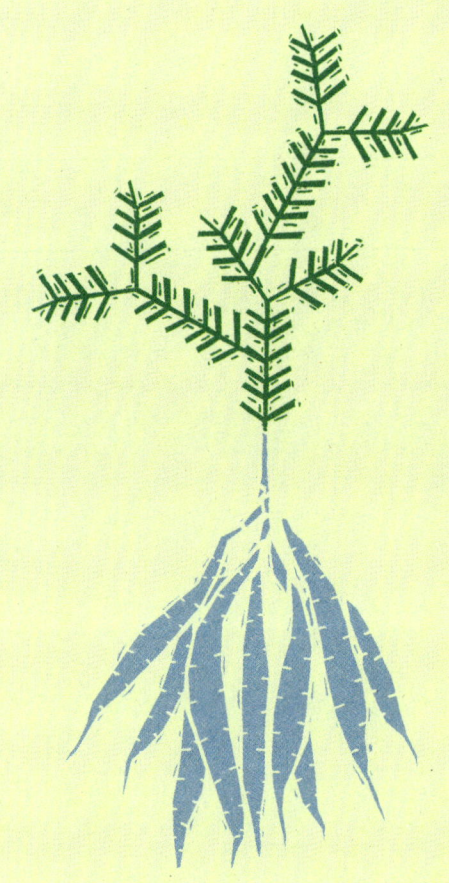

satavari

BUTTERMILK ROOT/CLIMBING ASPARAGUS/ WILD ASPARAGUS

Asparagus racemosus

SATAVARI *Hindi* . SHATAMULI *Bangla* . EKALKANTO SATAVARI
Gujarati . CHHOTARCU *Oriya* . AMMAIKODI *Tamil*

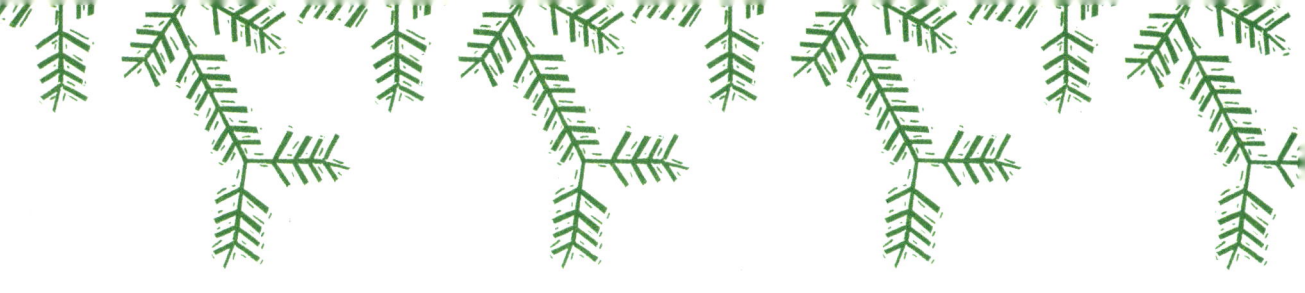

MEDICINAL PROPERTIES

A species of asparagus plant, satavari has been used in Ayurveda for various conditions. Its main use has been of the roots, to make a 'churna' (powder) that is a galactagogue to increase milk secretion in nursing mothers. It is known as the Indian 'female rejuvenative' as it is helpful in cases of low sex drive, menopause, PMS and infertility. It helps to balance hormonal system of women and regulates menstruation and ovulation. Satavari is also an excellent digestive herb as its roots' anti-flatulent property reduces the formation of gas, thereby also reducing indigestion. This herb is considered to be adaptogenic, which could mean that it helps regulate the body's systems and improve resistance to stress.

The herb is also useful in treating gastric ulcers, hyperacidity, dysentery, bladder infections, chronic fevers and rheumatism. A contemporary study showed that the herb strengthens the immune system by enhancing the functioning of macrophages – the immune cells responsible for digesting potentially destructive organisms.

CULINARY BENEFITS

With the help of satavari powder, one can prepare a nutritious and immunity-boosting beverage. Mix 500-1000 mg of the powder in a cup of milk with a pinch of turmeric, black pepper, and green cardamom. Bring to a simmer. Once cooled down, add honey and enjoy.

COSMETIC CURES

Satavari is a traditional Ayurvedic herb that can help re-balance levels of oestrogen, progesterone and testosterone, and help prevent acne and outbreaks. The constituents of the shatavari root help reduce the free-radical skin damage that cause wrinkles. The plant also helps prevent collagen breakdown, which maintains the skin's elasticity.

The name, Satavari, is sometimes translated to mean 'she who possesses a hundred husbands' in a reference to its fertility enhancing properties in women.

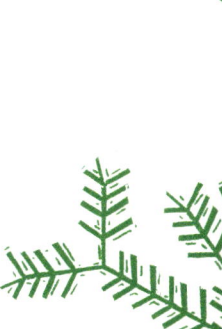

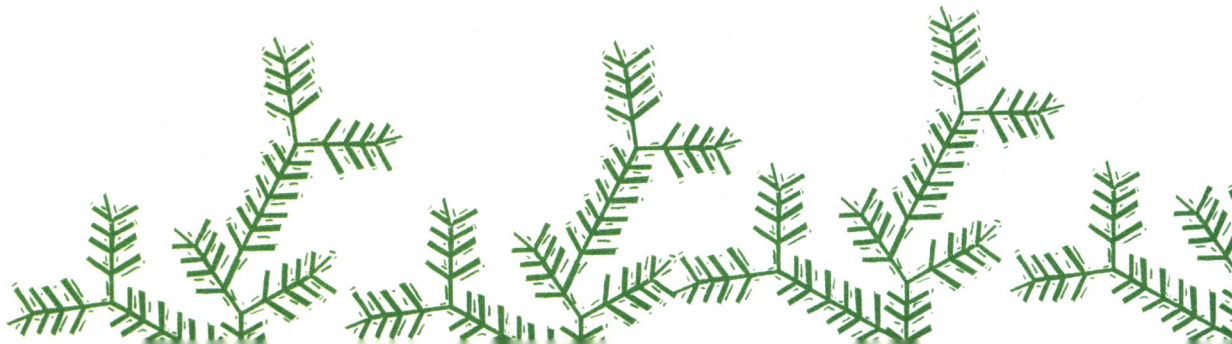

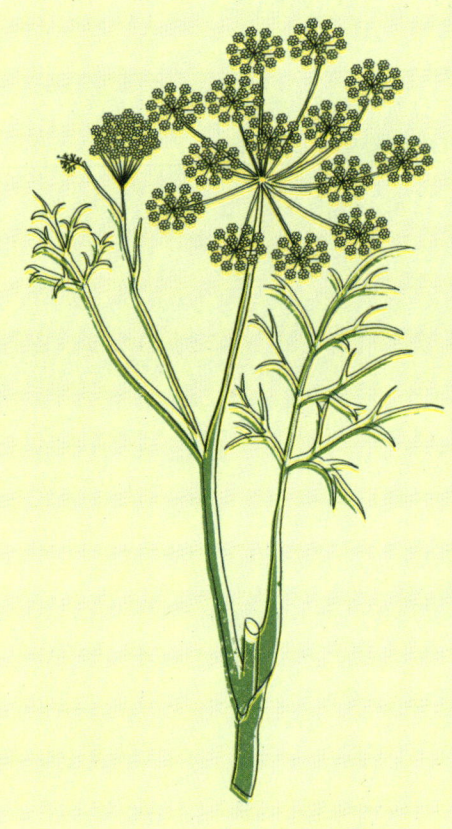

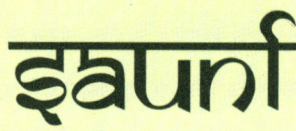

ANISEED/FENNEL

Foeniculum vulgare

SAUNF *Hindi* . **MOURI** *Bangla* . **VARIALI** *Gujarati* . **BADI SOPU** *Kannada* .
BADI SHEP *Marathi* . **SOMBU** *Tamil* . **SOPU/PEDDA JILA KURE** *Telugu*

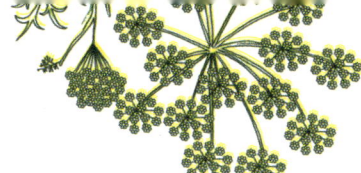
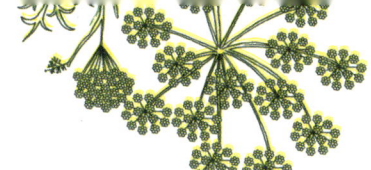

MEDICINAL PROPERTIES

Saunf is the fruit (not the seeds, as often cited) of the fennel plant. It is known to trigger the secretion of digestive juices and enzymes, and thus helps digestion. It is also an excellent laxative for constipation and other gastrointestinal maladies such as IBS. Saunf steeped in hot water makes an amazing tea that helps with menstrual cramps and hot flushes.

Saunf contains vitamin A and other nutrients that help with healthy vision and help treat respiratory ailments because they help fight mucus formation in the lungs. It improves the circulations of blood, hence is useful for those suffering from high blood pressure – its high potassium content balances the sodium level, enabling normal blood pressure. Drinking saunf water made by combining saunf seeds with a couple of ilaichi seeds, has many benefits: having a glass before bedtime, helps in a good night's sleep. A simple and effective remedy for bad breath, it is advised to suck on saunf seeds, not chew them. An amazing remedy for severe headaches can be made with making a decoction of saunf with adrak powder and putting four drops each, when just warm, into both nostrils. Additionally, warming a cotton cloth with some fennel leaves tied in it, is very effective to relieve joint pains.

CULINARY BENEFITS

Saunf is one of the most commonly used spices in Indian cuisine across different parts of the country. Due to its digestive properties, it is usually included in deep fried dishes to provide a balance. It is one of the main spices in the famous 'paanch phoran', used widely for tempering in Assamese, Bengali and Oriya cuisine. It is also an important component of the combination of spices used in pickles and chutneys. In powder form, saunf a very important component of Kashmiri cooking, often used in combination with adrak powder. Another very important use of saunf is in the preparation of a cooling drink called 'thandai', meaning 'that which cools'. This is a great antidote to the dry heat of Indian summers. Additionally, tea made from saunf is also a great digestive.

COSMETIC CURES

Saunf protects the skin from free radical damange, and improves skin longevity. It is widely used to treat conditions such as acne, rashes and dryness of skin.

Ishaq Ali of Sirohi, Rajasthan has earned himself the title of 'Saunf King' ever since he has demonstrated high yields in saunf production from his lands by continuously experimenting with using new methods of transplantation and cultivation on seeds saved from earlier generations, while applying new water-saving techniques in a dry area.

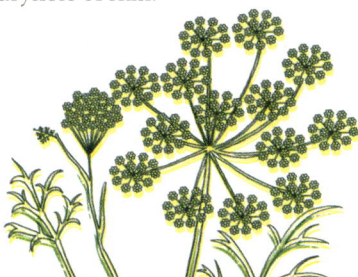
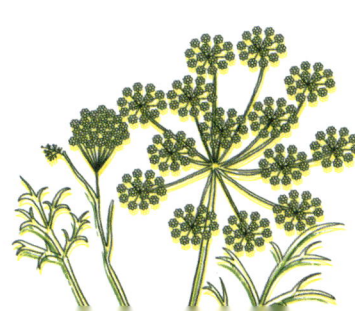

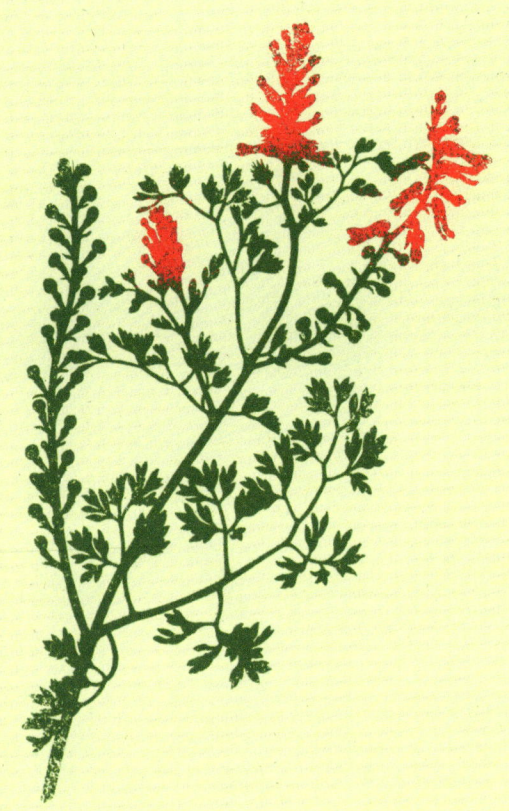

shahtar

COMMON FUMITORY
Fumaria officinalis Linn.

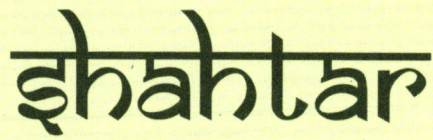

SHAHTAR/PITPAPRA *Hindi* . SHOTARA/PIPAPAPRA *Bangla* .
PITTAPAPRA *Marathi* . PITTAPAPDO *Gujarati* . PARPATAKA *Kannada* .
SHAHTERAH *Kashmiri* . PARPATA/PARPATAKA *Sanskrit* .
TURU/THUSHA *Tamil* . CHATA-RASHI *Telugu*

MEDICINAL PROPERTIES

The whole plant of shahtar is ascribed to possess medicinal virtues and is widely used in Ayurvedic and Unani systems of medicine. In traditional systems of medicine, the plant is reputed for its anthelmintic, diuretic, diaphoretic, laxative, cholagogue, stomachic and sedative activities, and is used to purify blood. The whole plant is also used in the preparation of important Ayurvedic medicinal preparations and polyherbal liver formulations. Shahtar possesses important pharmacological activities like smooth muscle relaxant, spasmogenic and spasmolytic, analgesic, anti-inflammatory, neuropharmacological and antibacterial activities.

Across different texts and commentaries written on Ayurveda over time, this plant has been extolled for its virtues. In Charaka and Sushruta texts, shahtar is recommended for treatment of fevers and blood disorders. In Sushruta, the plant has also been recommended in case of chronic skin diseases, urinary diseases and cough.

In Unani medicine, the plant is used as 'shaahtara' and is an important ingredient in a number of blood purifying compounds. Shahtar can be used to fight poison of any kind in the body. If available fresh, a couple of tea spoons of the juice from the crushed plant or a decoction of the powder of the dried plant can be used also to fight the side effects of strong medicines. Along with giloy, tulasi and some peppercorns, a decoction is used to reduce fevers, especially recurrent fevers – if had for a couple of months regularly.

Shahtar helps in treating nausea and is a strong digestive stimulant as it helps in breaking down food. Shahtar also has cold properties that helps in soothing areas with insect bites and reduce pain, itching and swelling.

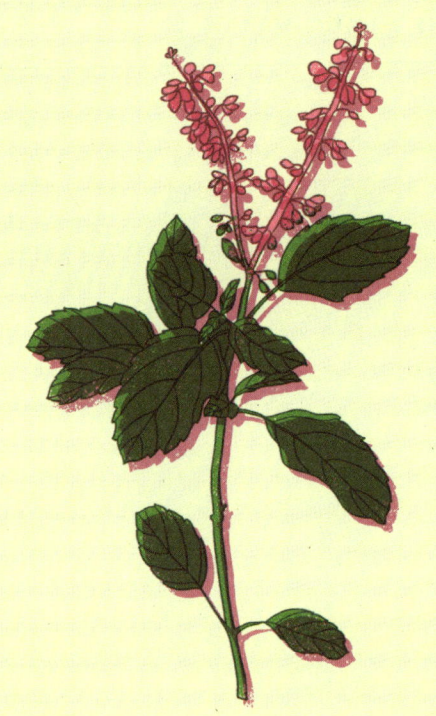

shyamtulasi

PURPLE LEAF BASIL

Aegeratum conyzoides Linn.

SHYAMTULASI *Hindi* . **BRINDA/AJUKA/MANJARI** *Sanskrit* .
TULASA *Marathi* . **VISHNU TULSI** *Kannada*

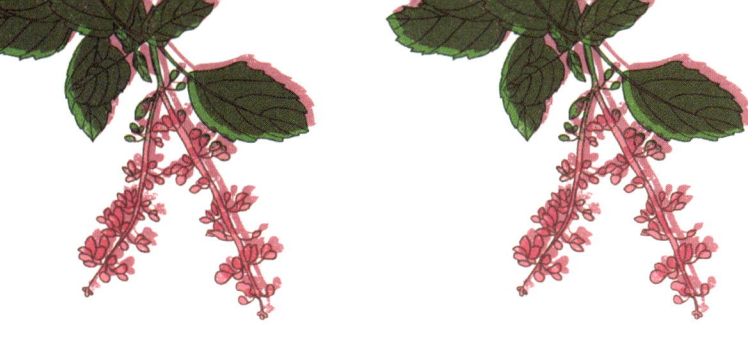
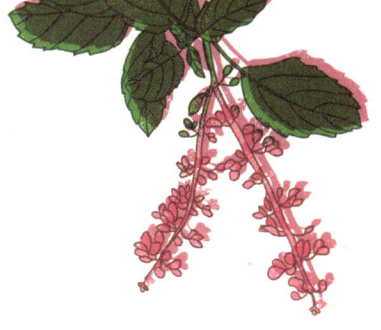

Shyamtulasi is a tropical, aromatic invasive annual herb mainly distributed over the tropical and subtropical regions of the world. Its virtues are so well known and used so widely that many households continue to have at least one plant growing in an open space somewhere.

It is one of those plants like the peepal (*Ficus religiosa*) that people offer a lamp in prayer to.

MEDICINAL PROPERTIES
This plant acts as a healing agent in various kinds of diseases which include dysentery, diarrhoea, skin diseases, cuts and sores, epilepsy, common cold, headaches, boils, eczema, and also act as an insecticide and nematodes. In fact, for open and long festering wounds, a paste of the leaves is very effective for healing. This is a great antidote to any kind of fever – just a spoonful juice from some leaves mixed with honey or a decoction of leaves mixed with honey works to reduce fevers immediately. Due to its antimicrobial property, it is used as a mouthwash and also in killing head lice. For children, it is a very effective deworming agent.

COSMETIC CURES
Once the leaves are boiled in rice water, the rice water can be used as a hair conditioning shampoo. It is also used as a base for skin-conditioning products in the cosmetic industry. Shyamtulasi also provides optimal nourishment to hair and rejuvenates them from root to tip. Apply the mixture of 10-15 ground tulasi leaves to your scalp and allow it to rest for an hour. Repeat this three times a week for a month to see visible results.

RITUAL USE
Shyamtulasi is used in some Hindu rituals along with the green tulasi. The plant is worshipped twice a day – once in the morning and then in the evening, when a lamp or candle is lit near the plant.

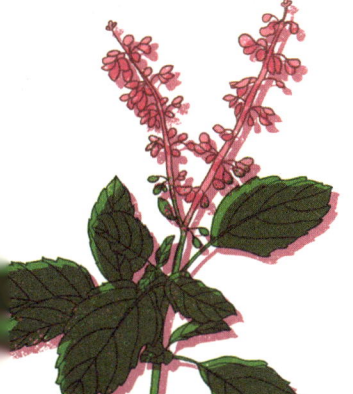
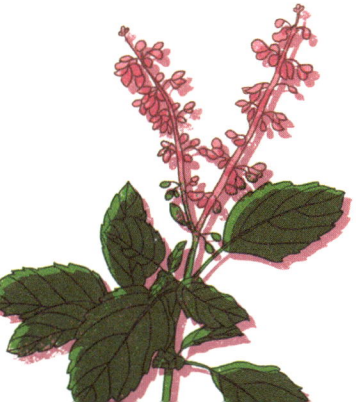
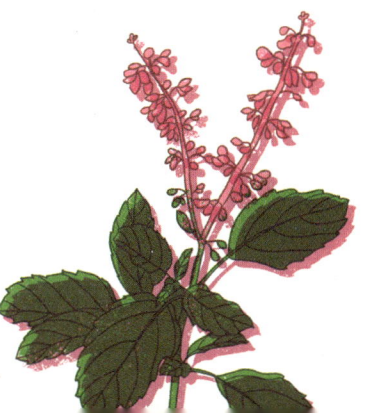

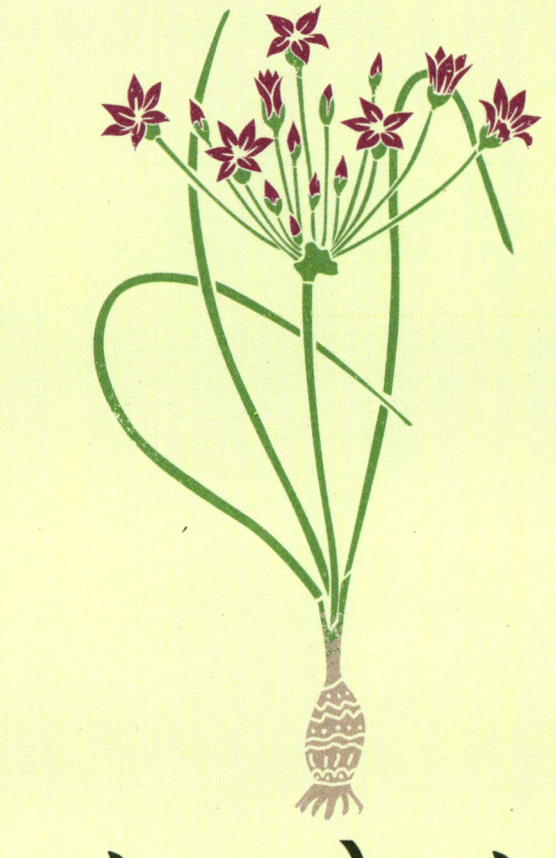

tej anglasing

CHINESE ONION

Allium chinensis

TEJ ANGLASING *Naga*

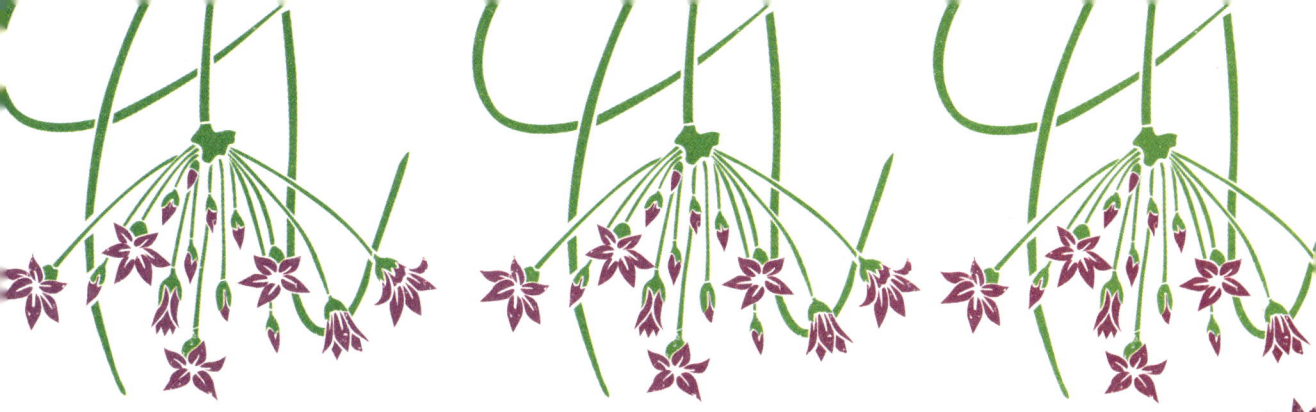

MEDICINAL PROPERTIES

Traditionally, local health practitioners boil the ground bulb in mustard oil and rub it on the body to reduce fever. They also use it to cure stomach ache and apply it on wounds to heal them. Tej anglasing possesses antimicrobial, anti-fungal, hemolytic, anxiolytic, antiviral, analgesic, anti-inflammatory, antioxidant, anthelmintic and antidiabetic activities.

COSMETIC CURES

It is understood to be a good cosmetic ingredient for skin conditioning as it contains a significant amount of vitamin C, though the same is not widely used yet.

CULINARY BENEFITS

Tej anglasing is an excellent source of essential minerals including calcium, magnesium and phosphorus – that support healthy bones and facilitate cellular energy metabolism. The bulbs and leaves are edible either raw or cooked. Utilized as spices and condiments either in dry or in fresh form for preparing almost all the traditional recipes. This herb can act as a supplementary food at the time of food scarcity. In hill areas of Manipur, the inflorescences are eaten raw with dry beef Ringneokashai or eaten in boiled vegetable soup. The bulbs and cloves are pickled in Northeast India, where it is popularly called Naga garlic.

Tej Anglasing contains compounds like allicin and other sulphurs which helps reduce blood cholesterol levels and acts as a tonic to the digestive system.

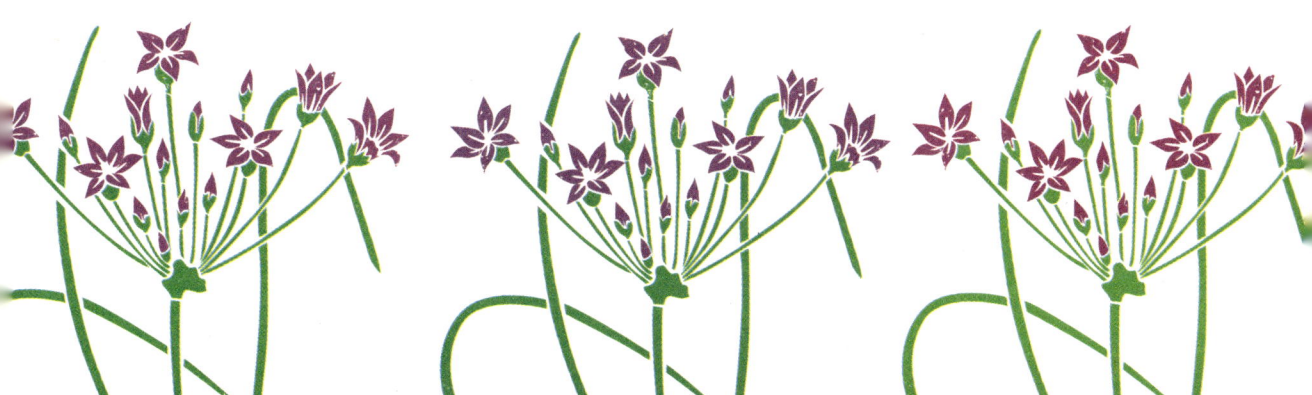

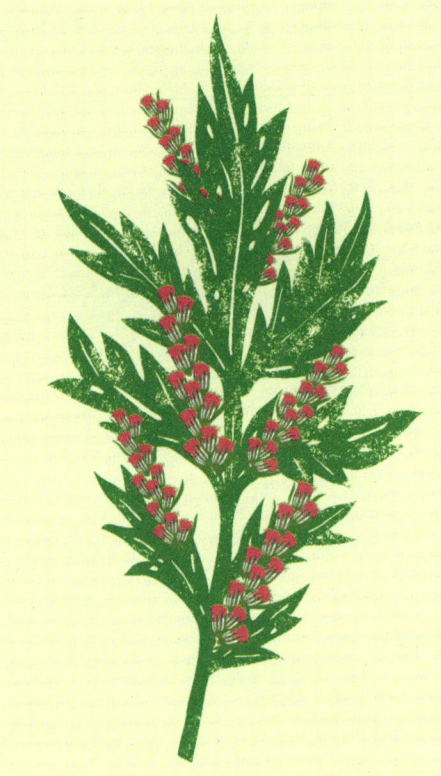

tetaypati

COMMON MUGWORT

Artemesia vulgaris L.

TETAYPATI *Nepali* . **DAMANAKA** *Sanskrit* . **DOUNA** *Hindi* .
DONA *Bangla* . **DEMORO** *Gujarati*

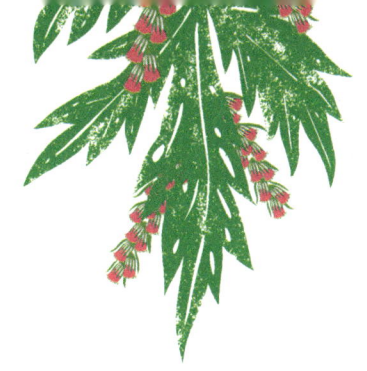
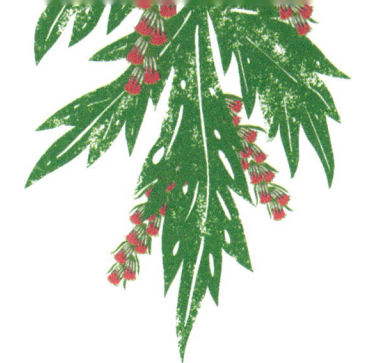

MEDICINAL PROPERTIES

Tetaypati is used in Ayurveda to primarily treat skin diseases, IBS, bleeding and several toxic conditions, along with maintaining the body tri-humours (Tridosaghna). It is medicinally used to cure headache, asthma and stomach ache. The leaf extract is used on cuts and bruises, to stop nose bleeding, curing measles amongst infants, and also used as an antiseptic.

COSMETIC CURES

It possesses a cleanser effect and is utilized as a purifying agent. The extract is denoted as skin conditioning, anti-oxidant and with anti-wrinkle agents.

CULINARY BENEFITS

Tetaypati is rich in vitamin C and unsaturated fatty acids. The young stems can be added to salads and the leaves can be cooked as a vegetable. The bruised leaves are used in the bath for sound skin, and the root is utilized as a tonic as well as a spice.

RITUAL USE

The plant is often used as an offering to the gods, or hung in a bundle at the doorway to the house, or used in a bundle to sweep and clean the floor.

Dried leaves of the plant are often smoked to promote lucid dreaming, and the smoke from the burnt leaves also help repulse mosquitoes and insects.

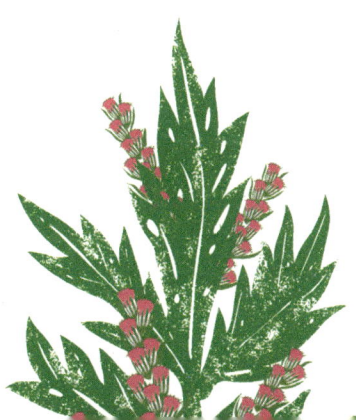
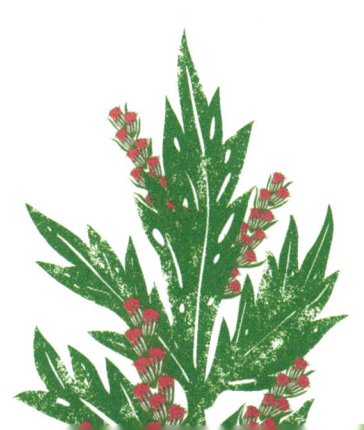

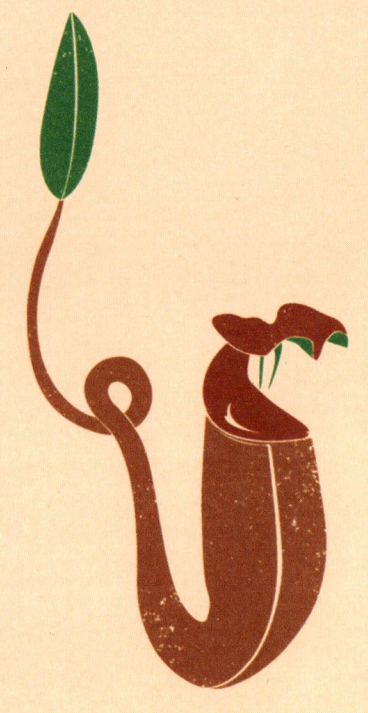

tiew rakot

MONKEY CUPS/INDIAN PITCHER PLANT
Nepenthes khasiana hook

TIEW RAKOT *Khasi*

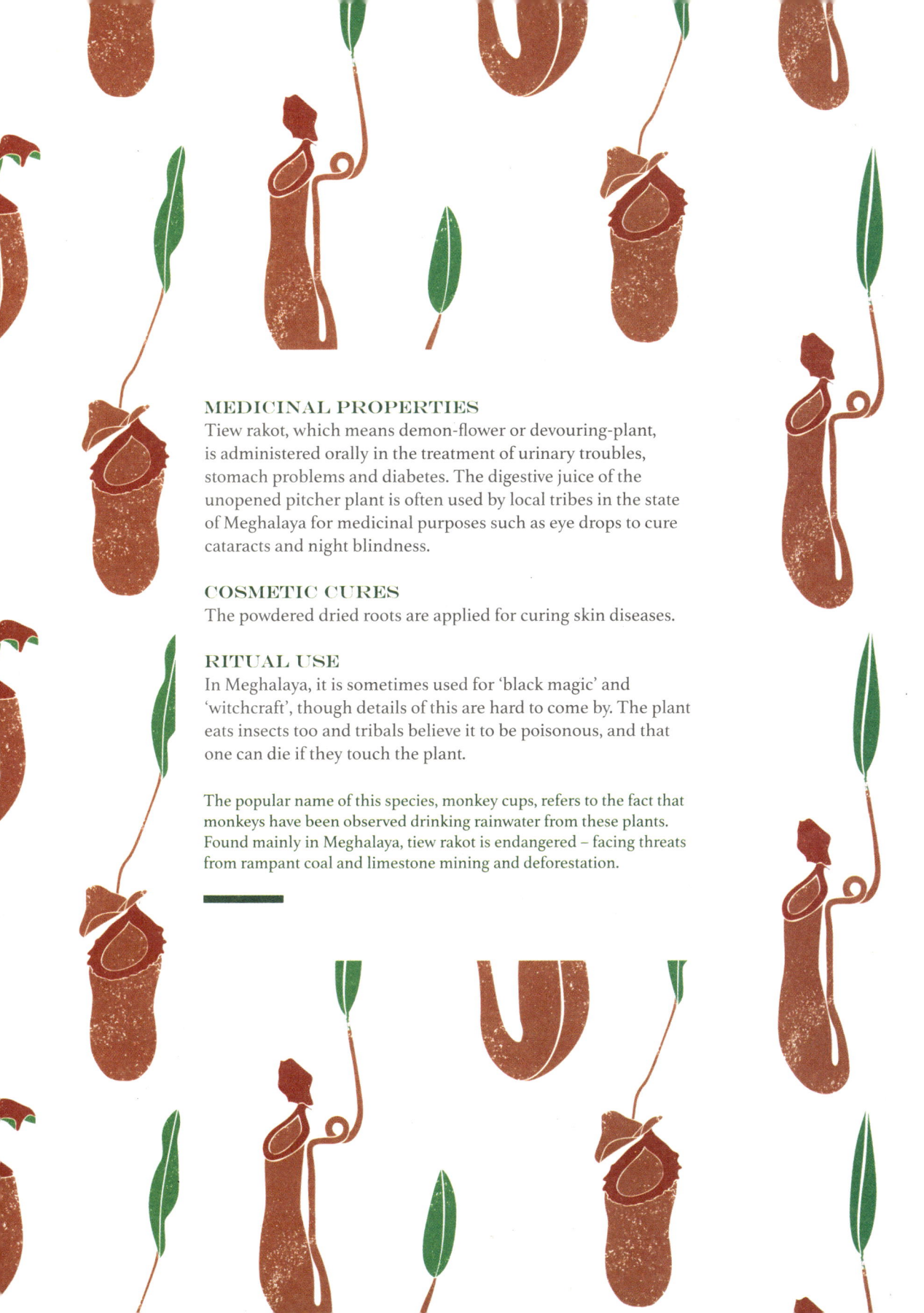

MEDICINAL PROPERTIES

Tiew rakot, which means demon-flower or devouring-plant, is administered orally in the treatment of urinary troubles, stomach problems and diabetes. The digestive juice of the unopened pitcher plant is often used by local tribes in the state of Meghalaya for medicinal purposes such as eye drops to cure cataracts and night blindness.

COSMETIC CURES

The powdered dried roots are applied for curing skin diseases.

RITUAL USE

In Meghalaya, it is sometimes used for 'black magic' and 'witchcraft', though details of this are hard to come by. The plant eats insects too and tribals believe it to be poisonous, and that one can die if they touch the plant.

The popular name of this species, monkey cups, refers to the fact that monkeys have been observed drinking rainwater from these plants. Found mainly in Meghalaya, tiew rakot is endangered – facing threats from rampant coal and limestone mining and deforestation.

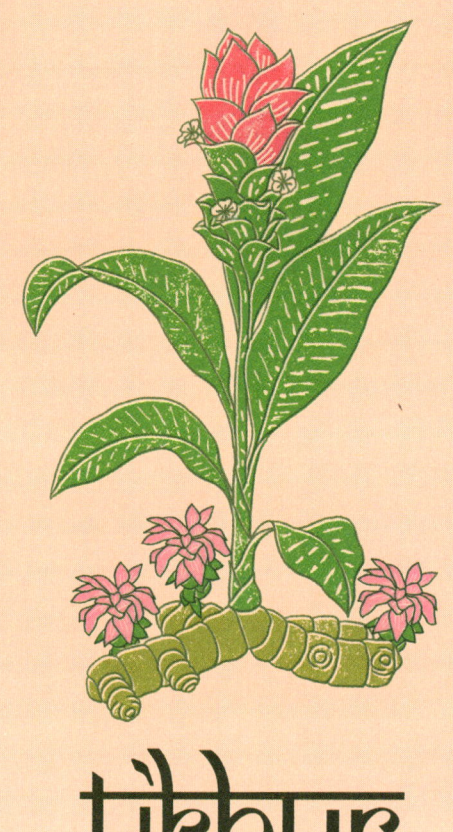

tikhur

WILD/EAST INDIAN ARROWROOT/ NARROW-LEAVED TURMERIC

Curcuma angustifolia Roxb.

TIKHUR *Hindi* . KEURI HALODHU *Bangla* . YAIPAN *Meitei* .
KOVVA *Malayalam* . TAVAKSIRA *Sanskrit* .
TAVAKILA *Marathi* . ARAKUT-KIZHAGU *Tamil*

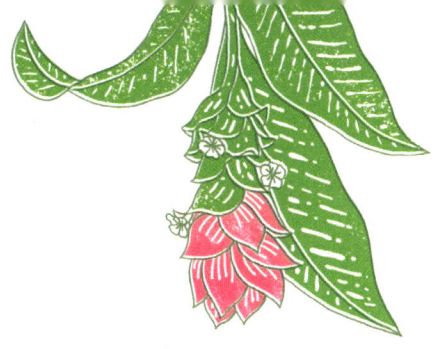
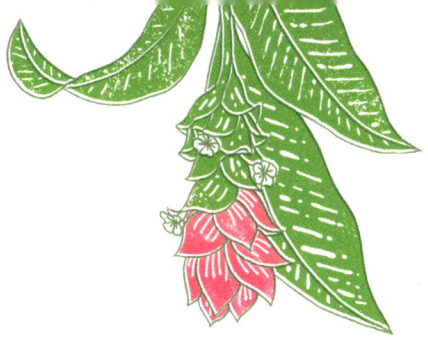

MEDICINAL PROPERTIES

The roots of this plant can be ground into flour, which is then mixed together with milk or water to form a meal that is highly nutritious and also easily digested. It is especially suitable for infants, children with weak constitution and invalids. It is used with milk to treat burning urination, fever, acidity, and gastric reflux disorder. It can also treat diarrhoea, when taken with hot water, and with honey, to treat cough and dyspnoea. Combining the juice of the roots with lime juice helps cure stomach aches.

The Rajbanshis of north Bengal use the rhizomes of this plant for the preparation of a weaning food for babies, locally called *Shotti*.

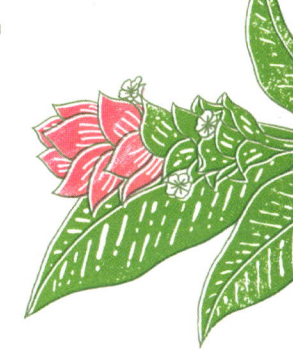

CULINARY BENEFITS

Several dishes are prepared using the rhizomes. Tikhur burfi is among the most popular, especially during fasts that require abstinence from cereals. The burfi removes extra heat from body and helps develop resistance against common diseases. In tribal belts of Chhattisgarh, which are rich in natural population of tikhur, the natives prepare its dishes in hot summer, including a sherbet, a cooling drink made with the starch of the plant.

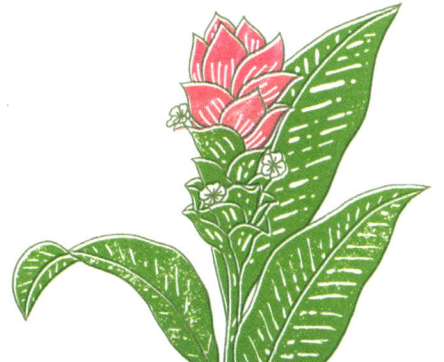
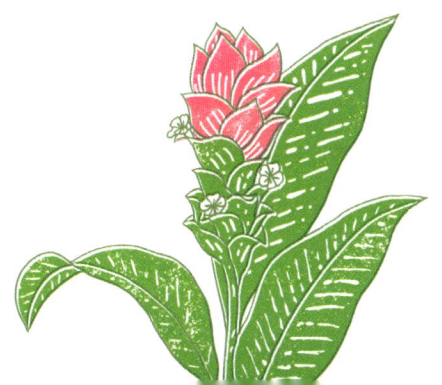

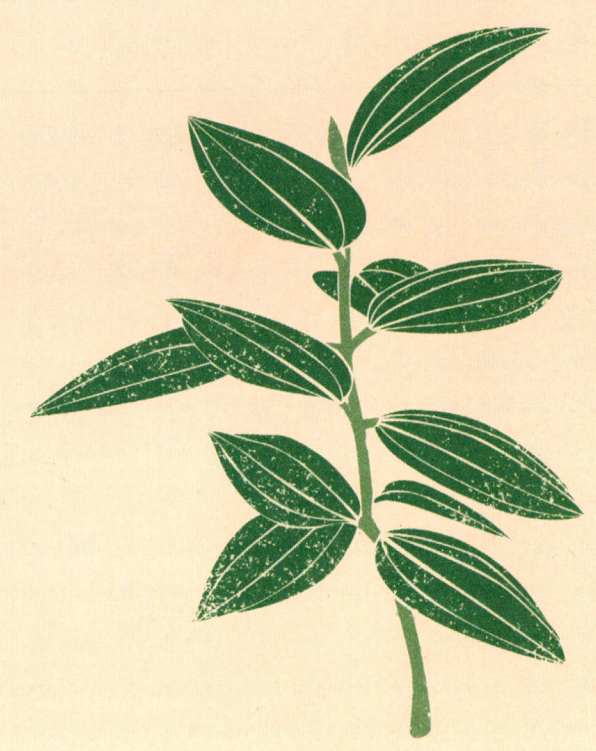

tincham

PENANGLANUS

Adenia penangiana

TINCHAM *Nicobarese*

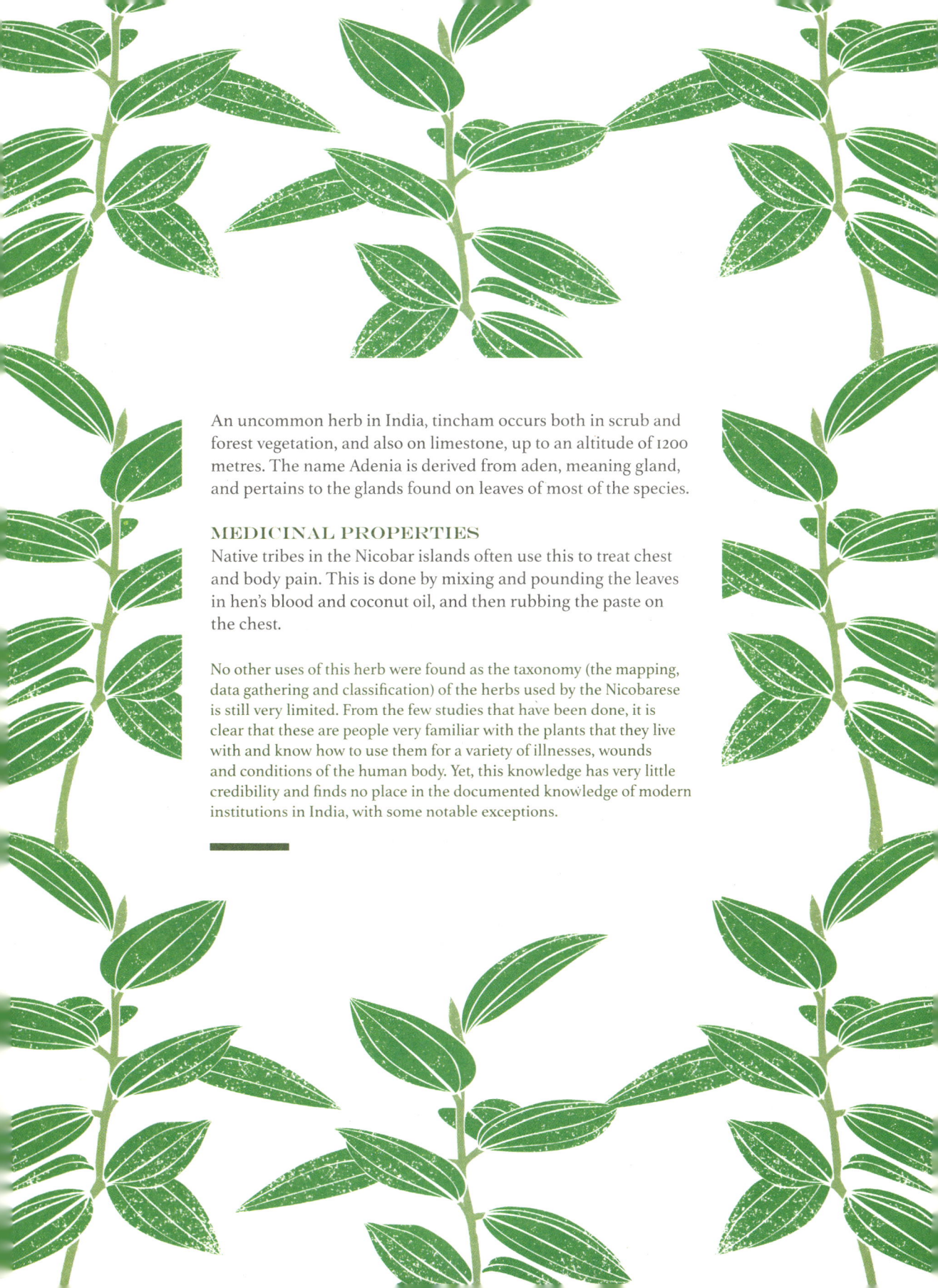

An uncommon herb in India, tincham occurs both in scrub and forest vegetation, and also on limestone, up to an altitude of 1200 metres. The name Adenia is derived from aden, meaning gland, and pertains to the glands found on leaves of most of the species.

MEDICINAL PROPERTIES

Native tribes in the Nicobar islands often use this to treat chest and body pain. This is done by mixing and pounding the leaves in hen's blood and coconut oil, and then rubbing the paste on the chest.

No other uses of this herb were found as the taxonomy (the mapping, data gathering and classification) of the herbs used by the Nicobarese is still very limited. From the few studies that have been done, it is clear that these are people very familiar with the plants that they live with and know how to use them for a variety of illnesses, wounds and conditions of the human body. Yet, this knowledge has very little credibility and finds no place in the documented knowledge of modern institutions in India, with some notable exceptions.

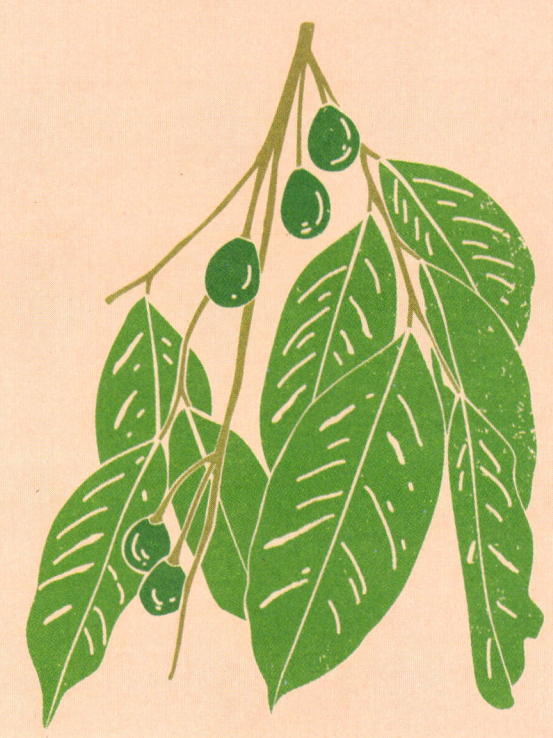

toirulelu

Drypetes a ndamanica

TOIRULELU *Andamanese*

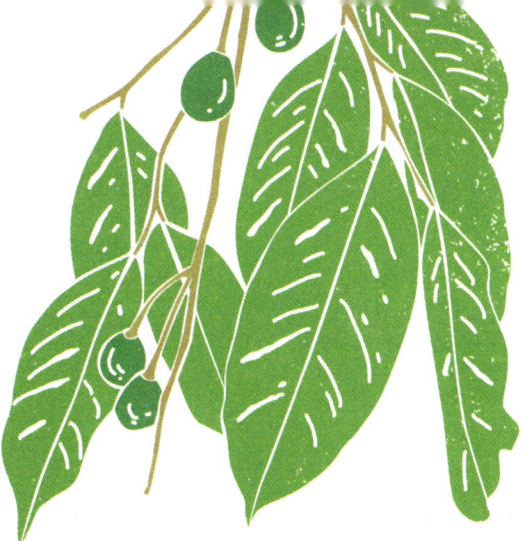
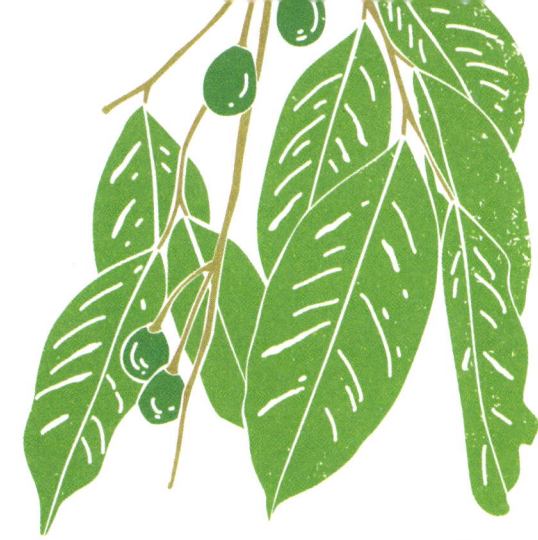
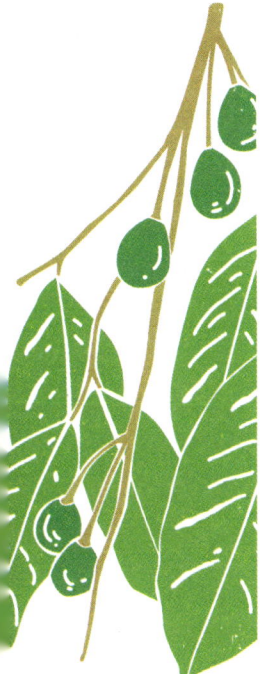

Another uncommon herb, toirulelu is an endangered plant, noted in the International Union for Conservation of Nature's list of endangered species since 1998.

MEDICINAL PROPERTIES

The leaves of this plant are used to treat chest pain. They are also used as an antidote for snake bites.

What is most evident is how little is really known about this herb or many of the others in the Andaman Nicobar islands. While there is a good documentation of the flowers of the region, medicinal plants are less well documented, and publication after publication by scientists (listed at the end of the book) rues this fact. Some have actually taken up very serious studies and sought to map their existence and condition but do believe that factors such as indiscriminate encroachments on many lands, felling and random building work pose grave danger to the delicate ecological balance of these species.

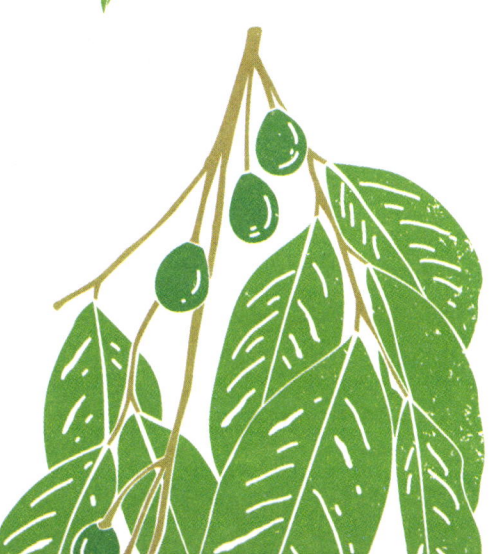
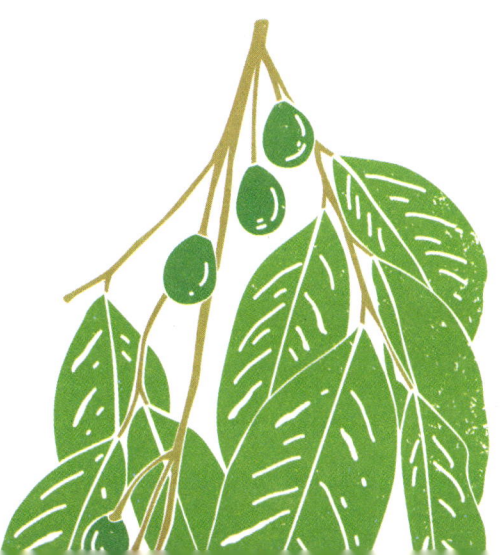

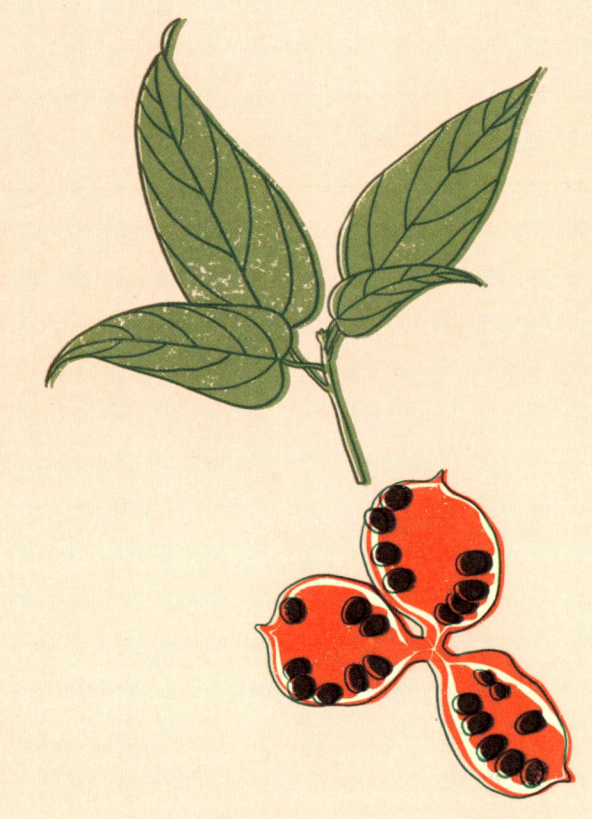

tosamu kantisembal

COMMON STERCULIA
Sterculia parviflora

TOSAMU KANTISEMBAL *Andamanese*

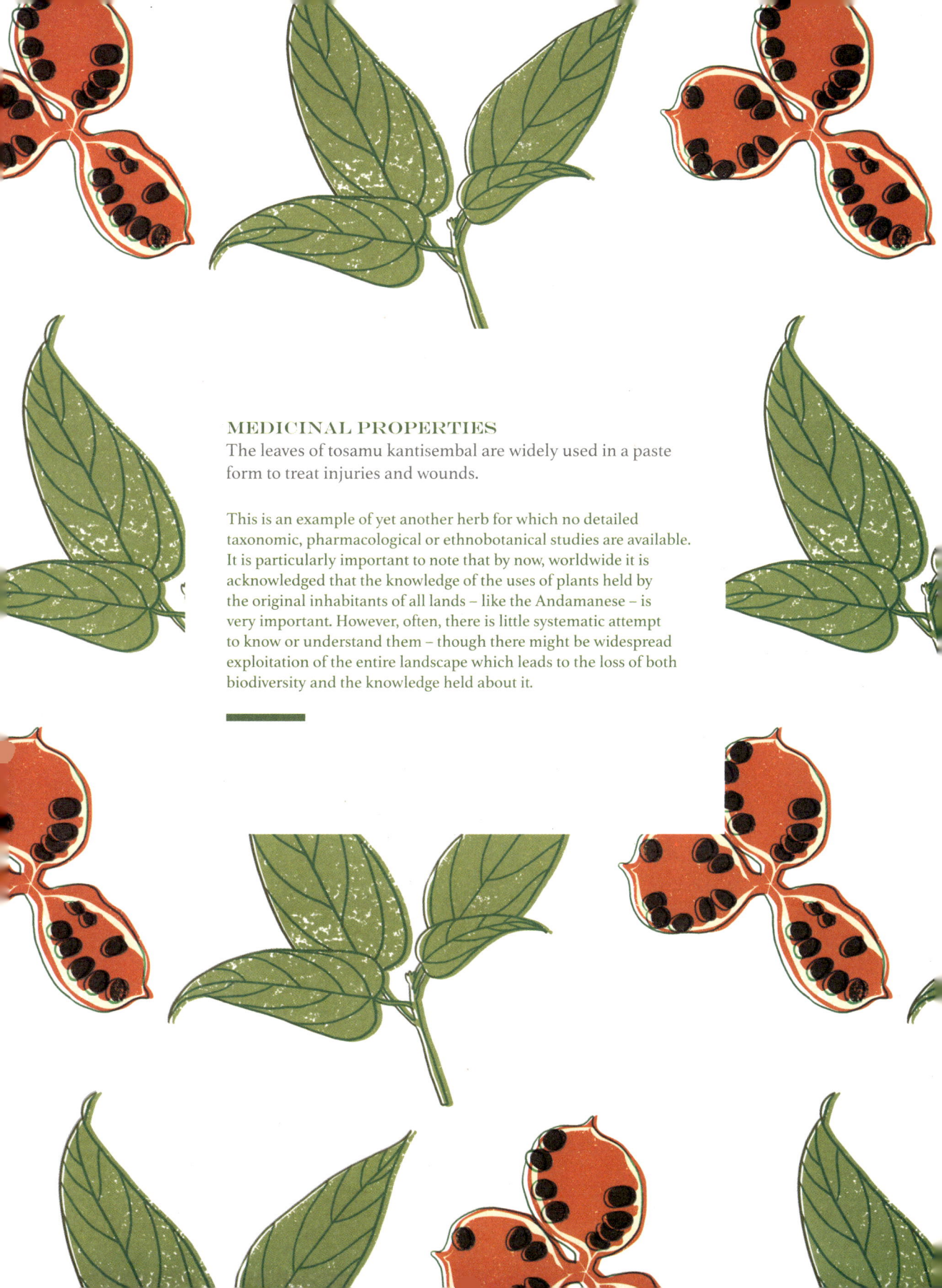

MEDICINAL PROPERTIES

The leaves of tosamu kantisembal are widely used in a paste form to treat injuries and wounds.

This is an example of yet another herb for which no detailed taxonomic, pharmacological or ethnobotanical studies are available. It is particularly important to note that by now, worldwide it is acknowledged that the knowledge of the uses of plants held by the original inhabitants of all lands – like the Andamanese – is very important. However, often, there is little systematic attempt to know or understand them – though there might be widespread exploitation of the entire landscape which leads to the loss of both biodiversity and the knowledge held about it.

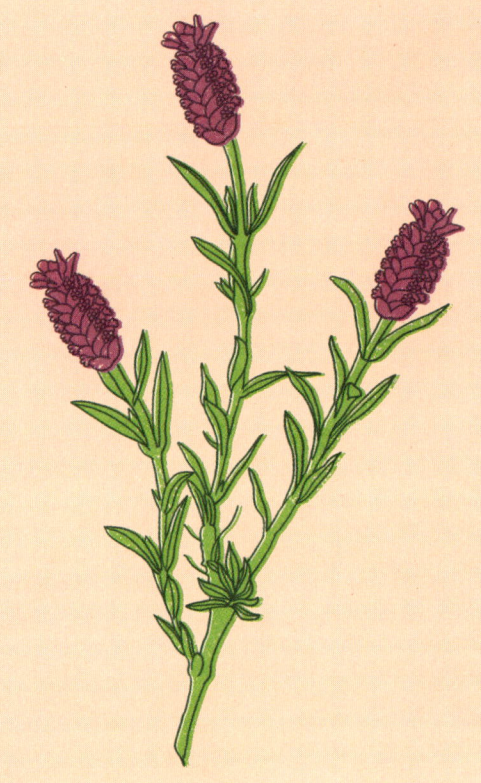

uste khadoos

COMMON LAVENDER/FRENCH LAVENDER

Lavandula stoechas

USTE KHADOOS *Urdu* . **TUNTUNA** *Bangla* . **DHARU/ ALPHAGANDHARU/PHULLARI** *Hindi* . **KALE WOUTH** *Kashmiri* . **LAVENDARABEPHULA** *Gujarati* . **PANIRAPPU** *Tamil*

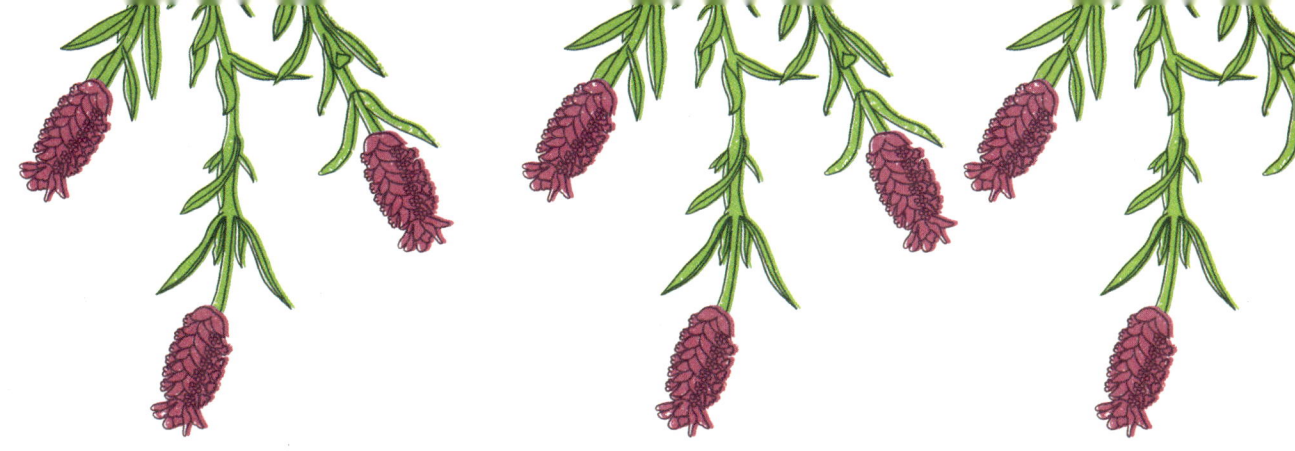

MEDICINAL PROPERTIES

In the Unani system of medicine, the plant is known as Jarub-i Dimagh (broom of brain) due to its scavenging property of evacuating morbid matters from the brain, especially ones that can cause neurological disorders like insomnia, amnesia and melancholia. Various studies on its effect on nervous system have been explored by researchers which can be attributed to the bioactive compounds present in it. It therefore helps manage depression and anxiety, apart from strengthening mind and curing mental fatigue.

Uste khadoos is used in combination with other herbs for headaches and migraine as it helps reduce the over activities of pain-sensitive areas of the brain. It is also given to provide relief from cough and is effective in sinusitis. A paste made from its flowers, when applied on the joints, helps relieve pain to a large extent.

This plant came to India from the Mediterranean region. Due to its limited area of growth, it is not deeply entrenched in folk use. However, in the different countries of the region where it comes from, it has uses for menstrual regularity (when drunk in the form of a tea) and also in wound healing, as an expectorant. Everywhere though, its principal use is in a range of nervous disorders, including epilepsy and migraine.

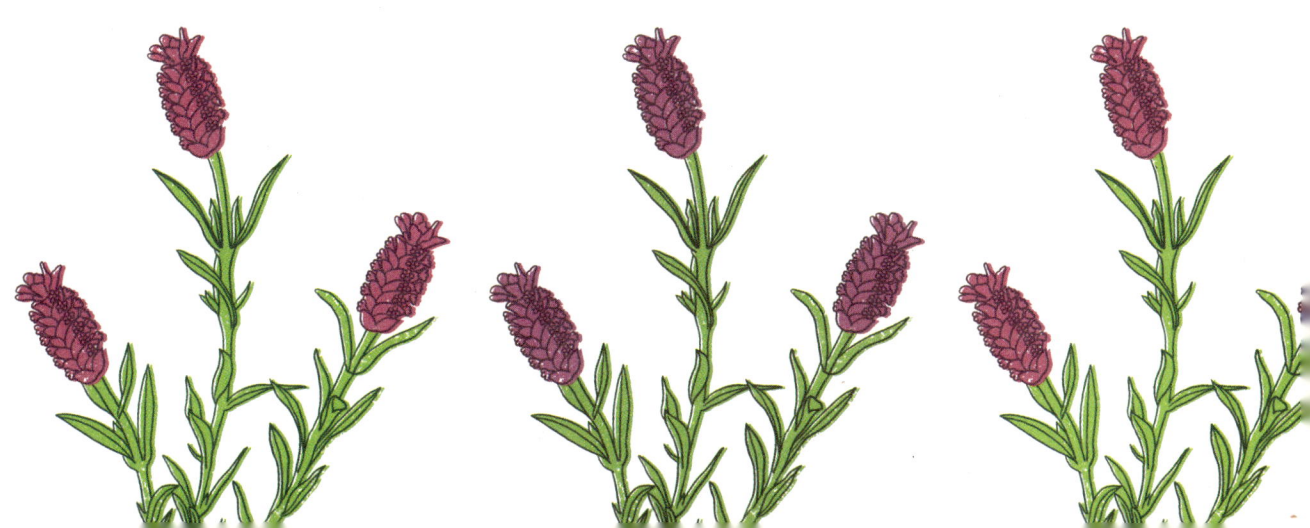

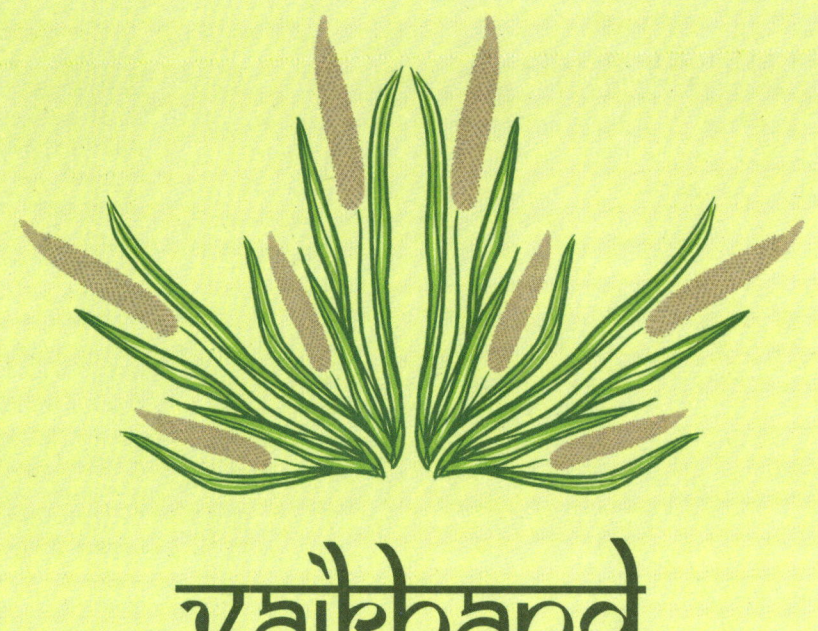

vaikhand

BEEWORT/MYRTLE GRASS/ GERMAN GINGER

Acorus calamus

VAIKHAND/ VACA/VEKHANDAS *Marathi* . BACH/GORA-BACH *Hindi* .
UGRAGANDHA/UGRA/SADGRANTHA *Sanskrit* . WAJA-E-TURKI *Urdu* .
VARCH/GHODAVACA *Punjabi* . GHODUVAJ/GHODVACH *Gujarati* .
ATHIBAJE/BAJE/ BAJE GIDA/DAGADE/KAVANA/NAARU BAERU/VASA
Kannada . VAYAMBU *Malayalam* . VASAMBU/PILLAI MARUNTHO *Tamil* .
VASA *Telugu*

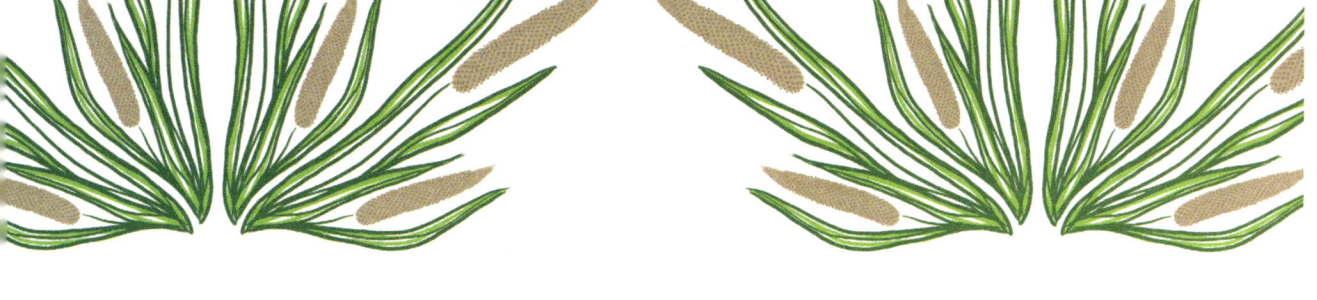

MEDICINAL PROPERTIES

Vaikhand is used for gastrointestinal ailments including ulcers, inflammation of the stomach lining (gastritis), flatulence, upset stomach and loss of appetite (anorexia). In Ayurveda, this is a rejuvenating herb due to its effect on the nervous system. Bitter in taste and often used in its dried form, one should take it along with honey to help manage speech disorders. Its consumption also helps in the management of cough by promoting the removal of sputum from the air passages due to its expectorant property.

Vaikhand also helps improve memory by fighting against cell damage caused by free radicals due to its antioxidant property, thereby improving behavioural changes, memory and mental performance.

It also provides relief in the case of kidney stones by increasing urine production due to its diuretic property. Its essential oil is considered useful in reducing pain and inflammation when applied externally.

COSMETIC CURES

A paste of powdered vaikhand and water can be applied on the skin for nourishment and to control various skin infections. Topical application of the powder with Triphala powder helps to reduce fat on the belly and thighs.

Vaikhand is often rubbed on a baby's stomach so that the toddler does not get a swollen tongue.

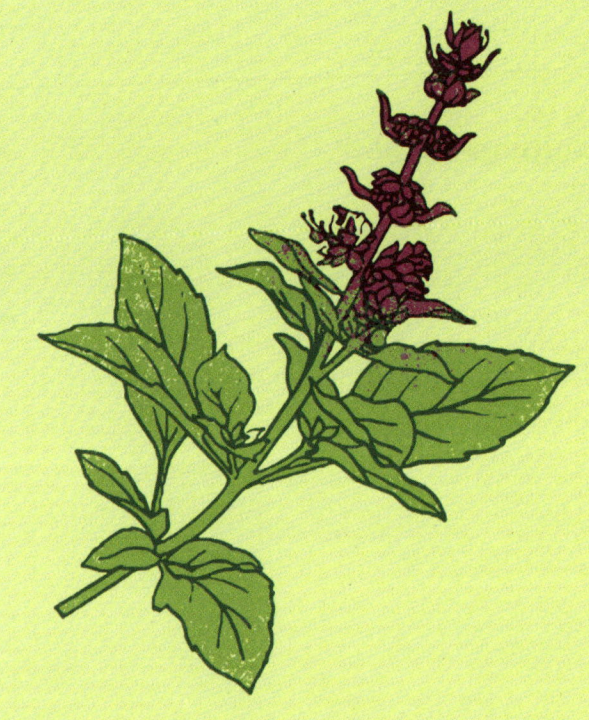

van tulasi/ ram tulasi

BASIL

Ocimum basilicum

VAN TULASI/RAM TULASI *Hindi, Bangla*

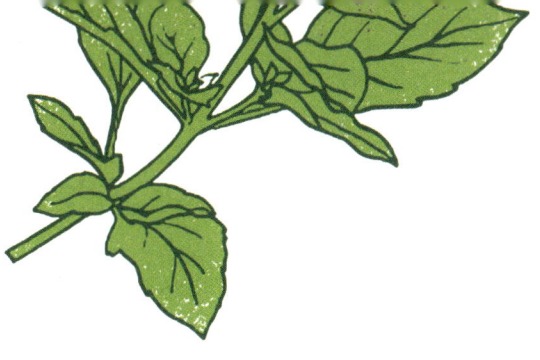
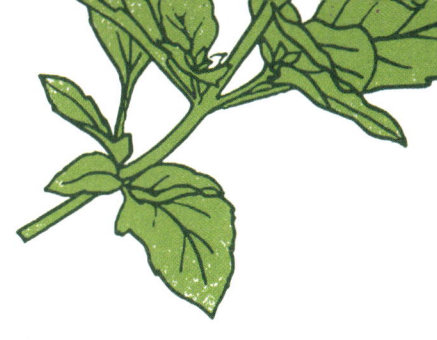

MEDICINAL PROPERTIES

Also known as sweet basil, van tulasi has been used for thousands of years as a culinary and medicinal herb. It acts principally on the digestive and nervous systems – easing flatulence, stomach cramps, colic and indigestion.

The leaves and flowering tops are antispasmodic, aromatic, carminative and digestive in nature. Boiled with water, it provides relief in the case of feverish illnesses, nausea and abdominal cramps. Applied topically, the paste made of leaves is used to treat acne, loss of smell, insect stings, snake-bites and skin infections. The fresh leaves, when chewed moderately, helps improve gum health and prevent mouth ulcers.

CULINARY BENEFITS

Van tulasi is an aromatic herb that is used extensively to add a distinctive aroma and flavour to food. Essential oils extracted from fresh leaves and flowers can be used as aroma additives in food, pharmaceuticals and cosmetics. When consumed in the form of tea, it provides increased physical and mental endurance by adding more oxygen to your bloodstream. For this, steep 3-4 tulasi leaves in warm water, and drink after adding a tablespoon of honey. The herb is also used in the preparation of pasta, pesto sauce and often as a pizza topping with others vegetables.

COSMETIC CURES

Van tulasi has antioxidants which help protect the skin from environmental stressors and reduce the appearance of wrinkles and fine lines. The plant can also help in providing relief from temporary itching. It also has great value when used as a soap base and for shampoos.

RITUAL USE

One among the four broad varieties used in India – rama tulasi, krishna tulasi, amrita tulasi and van tulasi – this plant, too, is planted in the courtyard of homes and worshipped every morning.

Van tulasi is used in a wide variety of home remedies on an everyday basis and as part of the complex medicines that are a hallmark of Ayurvedic and Unani medicines.

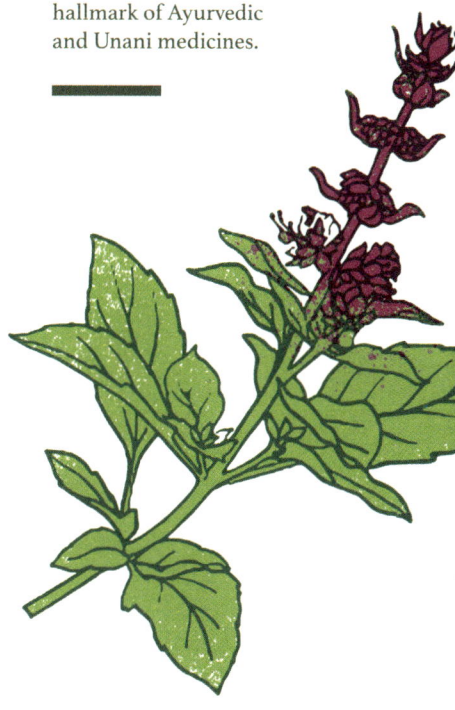
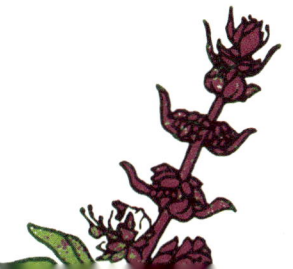
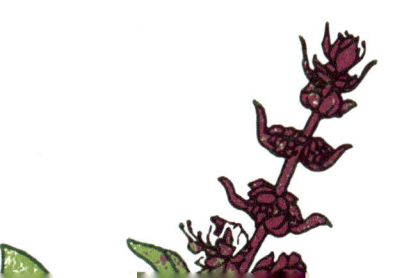

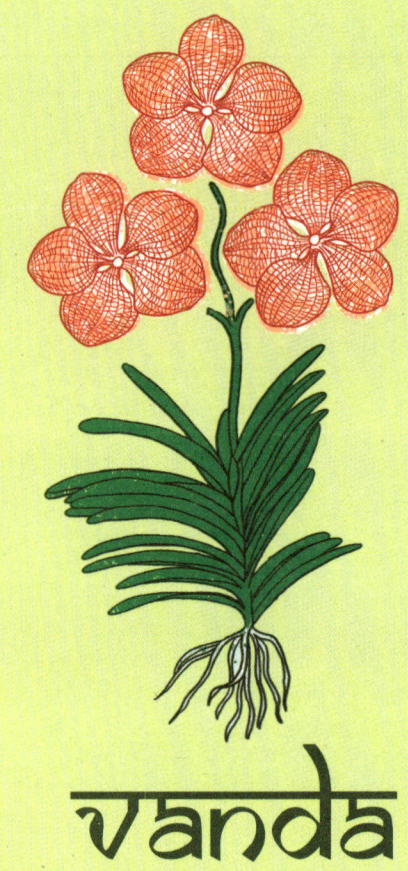

vanda

THE LATTICE-LIKE PATTERNED FLOWER
Vanda tessellata

VANDA/ BANDA/RASNA *Hindi* . RASNA *Bangla* .
RASNA *Marathi* . ATIRASA/GANDHANAKULI *Sanskrit* .
CHITTIVEDURI *Telugu*

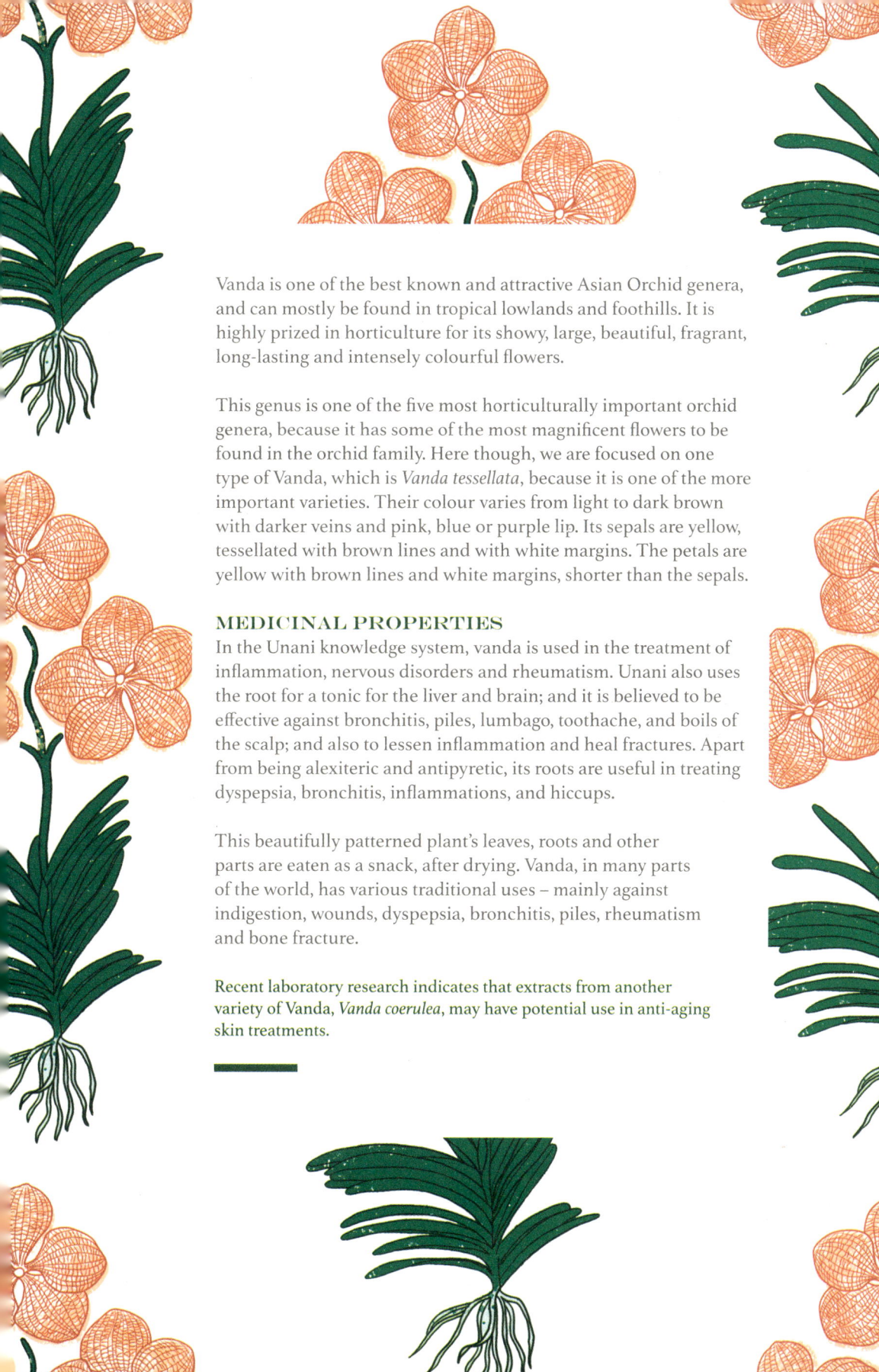

Vanda is one of the best known and attractive Asian Orchid genera, and can mostly be found in tropical lowlands and foothills. It is highly prized in horticulture for its showy, large, beautiful, fragrant, long-lasting and intensely colourful flowers.

This genus is one of the five most horticulturally important orchid genera, because it has some of the most magnificent flowers to be found in the orchid family. Here though, we are focused on one type of Vanda, which is *Vanda tessellata*, because it is one of the more important varieties. Their colour varies from light to dark brown with darker veins and pink, blue or purple lip. Its sepals are yellow, tessellated with brown lines and with white margins. The petals are yellow with brown lines and white margins, shorter than the sepals.

MEDICINAL PROPERTIES

In the Unani knowledge system, vanda is used in the treatment of inflammation, nervous disorders and rheumatism. Unani also uses the root for a tonic for the liver and brain; and it is believed to be effective against bronchitis, piles, lumbago, toothache, and boils of the scalp; and also to lessen inflammation and heal fractures. Apart from being alexiteric and antipyretic, its roots are useful in treating dyspepsia, bronchitis, inflammations, and hiccups.

This beautifully patterned plant's leaves, roots and other parts are eaten as a snack, after drying. Vanda, in many parts of the world, has various traditional uses – mainly against indigestion, wounds, dyspepsia, bronchitis, piles, rheumatism and bone fracture.

Recent laboratory research indicates that extracts from another variety of Vanda, *Vanda coerulea*, may have potential use in anti-aging skin treatments.

zafran

SAFFRON

Crocus sativus

ZAFRAN *Urdu* . **KESAR** *Hindi* . **KESARA** *Gujarati, Marathi* .
KESARI *Kannada* . **JAPHARANA** *Bangla* . **KUNKUMAM** *Malayalam* .
KUNKUMAPPU *Tamil* . **KAASHAAYAM** *Telugu* .
KOUNG/ZAFRAN *Kashmiri*

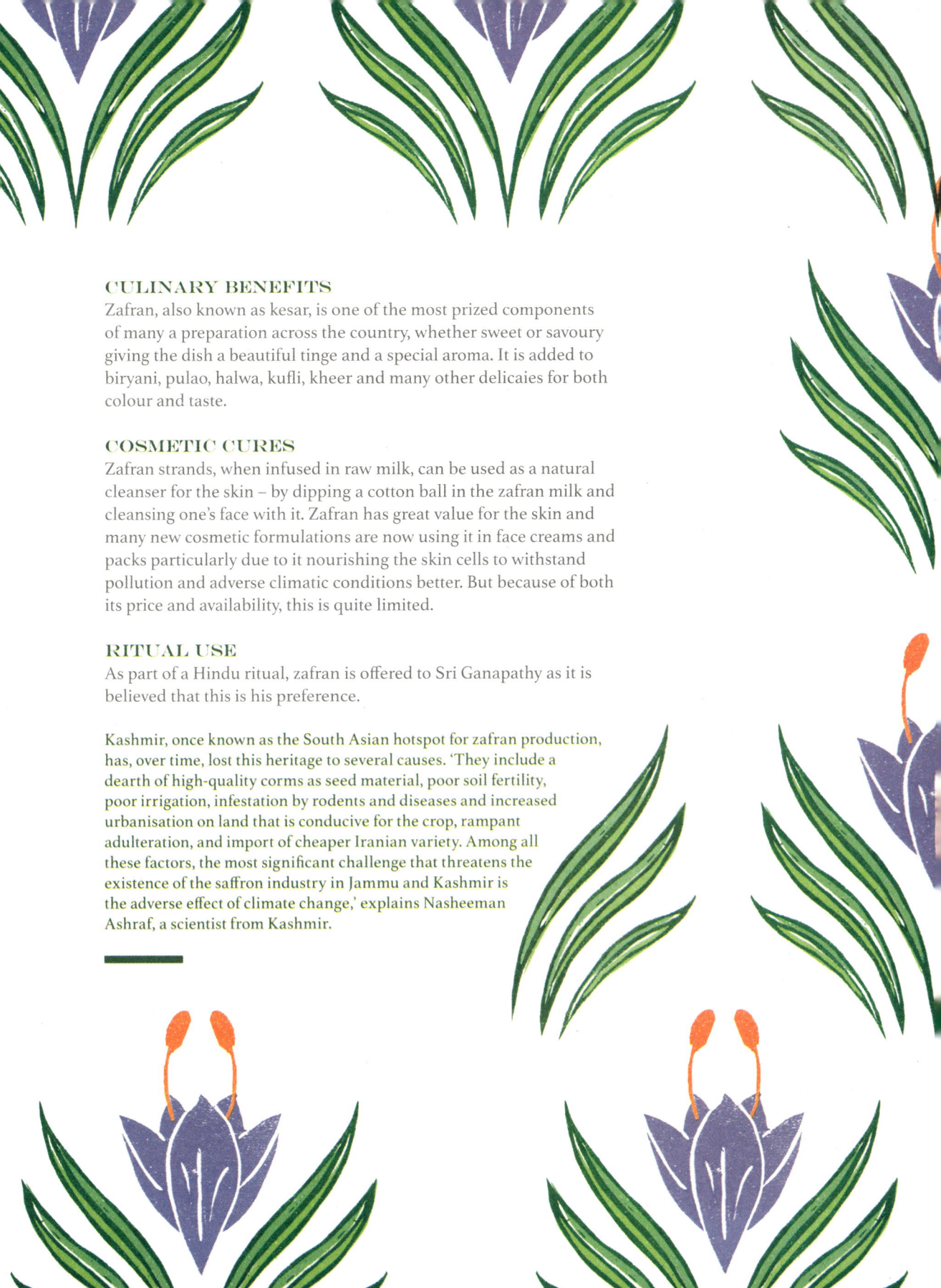

CULINARY BENEFITS

Zafran, also known as kesar, is one of the most prized components of many a preparation across the country, whether sweet or savoury giving the dish a beautiful tinge and a special aroma. It is added to biryani, pulao, halwa, kufli, kheer and many other delicaies for both colour and taste.

COSMETIC CURES

Zafran strands, when infused in raw milk, can be used as a natural cleanser for the skin – by dipping a cotton ball in the zafran milk and cleansing one's face with it. Zafran has great value for the skin and many new cosmetic formulations are now using it in face creams and packs particularly due to it nourishing the skin cells to withstand pollution and adverse climatic conditions better. But because of both its price and availability, this is quite limited.

RITUAL USE

As part of a Hindu ritual, zafran is offered to Sri Ganapathy as it is believed that this is his preference.

Kashmir, once known as the South Asian hotspot for zafran production, has, over time, lost this heritage to several causes. 'They include a dearth of high-quality corms as seed material, poor soil fertility, poor irrigation, infestation by rodents and diseases and increased urbanisation on land that is conducive for the crop, rampant adulteration, and import of cheaper Iranian variety. Among all these factors, the most significant challenge that threatens the existence of the saffron industry in Jammu and Kashmir is the adverse effect of climate change,' explains Nasheeman Ashraf, a scientist from Kashmir.

INDEX

REFERENCES

"Flora of Uttarakhand." 2018. Pahadi Direct. http://pahadidirect.com/flora-of-uttarakhand/

"National Register of Medicinal Plants." n.d. IUCN Portal. Accessed December 20, 2022. https://portals.iucn.org/library/sites/library/files/documents/2000-058.pdf

"Perilla frutescens (L.) Britton | Species." n.d. India Biodiversity Portal. Accessed 10 January 2022. https://indiabiodiversity.org/species/show/259348

"Proven Health Benefits of Black Stone Flower | Aka Kalpasi." n.d. Moolihai.com. Accessed 20 December 2022. https://www.moolihai.com/benefits-of-black-stone-flower/

"The Amazing and Mighty Ginger - Herbal Medicine - NCBI Bookshelf." n.d. NCBI. Accessed January 31, 2022. https://www.ncbi.nlm.nih.gov/books/NBK92775/

"जानीये औषधियों में कैसे निवास करती हैं मां दुर्गा – आयुर्वेद." 2019. आयुष दर्पण." https://ayushdarpan.com/religious-importance-of-herbs-with-navratri/

"वनस्पति." n.d. भारतकोष. Accessed December 20, 2022. https://bharatdiscovery.org/india/%E0%A4%B5%E0%A4%A8%E0%A4%B8%E0%A5%8D%E0%A4%AA%E0%A4%A4%E0%A4%BF

Acharya, Adithya. 2018. "Mahua – The tree of Elixir." Milaap. https://milaap.org/stories/mahua-the-tree-of-elixir

Alok, Shashi, Sanjay Kumar Jain, Amita Verma, Mayank Kumar, Alok Mahor, and Monika Sabharwal. "Plant profile, phytochemistry and pharmacology of Asparagus racemosus (Shatavari): A review." *Asian Pacific Journal of Tropical Disease* 3, no. 3 (2013): 242–251

Amalraj, Augustine, and Sreeraj Gopi. 2016. "Biological activities and medicinal properties of Asafoetida: A review." NCBI. https://www.ncbi.nlm.nih.gov/pmc/articles/PMC5506628/

Anwar, Farooq, Ali Abbas, and Khalid M. Alkharfy. "Cardamom (Elettaria cardamomum Maton) Oils." In *Essential Oils in Food Preservation, Flavor And Safety* edited by Victor R. Preedy, pp. 295-301. Academic Press, 2016

Bag, Anwesa, Subir Kumar Bhattacharyya, and Rabi Ranjan Chattopadhyay. "The development of Terminalia chebula Retz. (Combretaceae) in clinical research." *Asian Pacific Journal of Tropical Biomedicine* 3, no. 3 (2013): 244–252

Ballabh, Basant, and O. P. Chaurasia. "Traditional medicinal plants of cold desert Ladakh – used in treatment of cold, cough and fever." *Journal of Ethnopharmacology* 112, no. 2 (2007): 341-349. DOI:10.1016/j.jep.2007.03.020

Ballabh, Basant, and O. P. Chaurasia. "Traditional medicinal plants of cold desert Ladakh – used in treatment of cold, cough and fever." *Journal of Ethnopharmacology* 112, no. 2 (2007): 341–349

Bauman, Hannah, and Zachary Brown. n.d. "Food as Medicine Mustard (Brassica juncea and B. nigra, Brassicaceae)" American Botanical Council. Accessed December 20, 2022. https://www.herbalgram.org/resources/herbalegram/volumes/volume-14/number-3-march/food-as-medicine-mustard-brassica-juncea-and-b-nigra-brassicaceae/food-as-medicine-mustard/?t=1489589160

Begum, Samim Sofika, and Rajib Gogoi. "Herbal recipe prepared during Bohag or Rongali Bihu in Assam." (2007)

Bhawna, Kasna, Sharma Satish Kumar, Singh Lalit, M. Sharmista, and Singh Tanuja. "Cyperus scariosus: A Potential Medicinal Herb." *Int Res J Pharm* 4 (2013): 17–20

Bheemalingappa, Madiga, Madha Venkata Suresh Babu, and Boyina Ravi Prasad Rao. "Diversity and phytosociological attributes of trees of Baratang Island, Andaman and Nicobar Islands, India." *International Journal of Conservation Science* 9, no. 4 (2018)

Bode, Ann M., and Zigang Dong. "The amazing and mighty ginger." *Herbal Medicine: Biomolecular and Clinical Aspects. 2nd edition* (2011)

De Padua, L. S., N. Bunyapraphatsara, and R. H. M. J. Lemmens. *Plant Resources of South-East Asia*. Vol. 12, no. 1. Leiden: Backhuys Publ., 1999

Ghosh, Suvendu, Alak Kumar Syamal, and Debosree Ghosh. "Medicines from Indian Chillies: a mini review." Asian J Pharm Clin Res 9, no. 5 (2016): 1–3

Gilbert, Linda. n.d. "Spice Pages: Black Mustard Seeds (Brassica nigra/juncea)." Gernot Katzer. Accessed December 20, 2021. http://gernot-katzers-spice-pages.com/engl/Bras_nig.html

Hebbar, JV. "Mustard Benefits, Types, Usage, Side Effects, Research." Easy Ayurveda. https://www.easyayurveda.com/2015/03/19/mustard-benefits-types-side-effects-research/

Jadhav, V. M., R. M. Thorat, V. J. Kadam, and N. S. Sathe. "Hibiscus rosa sinensis Linn – Rudrapuspa: a review." *J Pharm Res* 2, no. 7 (2009): 1168-73.

Joshi, Hridayesh, and Sandhya Sekar. "The bugyals or Himalayan alpine meadows: a treasure trove endangered." Mongabay-India. https://india.mongabay.com/2020/08/the-bugyals-or-himalayan-alpine-meadows-a-treasure-trove-endangered/

Joshi, Pankaj N., Hiren B. Soni, SF Wesley Sunderraj, and Justus Joshua. "Distribution and conservation of less known rare and threatened plant species in Kachchh, Gujarat, India." *Our Nature* 11, no. 2 (2013): 152–167

Khan, Md Moniruzzaman, M. Sa dul Haque, and Md Saiful Islam Chowdhury. "Medicinal use of the unique plant Tinospora cordifolia: evidence from the traditional medicine and recent research." *Asian Journal of Medical and Biological Research* 2, no. 4 (2016): 508–512

Kirankumar H, Nataraj SK, Rajasekharan PE, Souravi K, Hanumanthappa M (2021). "An Insite into the Vanda Genera: Vanda's Natures Wonder." Advances in Crop Science and Technology. 9: 1000481

Kunnumakkara, Ajaikumar B et al. "Googling the Guggul (Commiphora and Boswellia) for Prevention of Chronic Diseases." *Frontiers in pharmacology* vol. 9 686. 6 Aug. 2018, doi:10.3389/fphar.2018.00686

Mali, Ravindra G. "Cleome viscosa (wild mustard): A review on ethnobotany, phytochemistry, and pharmacology." *Pharmaceutical Biology* 48, no. 1 (2010): 105–112

n.d. All Articles | Chopra. Accessed December 21, 2022. https://chopra.com/articles/

Narayan, Tara. 2020. "SOME IMPORTANT MEDICINAL PLANTS OF GOA." *Goan Observer*. https://www.goanobserver.in/2020/08/07/some-important-medicinal-plants-of-goa/

Neeraj, Vinita Bisht, and Vishal Johar. "Bael (Aegle marmelos) extraordinary species of India: a review." *Int. J. Curr. Microbiol. Appl. Sci* 6, no. 3 (2017): 1870–1887.

Patel, S., Soumitra Tiwari, P. S. Pisalkar, N. K. Mishra, R. K. Naik, and D. Khokhar. "Indigenous processing of Tikhur (Curcuma angustifolia Roxb.) for the extraction of starch in Baster, Chhattisgarh." (2015)

Pathak, Rashmi, and Himanshu Sharma. "A Review on Medicinal Uses of Cinnamomum verum (Cinnamon)." *Journal of Drug Delivery and Therapeutics* 11, no. 6-S (2021): 161–166

PRASAD, RCP, S. H. Raza, C. S. Reddy, and C. B. S. Dutt. "Euphorbiaceae of North Andaman forest – An ecological and phytosociological perspective." *The Journal of Indian Botanical Society* 87, no. 1&2 (2008): 1–3

Prasad, Sahdeo, and Bharat B. Aggarwal. "Turmeric, the golden spice." *Herbal Medicine: Biomolecular and Clinical Aspects.* 2nd edition (2011)

Raja, Vidya. 2021. "India's 'Saunf King' Grows 25 Tonnes of Fennel on 15 Acres While Also Saving Water." *The Better India.* https://www.thebetterindia.com/248594/saunf-king-fennel-farmer-earns-lakhs-ishaq-ali-rajasthan-agriculture-drip-irrigation-method-success-story-information-vid01

Sharma, Bharat, Neeru Vasudeva, and Sunil Sharma. "Essential oil composition and anti-scabies potential of Amomum subulatum Roxb. leaves." *Anti-Infective Agents* 18, no. 3 (2020): 261–267

Shrikant Baslingappa, Swami, Thakor Nayan Singh J, Patil Meghatai M, and Haldankar Parag M. "Jamun (Syzygium cumini (L.)): a review of its food and medicinal uses." *Food and Nutrition Sciences* 2012 (2012)

Singh, K. A., R. N. Rai, and D. T. Bhutia. "Large cardamom (Amomum subulatum Roxb.) plantation – An age old agroforestry system in Eastern Himalayas." *Agroforestry Systems* 9, no. 3 (1989): 241–257

Srinivasan, Krishnapura. "Cumin (Cuminum cyminum) and black cumin (Nigella sativa) seeds: traditional uses, chemical constituents, and nutraceutical effects." *Food quality and safety* 2, no. 1 (2018): 1–16

Sureshbabu, P., and N. Ramakrishna. "Traditional botanical knowledge of local people of Anantagiri and Dhamagundam forest area, Vikarabad district Telangana state." *Journal of Scientific and Innovative Research* 7, no. 4 (2018): 92–99

Telangana Today. "The secret magic of coriander in skincare." March 22, 2021. https://telanganatoday.com/the-secret-magic-of-coriander-in-skincare

Tsering, Jambey, Ngilyang Tam, Hui Tag, Baikuntha Jyoti Gogoi, and Ona Apang. "Medicinal orchids of Arunachal Pradesh: a review." *Bulletin of Arunachal Forest Research* 32, no. 1-2 (2017): 1–16

Verma, Abhinav. "Summer respite for Delhiites: The enchanting Amaltas tree." *Hindustan Times.* https://www.hindustantimes.com/more-lifestyle/summer-respite-for-delhiites-the-amaltas-tree/story-kXFNKj9qKPnPn7z1ONR2xN.html

Verma, R. K., and V. P. Tewari. "Some important medicinal plants of cold desert regions of District Kinnaur of Himachal Pradesh state in India: Their uses and chemical ingredients." *J. Plant Chemist Ecophysiol* 1 (2016): 1009

Ware, Megan, and LD RDN. "How can antioxidants benefit our health." *Medical News Today* (2018)

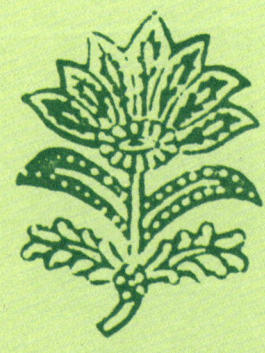